CURRENT CONTROVERSIES IN BONE MARROW TRANSPLANTATION

CURRENT CLINICAL ONCOLOGY

Maurie Markman, MD, SERIES EDITOR

Current Controversies in Bone Marrow Transplantation, edited by BRIAN J. BOLWELL, 2000

Regional Chemotherapy: *Clinical Research and Practice,* edtied by MAURIE MARKMAN, 2000

Intraoperative Irradiation: *Techniques and Results,* edited by L. L. GUNDERSON, C. G. WILLETT, L. B. HARRISON, F. A. CALVO, 1999

CURRENT CONTROVERSIES IN BONE MARROW TRANSPLANTATION

Edited by

BRIAN J. BOLWELL, MD

Director, Bone Marrow Transplant Program
The Cleveland Clinic Foundation, Cleveland, OH

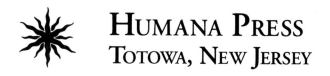

HUMANA PRESS
TOTOWA, NEW JERSEY

Library of Congress Cataloging-in-Publication Data

Current controversies in bone marrow transplantation / edited by Brian J. Bolwell.
        p.   cm. -- (Current clinical oncology)
    Includes index.
    ISBN 0-89603-782-7 (alk. paper)
    1. Hematopoietic stem cells--Transplantation. 2. Cancer-Immunotherapy. 3. Bone
marrow--Transplantation. I. Bolwell, Brian J. II. Series.
    [DNLM: 1. Neoplasms--therapy. 2. Bone Marrow Transplantation.
 3. Hematopoietic StemCell Transplantation.   QZ 266 C975 2000]
    RC271.B59C87 2000
    617.4'4--dc21
    DNLM/DLC
    for Library of Congress   99-38948
                                                                  CIP

*To the Bone Marrow Transplant Program
at the Cleveland Clinic Foundation,
and to transplant patients everywhere*

Preface

During my hematology/oncology fellowship, I remember a conversation I had with one of my professors about medical textbooks. He stated that most textbooks were, in his opinion, limited and inadequate. He said textbook chapters generally give an exhaustive summary of data and studies, but rarely provide an expert commentary and interpretation of the data. He felt that the best book chapters were those in which the author stated his or her opinion, and made liberal use of expert commentary analyzing scientific data.

That conversation reflects the philosophy of this book. This is not a textbook of bone marrow transplantation. Rather, this book examines many aspects of clinical bone marrow/hematopoietic cell transplantation that are controversial, and invites the authors not only to synthesize available published data, but also to offer their opinions and interpretations of those data. All authors are members of leading bone marrow transplant programs in the United States, and bring a pragmatic and clinical perspective to this book. The contributors to this book are also fairly young. We grew up with transplantation and do not view it as an oddity; rather, we embrace its therapeutic potential while acknowledging its limitations.

This book is entitled *Current Controversies in Bone Marrow Transplantation*. I am sure many oncologists would argue that the entire field of bone marrow transplantation is controversial! Certainly some areas are more controversial than others: the field of autologous transplantation for solid tumor tends to generate more "controversy" than does allogeneic bone marrow transplantation for leukemias. However, even within an accepted indication for bone marrow transplantation, such as allogeneic bone marrow transplant for refractory leukemia, there are certainly many opinions concerning aspects of transplant strategies and transplant outcomes that differ among experts in the field. Twenty-one such topics of potential controversy and clinical challenges are examined in this book.

Part I is entitled Transplant Strategies. The first chapter discusses how many cells are sufficient for engraftment of allogeneic, autologous bone marrow, autologous peripheral blood progenitor cell, and umbilical cord blood cells. As one reads this chapter it is fascinating how much of the current dogma is based on dated literature. The next chapter discusses whether older patients should be routinely excluded from bone marrow transplant protocols. Again, much of the literature concerning the outcome of older patients in bone marrow transplantation is not current, and I attempt to make the point that the decision to perform a bone marrow transplant should be more of a question of physiologic health, rather than chronological health. The controversial role of umbilical cord blood cell transplantation in both children and adults is discussed in a single chapter; this is clearly an area of intensive investigation. Finally, a great deal of bias exists concerning physician preference for total body irradiation versus nontotal body irradiation preparative regimens, and Chapters 4 and 5 analyze the pros and cons of each for adults (Chapter 4) and children (Chapter 5) in an articulate and thoughtful manner.

Part II discusses controversies and challenges of BMT in the treatment of hematologic malignancies. The first chapter discusses the timing of transplantation for chronic myelogenous leukemia (CML), using both related and unrelated donors, as well as other alternative treatment strategies. The next chapter is an examination of adult acute lymphoblastic leukemia (ALL). There is a significant discrepancy in results of conventional chemotherapy in adult ALL from different parts of the world; this chapter discusses the realistic outcomes of adult ALL with conventional chemotherapy and the therapeutic potential of the early use of allogeneic bone marrow transplant. Chapter 3 discusses the outcome of refractory leukemia with bone marrow transplantation. Though patients with AML or ALL in second or third complete remission are uniformly felt to be excellent BMT candidates with favorable outcomes, this chapter details the realistic clinical outcome of allogeneic BMT for those unfortunate patients who have refractory disease. Chapter 4 examines the role of autologous transplantation in the management of leukemia. Autologous bone marrow transplant has fallen into disfavor in the United States based on some negative clinical results; this chapter discusses all of the available data and defines potential therapeutic strategies for autologous transplantation in this setting. The next three chapters address the role of BMT in the management of lymphomas. The fifth chapter of this Part is a thoughtful analysis of different subsets of patients with Hodgkin's disease who may or may not be transplant candidates, and it also discusses the potential benefit of post-transplant radiation therapy. Chapter 6 discusses mantle cell non-Hodgkin's lymphoma and reviews currently available conventional therapies, as well as the potential therapy role of transplantation. The last chapter of this Part analyzes the efficacy of autologous transplantation for non-Hodgkin's lymphoma, both for relapsed patients, as well as those who are at high risk at diagnosis, and for those with follicular non-Hodgkin's lymphoma. My belief is that a minority of appropriate transplant candidates are currently being referred to transplant centers, and I attempt to make this point in several commentary sections of this chapter.

Part III discusses transplantation for solid tumors. The first three chapters provide a critical analysis of two of the more controversial disease indications, namely ovarian cancer and breast cancer. The timing of autologous transplantation for patients with breast cancer is increasingly controversial and is reviewed in the second chapter. The poor prognosis of inflammatory carcinoma of the breast with conventional therapy is covered in depth in the next chapter. Finally, an analysis of various risk groups of germ cell tumors and the potential therapeutic application of transplantation in these settings is discussed in the fourth chapter.

Complications of transplantation are discussed in Part 4. The most vexing complication of allogeneic BMT is graft-versus-host disease (GVHD). Therapeutic progress has not happened at a rapid pace and the first chapter of this Part covers what, if any, progress has been made in the past decade in the treatment of GVHD. Another challenge of both allogeneic and autologous transplantation is the management of veno-occlusive disease of the liver. While many therapeutic interventions have been attempted, few have shown clear-cut efficacy, as is discussed in the second chapter. Post transplant myelodysplasia, a very serious complication that has been increasingly recognized over the past five years, is reviewed in depth in the third chapter. Finally, the book closes with two chapters concerning challenges in the prevention and management of two common and potentially life threatening infectious complications of allogeneic BMT, aspergillosis and cytomegalovirus infections.

This preface was written one week after the 1999 American Society of Clinical Oncology meetings. Several abstracts were presented at that meeting in May 1999 that discussed early results of transplantation for breast cancer. I believe it is premature to include a commentary of those abstracts in this book until the data are published in peer-reviewed journals. For the same reason, this book does not discuss non-myeloablative allogeneic BMT, as most of the available data at the present time are scanty and based on extremely small numbers of patients. Studies examining this exciting potential therapeutic modality will clearly be of interest in the next several years.

Bone marrow transplantation is a constantly evolving therapy. Autologous transplantation was revolutionized by the use of primed peripheral blood progenitor cells in the 1990s, and undoubtedly there will be other new strategies in the near future. This book represents a snapshot of many current issues in the field of transplantation as we enter the new millennium. All of the authors of this book are committed to the belief that answers to the controversies presented will ultimately be achieved, for the benefit of patients everywhere.

Brian J. Bolwell, MD

Contents

Contributors

KARIM A. ADAL, MD, *Staff Physician, Department of Infectious Disease, Cleveland Clinic Foundation, Cleveland, OH*

BELINDA R. AVALOS, MD, *Associate Professor of Medicine, Bone Marrow Transplant Program, The Arthur G. James Cancer Hospital and Richard J. Solove Research Center, Ohio State University, Columbus, OH*

ROBIN K. AVERY, MD, *Staff Physician, Department of Infectious Disease, Cleveland Clinic Foundation, Cleveland, OH*

SCOTT I. BEARMAN, MD, *Professor of Medicine, Clinical Director, Bone Marrow Transplant Program, University of Colorado Health Sciences Center, Denver, CO*

MICHAEL R. BISHOP, MD, *Head, Bone Marrow Transplant Unit, Department of Experimental Transplantation and Immunology, National Cancer Institute, National Institute of Health, Bethesda, MD*

BRIAN J. BOLWELL, MD, *Director, Bone Marrow Transplant Program, Staff Physician, Department of Hematology/Medical Oncology, Cleveland Clinic Foundation, Cleveland, OH*

E. RANDOLPH BROUN, MD, *Medical Director, Bone Marrow Transplant Program, Jewish Hospital/University of Cincinnati Stem Cell Transplant Program, The Jewish Hospital of Cincinnati, Cincinnati, OH*

EDWARD A. COPELAN, MD, *Associate Professor of Medicine, Director, Bone Marrow Transplant Program, The Arthur G. James Cancer Hospital and Richard J. Solove Research Institute, Ohio State University, Columbus, OH*

PATRICK J. ELDER, MS, *Technical Supervisor, Bone Marrow Transplant Processing Lab, The Arthur G. James Cancer Hospital and Richard J. Solove Research Institute, Ohio State University, Columbus, OH*

MATT E. KALAYCIO, MD, *Director, Leukemia Program, Staff Physician, Department of Hematology/Medical Oncology, Cleveland Clinic Foundation, Cleveland, OH*

MARY J. LAUGHLIN, MD, *Director, Allogeneic Transplant Program, Ireland Cancer Center, University Hospital of Cleveland, Cleveland, OH*

DAVID L. LONGWORTH, MD, *Chairman, Department of Infectious Disease, Cleveland Clinic Foundation, Cleveland, OH*

SELINA M. LUGER, MD, *Director, Leukemia Program, Assistant Professor of Medicine, University of Pennsylvania Cancer Center, Philadelphia, PA*

DEAN S. McGAUGHEY, MD, *Fellow, Hematology/Oncology Department of Medicine, Adult Bone Marrow Transplantation, Duke University Medical Center, Durham, NC*

CRAIG H. MOSKOWITZ, MD, *Assistant Attending, Hematology/Oncology, Lymphoma Service, Memorial Sloan-Kettering Cancer Center, New York, NY*

SHERIF B. MOSSAD, MD, *Staff Physician, Department of Infectious Disease, Cleveland Clinic Foundation, Cleveland, OH*

STEPHEN D. NIMER, MD, *Head, Division of Hematologic Oncology; Chief, Hematology Service, Memorial Sloan-Kettering Cancer Center, New York, NY*

LYNN C. O'DONNELL, PHD, *Scientific Director, Bone Marrow Transplant Processing Lab, The Arthur G. James Cancer Hospital and Richard J. Solove Research Center, Ohio State University, Columbus, OH*

BETH A. OVERMOYER, MD, *Director, Clinical Trials in Breast Cancer, Assistant Professor of Medicine, Ireland Cancer Center, University Hospitals of Cleveland, Case Western Reserve University, Cleveland, OH*

SAM L. PENZA, MD, *Assistant Professor of Clinical Medicine, Bone Marrow Transplant Program, The Arthur G. James Cancer Hospital and Richard J. Solove Research Center, Ohio State University, Columbus, OH*

BRAD POHLMAN, MD, *Director, Lymphoma Program, Staff Physician, Department of Hematology/Medical Oncology, Cleveland Clinic Foundation, Cleveland, OH*

JANET RUZICH, DO, *Fellow, Division of Hematology-Oncology, Department of Medicine, Loyola University Medical Center, Maywood, IL*

ROBERT SACKSTEIN, MD, PHD, *Associate Scientific Director, Bone Marrow Transplant Program, Massachusetts General Hospital, Harvard Medical School, Boston, MA*

SUSAN B. SHURIN, MD, *Chief, Pediatric Hematology/Oncology, Rainbow Babies and Children Hospital, University Hospitals of Cleveland; Professor, Case Western Reserve University, Cleveland, OH*

THOMAS R. SPITZER, MD, *Director, Bone Marrow Transplant Program, Massachusetts General Hospital, Harvard Medical School, Boston, MA*

EDWARD A. STADTMAUER, MD, *Associate Professor of Medicine, Director, Bone Marrow and Stem Cell Transplant Program, University of Pennsylvania Cancer Center, Philadelphia, PA*

PATRICK J. STIFF, MD, *Professor of Medicine, Director, Bone Marrow Transplant Program, Loyola University Medical Center, Maywood, IL*

JAMES J. VREDENBURGH, MD, *Associate Professor of Medicine, Department of Medicine, Adult Bone Marrow Transplantation, Duke University Medical Center, Durham, NC*

SUSAN R. WIERSMA, MD, *Associate Professor, Pediatrics and Oncology, Case Western Reserve University; Associate Director, Pediatric Blood and Marrow Program, Rainbow Babies and Children Hospital, University Hospitals of Cleveland, Cleveland, OH*

STEPHANIE F. WILLIAMS, MD, *Associate Professor of Medicine, Section of Hematology/Oncology, University of Chicago Medical Center, Chicago, IL*

I   TRANSPLANT STRATEGIES

1

How Many Stem Cells Are Sufficient for Engraftment?

Lynn C. O'Donnell, PhD, Patrick J. Elder, MS, and Belinda R. Avalos, MD

CONTENTS

1. INTRODUCTION

The past 15 yr have witnessed an explosion of advances leading to important information regarding hematopoietic stem cells (HSCs), which has been directly applicable to the clinical setting. Mobilized peripheral blood (PB) and umbilical cord blood (CB)

From: *Current Controversies in Bone Marrow Transplantation*
Edited by: B. Bolwell © Humana Press Inc., Totowa, NJ

have been identified as alternatives to bone marrow (BM) as sources of human HSCs for clinical transplantation. Currently, BM remains the predominant stem cell source for allogeneic transplants (allotransplant); most autologous transplants (autotransplants) are now performed solely with mobilized PB stem cells (PBSC). Although experience with CB as a source of stem cells has been limited, it is expected to have its greatest application in the unrelated allotransplant setting. Recent observations that stem cells from each of these sources have biologically distinct properties, and that stem cell doses affect outcomes in clinical transplantation, underscore the importance of stem cell enumeration in predicting transplant outcomes.

2. HSC ASSAYS

HSCs are self-renewing pluripotent cells that have the ability to engraft upon transplantation, to proliferate, and to sustain multilineage hematopoiesis in vivo. A variety of approaches have been used to characterize HSCs. Functional assays for human stem cells have, until recently, been limited to various in vitro colony-forming assays. Cells that give rise to colonies in semisolid media, termed colony-forming units (CFU), typically display limited self-renewing potential, and are thought to represent committed progenitors responsible for early engraftment in vivo. Cells that can form colonies in stromal-cell-supported cultures, called long-term culture-initiating cells (LTC-ICs), represent self-renewing stem cells, which are believed to be required for sustained engraftment in vivo. The most conclusive assay for HSCs is their repopulation potential in conditioned recipients. The nonobese diabetic/severe combined immunodeficient (NOD/SCID) mouse has recently provided a novel in vivo model system for assaying human stem cells for their repopulation potential.

2.1. Colony Assays

HSCs can proliferate and differentiate to form colonies in vitro. A wide variety of conditions have been established to assess HSC populations for the presence of immature multipotent or specific lineage-committed progenitors. Colony-forming cells (CFC) with self-renewing potential can be identified by their ability to form colonies in both stromal-cell-supported cultures (LTC-ICs) and in semisolid media (blast-CFUs). Assays for CFUs of granulocyte-macrophage colony-forming units (GM-CFU) have been extensively used in the clinical setting. However, the GM-CFU and other colony-forming assays have not been well standardized. The use of undefined biological supplements, such as fetal bovine serum or conditioned medium, as sources of growth factors, requires stringent quality-control procedures to minimize lot-to-lot variability. Because of the subjective nature of data interpretation and the imprecision of quantitation when progenitor cell content is low, variability in GM-CFU assays is high, both within and between institutions (1). The usefulness of clonogenic assays in the clinical setting is also limited by the requirement for expensive biological reagents, and by an approximate 2-wk delay before results are obtained.

2.2. Cell Surface Markers

In contrast to clonogenic assays, expression of specific cell surface markers can be rapidly assessed within a few hours by flow cytometry. Thus, much effort has been expended to functionally characterize stem cells, based on expression patterns of the CD34 surface marker. CD34 is a surface glycoprotein, discovered in the 1980s, which is expressed on HSCs and early committed progenitor cells from all hematopoietic lineages. In the clinical setting, the CD34$^+$/CD33$^{+/-}$ and CD34$^+$/CD38$^{+/-}$ subpopulations have been most extensively analyzed for stem and progenitor cell content. Many investigators have characterized these subsets using in vitro colony assays.

CD33 is expressed on immature myeloid cells and its expression correlates with myeloid lineage commitment. For BM or mobilized PB, LTC-ICs and blast-CFUs have been shown to segregate within the CD34$^+$/CD33$^-$ subset, which also contains multilineage progenitors *(2–4)*. In contrast, the CD34$^+$/CD33$^+$ subset is enriched for GM-CFUs, and lacks LTC-ICs *(2,4)*. The CD38 antigen (Ag) is coexpressed with multiple lineage markers, including CD33, and its expression is an early event associated with differentiation along the erythroid, myeloid, and lymphoid lineages. CD34$^+$ cells that lack CD38 expression also lack lineage markers, and are designated "Lin$^-$" *(5)*. Although both CD34$^+$/CD38$^-$ and CD34$^+$/CD38$^+$ subsets from BM have been shown to contain committed multilineage progenitors, only the CD34$^+$/CD38$^-$ fraction is enriched for self-renewing stem cells (LTC-ICs and bl-CFUs) *(4–6)*.

Differences in CD34$^+$ cell populations have been reported between stem cells isolated from BM, PB, and CB. CB CD34$^+$ cells express lower levels of CD38, and contain a higher proportion of CD38$^-$ cells than BM or PB, indicating the presence of a more primitive population of progenitor cells in CB *(7,8)*. CB CD34$^+$/CD38$^-$ cells have a higher cloning efficiency than the same cell subpopulation from BM or mobilized PB, and yield higher numbers of GM-CFU and LTC-IC *(9,10)*. In addition, CB LTC-IC can be maintained in vitro for significantly longer periods of time than adult BM LTC-IC *(9,11)*. Thus, the proliferative potential of CB HSC is higher, compared to adult stem cells. Expression of the CD11a and CD62L cell adhesion molecules has also been reported to be higher on the CB CD34$^+$/CD38$^-$ subset of cells, compared to the same subset in BM, suggesting a possible advantage in homing and engraftment of CB cells *(12)*. The c-kit receptor for stem cell factor (SCF) (CD117) has been shown to be strongly expressed on CB CD34$^+$/CD38$^-$ cells, but not in the same cell subset from BM or PB *(13)*. These properties make CB stem cells ideal for ex vivo expansion, for use in transplantation of larger adults, to speed engraftment, and for gene transfer.

2.3. Technical Aspects Related to CD34 Quantitation

Although intralaboratory precision for CD34$^+$ cell enumeration is good, interlaboratory variability is significant and directly related to several variables. This topic was recently reviewed by the European Working Group on Clinical Cell Analysis (EWG-CCA), resulting in their recommendation of the adoption of standard protocols for CD34 quantitation by all laboratories *(14)*. The EWGCCA found that only two of 11 published interlaboratory protocol comparisons, the Nordic and Becton Dickinson's ProCOUNT™ (Becton Dickinson Immunocytometry Systems, San Jose, CA) protocols, achieved coefficients of variation (CVs) between institutions below 15%. The highest CV was reported at 235% by a study in the United States, although sample deterioration and the participation of some inexperienced centers may have contributed to the poor CV.

Interlaboratory variability in determination of CD34$^+$ cell content can be affected by many factors, including the gating strategy used, the method of sample preparation, and the specific CD34 antibody utilized for analysis. The EWGCCA has made the following general recommendations aimed at reducing interlaboratory variation.

1. Utilization of bright fluorochrome (e.g., Phycoerythrin) conjugates of class II or III monoclonal antibodies (mAbs) that recognize all glycosylated forms of CD34.
2. Use of a vital nucleic acid dye to exclude platelets, unlysed red cells, and debris.
3. Counterstaining with CD45 mAb to define CD34⁺ progenitor cells, on the basis of low CD45 expression and low sideward light-scatter signals.
4. Inclusion of both CD34^{dim} and CD34^{bright} populations in the CD34⁺ cell count.
5. Elimination of isotype control staining for nonspecific mAb binding.
6. Enumeration of at least 100 CD34⁺ cells in apheresis products, to ensure a precision of 10%.

This group also suggested the use of control specimens to validate protocol accuracy and hands-on training of laboratory technicians at centralized workshops to reduce interlaboratory variation.

It may not be feasible for all laboratories to adhere to the same protocol for CD34⁺ cell enumeration, but there are several established protocols that have been shown to produce similar CD34⁺ cell counts in single-center comparisons *(14)*. The single-platform ProCOUNT™ protocol and the International Society of Hematotherapy and Graft Engineering (ISHAGE) protocol and its single-platform version, Stem-Kit™ (Beckman Coulter, Fullerton, CA), have yielded similar single-center results that closely conform to the recommendations of the EWGCCA. However, these protocols have not yet been compared in multicenter studies to determine which yields the highest reproducibility between laboratories. Protocols that produce low interlaboratory variability should be used as standard backbone protocols. Any modifications to standard protocols (e.g., addition of lineage and/or viability markers) will need to be compared to standard methods, and shown to produce a high degree of concordance over a wide range of CD34⁺ cell counts, before being implemented. As knowledge of stem cell surface markers continues to increase, protocols for stem cell enumeration will probably change to incorporate new information and technologies.

2.4. HSC Characterization in Xenotransplant Models

Studies of human stem cells in immunodeficient mice have revealed important differences in the hematopoietic repopulation capacities of stem cells derived from BM, PB, and CB. High-level engraftment of human stem cells from adult BM into SCID mice has been shown to require additional treatment of transplanted mice with human growth factors *(15)*. In contrast, injection with human cytokines, or other additional treatments, is not required to establish high-level human cell engraftment after transplantation of CB cells into immunodeficient mice *(16–18)*, or for engraftment of mobilized human PB progenitor cells *(19)*. This difference in the xenotransplantation requirements of human stem cells is also observed when immunodeficient mice are transplanted with purified human CD34⁺ cell populations from adult BM, PB, and CB. In addition, CD34⁺ cells from CB have not only been shown to engraft in immunodeficient mice, but to significantly proliferate in the hematopoietic tissues of NOD/SCID mice, with a 5–500-fold increase in CD45⁺ cells, compared to no increase after transplantation with CD34⁺ cells from BM *(20,21)*. Thus, the CD34⁺ cell population must contain an as-yet-undefined subpopulation of stem cells that is responsible for this difference.

2.5. HSC Quantification for Clinical Application

In the absence of a more precisely defined population of HSCs present in BM, PB, or CB which is capable of rapid and sustained engraftment, investigators have used surrogate parameters, such as graft content of nucleated cells (NCs), mononuclear cells (MNCs), GM-CFUs, and CD34$^+$ cells, to determine the optimal and minimal dose of HSCs derived from each source that is required for successful engraftment. The presence of multilineage CFUs in CD34$^+$/CD33$^-$, CD34$^+$/CD33$^+$, CD34$^+$/CD38$^-$, and CD34$^+$/CD38$^+$ subsets suggests that quantitation of any or all of these subsets in infused cells could be predictive of the speed of engraftment. Sustained hematopoiesis might be expected to correlate more significantly with the CD34$^+$/CD33$^-$ and CD34$^+$/CD38$^-$ subsets, which contain most of the LTC-ICs. However, the contribution of CD34 subsets to sustained hematopoiesis has been difficult to assess in the autologous setting, because of the potential for autologous marrow reconstitution and the low success rates currently obtained with gene transduction into human cells for genetic marking studies. This may therefore be more easily addressed in the future in the allogeneic setting.

3. BONE MARROW

Estimation of BM stem cell numbers needed to regenerate the marrow after ablative therapy and BM transplant (BMT) has not been reported in great detail. Even less has been published about the quality of BM grafts. In 1970, Thomas et al. *(22)* reported that 5×10^8 NC/kg recipient body wt was a reasonable estimate of the number of allogeneic BM cells required for a successful transplant. Storb et al. *(23)* subsequently performed a multivariate analysis to identify factors predisposing aplastic anemia patients to rejection of allogeneic BM grafts. They reported that a dose $<3 \times 10^8$ NC/kg recipient body wt correlated with an increased risk of graft rejection. The results of these studies became the basis for the initial widespread use of NC content as an indicator of the stem cell content of BM grafts.

Unfortunately, subsequent studies assessing the predictive value of BM NC dose, or dose of CFU or CD34$^+$ cells, on engraftment and other outcome measures with BMT have not yielded consistent results. Difficulties in establishing the number of cells needed for rapid engraftment in BMT may reflect the fact that some minimum threshold number of cells is required for engraftment, above which there is no correlation with speed of engraftment. Failure to engraft or delays in engraftment may also be related to factors other than stem cell dose, such as the effects of ex vivo graft manipulation, conditioning regimens, and underlying disease or prior treatment. In the allogeneic setting, histocompatibility factors, graft-vs-host disease (GVHD), and the posttransplant immunosuppression regimen used may also affect engraftment. In addition, the general inability to control the number of cells a patient receives, especially in the allotransplant setting, and the widespread practice of infusing as many cells as possible to give the recipient the best possible chance of complete recovery have made it difficult to analyze the effect of BM cell dose on engraftment outcome. Thus, in any discussion of stem cell dose requirements, it is important to clearly distinguish between studies done in the allogeneic and autologous settings, as donor–host interactions probably contribute to engraftment and outcome. Unfortunately, this has not always been done, and has led to some confusion regarding stem cell doses required for BMT.

3.1. Autotransplants

Autotransplants provide a simpler model for studying the relationship between stem cell numbers and transplant course than allotransplants, because of elimination of confounding factors, such as histocompatibility and graft rejection. Autotransplants are generally performed when the BM is not involved with disease, or when contaminating tumor cells can be removed by purging. Studies by several groups examining the predictive value of NC or MNC dose, GM-CFU content, or both, on the kinetics of hematopoietic recovery following autologous BMT (ABMT), have demonstrated no statistically significant correlation between infused numbers of NC/kg or MNC/kg and time to neutrophil or platelet engraftment (24,25). These results may reflect the limited range of cell doses given in these studies, or a loss of stem cell function in the NC pool caused by marrow toxicity from multiple rounds of chemotherapy (CT). In contrast, most groups have a reported significant correlation between GM-CFU numbers in autografts and the speed of neutrophil or platelet recovery. Threshold doses below $0.1–3 \times 10^4$ GM-CFU/kg have been reported to result in significant delays in engraftment (24,26). The broad range in optimal GM-CFU doses reported may result from imprecision with GM-CFU assays as previously discussed in Subheading 2.1.

3.1.1. EFFECTS OF EX VIVO MANIPULATION OF AUTOGRAFTS

Ex vivo manipulation of autologous BM harvests, to remove contaminating tumor cells, is currently being investigated, using methods that result in either destruction or physical separation of unwanted cells. A variety of techniques have been used, including pharmacological, biophysical, and immunological methods. However, it is not clear that the removal of tumor cells by currently available methods will affect disease-free survival rates (27).

Pharmacological purging techniques involve treatment of harvested cells with a CT agent to destroy tumor cells that may be hypersensitive to the purging agent. Some agents that have been used to purge BM include 4-hydroxyperoxycyclophosphamide (4-HC), etoposide, vincristine, and mafosfamide. A potential disadvantage of purging is delayed engraftment caused by nonspecific toxicity of the purging agent to the stem cell population, and the loss of stem cells during the procedure itself.

GM-CFU doses have been shown to correlate with outcome in ABMT using purged grafts, although no threshold GM-CFU doses have been reported (28,29). Investigators at Johns Hopkins (29) showed that the number of GM-CFU in 4-HC-purged autografts is predictive of time to neutrophil and platelet engraftment, in both univariate and multivariate analyses. In contrast, only the prepurging GM-CFU yield, and not the infused GM-CFU dose from mafosfamide-purged BM, was shown to correlate with days to neutrophil and platelet recovery or transplant-related mortality (28). These conflicting results may reflect the low recovery of GM-CFU observed after mafosfamide purging (median 0.4%), and suggest that prepurging GM-CFU may be a measure of marrow function or graft quality.

Another approach to tumor removal from autografts has been the positive selection of CD34+ cells, which can effectively reduce, by 1–2 logs, contaminating tumor cells that do not express the CD34 Ag. Positive selection also decreases the volume of stem cell products, which may reduce the incidence of dimethyl sulfoxide (DMSO)-associated infusional toxicity. Several groups have utilized the Ceprate SC™ stem cell concentration system (Cellpro, Bothwell, WA), which uses a biotinylated mAb to CD34 to immobilize and isolate cells expressing the CD34 Ag. In a preliminary analysis of the safety and efficacy of positively selected CD34+ cells for ABMT in 15 lymphoma patients, Gorin et al. *(30)* observed a trend toward slower neutrophil and platelet engraftment with lower doses of GM-CFUs or CD34+ cells. The small number of patients in this study may have contributed to the lack of statistical significance observed. However, based on their preliminary data, these investigators suggested a cell dose $>0.5 \times 10^6$ CD34+ cells/kg and $>1 \times 10^4$ GM-CFU/kg. The results from a randomized trial of CD34+ cell selection for ABMT in 89 high-risk breast cancer patients have recently been published *(31)*. Compared to patients receiving unselected cells, patients receiving selected CD34+ cells tended to experience delayed engraftment of neutrophils and platelets ($p = 0.218$ and $p = 0.051$, respectively). However, no significant delays in engraftment were seen in these patients when $>1.2 \times 10^6$ CD34+ cells/kg were infused. Moreover, platelet engraftment was reported to be delayed, irrespective of CD34+ cell selection, when $<1.2 \times 10^6$ CD34+ cells/kg were transplanted.

3.1.2. BM Stem Cell Viability

Current studies in BM cryopreservation are aimed at examining the effect of long-term storage (i.e., longer than 2 yr) on engraftment parameters following transplantation. Attarian et al. *(32)* retrospectively compared 36 patients, whose BM had been stored longer than 2 yr prior to BMT, with a historical control group, matched for diagnosis and date of storage, whose BM was stored less than 2 yr. No statistically significant differences were found between the study group (median 2.7 yr storage, range 2.0–7.8) and the control group (median 0.3 yr storage, range 0.04–1.7) for recovery of GM-CFU or time to engraftment of neutrophils or platelets. Thus, it appears that BM cells can be stored at early points in treatment, before cumulative marrow damage occurs from multiple rounds of CT and/or radiation, and can subsequently be used years later for transplantation.

3.2. Allotransplants

Allotransplants are significantly more complicated than autotransplants. These transplants involve infusion of cells from an human leukocyte antigen (HLA)-compatible, related or unrelated donor. Complications such as graft rejection and GVHD, which are inherent to allotransplantation, and the use of immunosuppressive agents to prevent these complications, can affect the outcome of allogeneic BMT (allo-BMT). In contrast to the results reported with ABMT, analysis of the GM-CFU content in allografts has generally been found to be of no predictive value for speed of engraftment *(33–35)*. However, two groups have reported that a low GM-CFU dose increases the risk of transplant-related mortality due to infections *(35,36)*.

A correlation between NC or MNC numbers and engraftment kinetics and transplant outcome has been observed with allo-BMT. The International Bone Marrow Transplant Registry has reported that, in patients with acute myeloid leukemia, a NC dose $>2.3 \times 10^8$/kg was significantly associated with decreased risk of interstitial pneumonitis or moderate-to-severe GVHD, and with increased survival in the first 6 mo posttransplant *(37)*. In an analysis of allo-BMT from matched unrelated donors (MUD), investigators in Seattle *(38)* reported that a NC dose $>3.7 \times 10^8$/kg was associated with faster engraftment of neutrophils, platelets, and lymphocytes, and with a decreased risk of developing severe acute GVHD. In addition, in patients transplanted in remission,

Table 1
Summary of HSC Doses in BMT

HSC enumeration		Patients	
		Autologous	Allogeneic
NC	Correlation	−	+
	Threshold		$2.3–3.7 \times 10^8$/kg
GM-CFU	Correlation	+	−
	Threshold	$0.1–3 \times 10^4$/kg	
CD34$^+$ cells	Correlation	+	+
	Threshold	1.2×10^6/kg	$1–2 \times 10^6$/kg

higher NC doses were associated with a decreased risk of nonleukemic death and increased leukemia-free survival.

Very few studies have reported the relevance of CD34$^+$ cell doses on engraftment or outcome in allo-BMT. Using elutriation as a method for depleting T-cells from allografts, Mavroudis et al. (39) reported that the CD34$^+$ cell dose correlated with speed of engraftment for all lineages except neutrophils. The lack of correlation with neutrophil engraftment may have resulted from the use of granulocyte colony-stimulating factor (G-CSF) posttransplant. Patients in this study receiving $>2 \times 10^6$ CD34$^+$ cells/kg achieved red blood cell and platelet transfusion independence sooner, required less G-CSF administration for white blood cell support, and spent fewer days in the hospital during the first 100 d posttransplant. Patients receiving $<1 \times 10^6$ CD34$^+$ cells/kg were found to have a significantly higher risk of transplant-related mortality caused by infections (65 vs 7%) and a lower survival rate (31 vs 74%) than the group receiving $>1 \times 10^6$ CD34$^+$ cells/kg.

3.3. Summary

NC or MNC doses have historically been used to assess stem cell content in BM grafts. In the allogeneic setting, a dose of $2–4 \times 10^8$ NC/kg appears to be a valid threshold (Table 1). However, in the autologous setting, GM-CFU and not NC dose appears to be a better predictor of engraftment kinetics. Limited information has been published regarding CD34$^+$ cell doses and outcomes in patients undergoing transplants with BM as the stem cell source, particularly in the unrelated allotransplant setting. The available data suggest a threshold of $1–1.2 \times 10^6$ CD34$^+$ cells/kg for patients undergoing auto- or allotransplants from matched sibling donors. Additional studies are clearly needed to better define CD34$^+$ cell thresholds for patients undergoing related and unrelated allotransplants. However, current difficulties in obtaining CD34$^+$ cell counts in a timely manner, during the time of marrow harvest, will limit its use in determination of the volume of BM to be harvested from a given donor, and hence the cell dose a patient receives.

4. PERIPHERAL BLOOD

In the autologous setting, PBSC transplants (PBSCT) are now much more common than BMT, mostly because of the faster engraftment kinetics observed with PBSC. Transplantation with PBSC is also being investigated in the allogeneic setting. As with

BM, a variety of surrogate parameters have been utilized to assess HSC content in PBSC collections, in an attempt to determine reliable predictors of rapid and sustained hematopoietic engraftment.

4.1. MNC and CFU Content

MNC content generally does not reliably predict the speed of engraftment of PBSC, chiefly because of the highly variable frequency of progenitor cells in the total NC population of PB (40,41). However, two groups have demonstrated that, for patients with lymphoma mobilized with cyclophosphamide + G-CSF, and subsequently treated with BEAM (carmustine, etoposide, cytosine arabinoside, melphalan) and PBSC rescue, a threshold of $\geq 3 \times 10^8$ MNC/kg reliably predicts multilineage recovery (42,43). A significant correlation between GM-CFU numbers in PBSC and recovery of neutrophils after transplantation has been reported (40,41,43–45). However, a correlation between GM-CFU and platelet recovery has not been consistently observed. Enumeration of megakaryocyte-CFU (MK-CFU) in PBSC products appears to be no better at predicting time to platelet engraftment (46). The lack of standardization and poor precision of clonogenic assays probably account for the wide range of threshold GM-CFU doses that have been reported for PBSC, which range from 8 to 50×10^4 GM-CFU/kg.

4.2. CD34+ Cell Dose

The relationship between CD34+ PBSC dose and engraftment kinetics first reported by Bender et al. (40) is nonlinear, and threshold values, below which there is a higher risk of delayed engraftment, have been identified. However, different transplant centers associate varying levels of risk with the number of days patients experience specific cytopenias, which has led to variability in the meaning of "delayed engraftment" and "optimal cell dose" between transplant centers. This, as well as interlaboratory variability in CD34+ cell counts, and the lack of information regarding the functional equivalence of CD34+ cell populations mobilized in different patient populations or by various mobilization regimens, would be expected to result in a wide range of optimal CD34+ cell doses reported. However, most groups have reported optimal CD34+ cell doses that fall within the narrow range between 2 and 5×10^6 CD34+ cells/kg. Shown in Table 2 is a compilation of threshold CD34+ cell doses derived from recent data reported from studies with patients with a variety of underlying diseases treated at multiple centers, or from studies with large cohorts of patients with a single disease treated with defined mobilization regimens. Most groups have observed prompt engraftment of neutrophils and an effect of CD34+ cell dose on the time to engraftment of platelets, but not of neutrophils (43,47,48). Weaver et al. (49) have reported a lower threshold for neutrophil recovery than for platelet recovery, with thresholds of 2.5×10^6 CD34+ cells/kg and 5×10^6 CD34+ cells/kg, respectively. This group has therefore recommended infusion of the higher dose, when possible.

Several investigators have also analyzed the effects of CD34+ cell doses on sustained hematopoiesis, by determination of the time required for return of normal hematologic values and assessment of blood count values at later time intervals. Haas et al. (44) suggested that the CD34+ cell dose affected long-term hematopoiesis, and correlated with the same threshold dose for engraftment (Table 2). However, in multivariate analyses, other groups have not demonstrated a significant correlation between CD34+ cell dose and long-term reconstitution (50,51). These groups have therefore suggested

Table 2
Summary of PBSC CD34+ Cell Doses in Recent Large Studies

| Ref. (no.) | Single or multi-center | Patients | | Optimal CD34+ cell dose | | Minimal CD34+ cell dose | Other analysis |
		N	Disease	Neutrophil recovery[a]	Platelet recovery[b]		
Haas et al., 1995 (44)	Single	145	Mixed	$\geq 2.5 \times 10^6$/kg	$\geq 2.5 \times 10^6$/kg	–	Sustained hematopoiesis
Bensinger et al., 1995 (52)	Multi	243	Mixed	$\geq 2.5 \times 10^6$/kg	$\geq 2.5 \times 10^6$/kg or $\geq 5 \times 10^6$/kg[d]	NS	Posttransplant myeloid growth factors
Weaver et al., 1995 (49)	Multi	692	Mixed	$\geq 2.5 \times 10^6$/kg	$\geq 5 \times 10^6$/kg	NS	
Tricot et al., 1995 (47)	Single	225	Multiple Myeloma	NS[c]	$\geq 2 \times 10^6$/kg or $\geq 5 \times 10^6$/kg[e]	–	Duration of prior CT
Watts et al., 1997 (43)	Single	101	Lymphoma	NS	$\geq 3.5 \times 10^6$/kg	$\geq 1 \times 10^6$/kg	
Glaspy et al., 1997 (48)	Multi	215	Breast cancer	NS	$\geq 5 \times 10^6$/kg[f] or $\geq 2 \times 10^6$/kg[g]	–	SCF during mobilization

[a] ANC > 0.5×10^9/L for 1–7 d.

[b] Platelets > $20–50 \times 10^9$/L or platelet transfusion independence for 1–7 d.

[c] NS, not statistically significant.

[d] $\geq 5 \times 10^6$/kg in patients receiving posttransplant G-CSF or GM-CSF.

[e] $\geq 5 \times 10^6$/kg in patients who received >24 mo prior CT.

[f] Gives 85% chance of engraftment by d 14 and 98% by d 28.

[g] Gives 65% chance of engraftment by d 14 and 90% by d 28.

that other variables, including age, diagnosis, quality of mobilization, and speed of engraftment, are more important factors affecting long-term hematopoiesis. Duration of prior CT has also been found to affect engraftment kinetics and CD34$^+$ cell thresholds. Tricot et al. *(47)* reported that multiple myeloma patients, mobilized with CT + GM-CSF, who had received more than 24 mo of prior cytotoxic therapy, required a larger CD34$^+$ cell dose to ensure rapid engraftment than those who received less than 24 mo of prior therapy (Table 2). In addition, they observed that only 28% of the heavily pretreated patients in their study reached the target dose of 5×10^6 CD34$^+$ cells/kg. These data suggest that heavily treated patients with myeloma might benefit from the use of alternative mobilization strategies, such as those utilizing SCF *(48)*, to increase yields of PBSC. These observations may also be applicable to mobilization in other heavily pretreated patients with different malignant disorders.

The minimum PBSC dose required to achieve engraftment has been difficult to determine due to the paucity of patients in reported studies who either received low cell doses or experienced unacceptably delayed engraftment *(49,52)*. Watts et al. *(43)* reported a minimum cell dose below which they would not recommend PBSCT after myeloablative therapy. In a study of 101 lymphoma patients, these investigators found that when patients received $<1 \times 10^6$ CD34$^+$ cells/kg there was a 40% chance of delayed platelet engraftment, defined as engraftment that occurred beyond 28 d. In a retrospective analysis, Weaver et al. *(53)* reviewed the records of 2079 nonleukemia patients transplanted at multiple institutions, and identified 48 (2.3%) who were infused with $<2.5 \times 10^6$ CD34$^+$ cells/kg: 36 because of poor harvests, and 12 who elected to reserve a fraction of their harvested cells for future treatment options *(53)*. In this analysis, the median dose infused was 2.12×10^6 CD34$^+$ cells/kg, with the lowest dose still in excess of 1×10^6 CD34$^+$ cells/kg. Engraftment was compared to a large historical group of control patients, matched to the study group by disease and regimen, who received $>2.5 \times 10^6$ CD34$^+$ cells/kg. The entire study group achieved neutrophil engraftment (median 11 d vs control 10 d), and 98% achieved platelet engraftment (median 14 d vs control 10 d). None of the 12 patients who had adequate harvests, but who elected to receive only a fraction of their collected cells, experienced delayed platelet engraftment beyond 28 d. However, five of the 36 patients who received $<2.5 \times 10^6$ CD34$^+$ cells/kg because of poor yields either experienced delayed platelet engraftment after 28 d or died without achieving platelet engraftment. Based on these data, it is possible that the delayed platelet engraftment observed in patients receiving low CD34$^+$ cell does may have been related more to poor quality of the CD34$^+$ cells harvested or to damage of the BM stroma than to the number of CD34$^+$ cells infused. Thus, there may not be an absolute value for the minimum CD34$^+$ cell dose required to achieve engraftment in the autologous setting. For patients with low CD34$^+$ cell yields, the relative risks of disease progression and the requirement for increased supportive care due to delayed platelet engraftment need to be heavily weighed prior to proceeding with myeloablative therapy and PBSCT.

4.2.1. CD34$^+$ Subsets

In an effort to determine better predictors of PBSC engraftment kinetics, several groups have examined specific CD34$^+$ cell subsets in PBSC products. Table 3 summarizes the results from several of these studies. In a univariate analysis of various CD34$^+$ cell subsets, Dercksen et al. *(54)* found that only CD33$^-$ and CD41$^+$ subsets correlated

Table 3
Subset Analysis of PBSC CD34$^+$ Cell Doses

	Patients		Optimal CD34$^+$ subset and cell dose		Observations
Ref. (no.)	N	Disease	Neutrophil recovery[a]	Platelet recovery[b]	
Dercksen et al., 1995 (54)	59	Mixed	CD34$^+$/CD33$^-$ 2.8 × 10^6/kg	CD34$^+$/CD41$^+$ 0.5 × 10^6/kg	Others no better (CD38$^{+/-}$, 45$^+$, 33$^+$, 13$^{+/-}$, 71$^+$, 61$^+$, HLA-DR$^{+/-}$, c-kit$^+$)
Copelan et. al., 1997 (55)	169	Mixed	CD34$^+$ 4 × 10^6/kg	CD34$^+$/CD33$^-$ 1.2 × 10^6/kg	CD34$^+$/CD33$^-$ dose not predictive for neutrophil recovery
Miller et. al., 1998 (56)	68	Mixed	NS[c]	CD34$^+$/CD33$^-$ 1.4 × 10^6/kg	Only CFU-GM predictive for neutrophil recovery
Pecora et. al., 1998 (57)	410	Mixed	CD34$^+$/CD33$^-$ 1 × 10^6/kg	CD34$^+$/CD33$^-$ 1 × 10^6/kg	Percent CD34$^+$ that were CD33$^-$ is independently predictive for both neutrophil and platelet recovery
Mayol et. al., 1998 (58)	67	Mixed	CD34$^+$/CD33$^-$ 0.9 × 10^6/kg	CD34$^+$ 2.7 × 10^6/kg	In univariate analysis CD34$^+$/CD33$^-$ is also predictive of platelet recovery
Hénon et. al., 1998 (60)	45	Mixed	CD34$^+$/CD38$^-$ 0.05 × 10^6/kg	CD34$^+$/CD38$^-$ 0.05 × 10^6/kg	CD34$^+$/CD33$^-$ only predictive for recovery to ANC > 2 × 10^9/L

[a]ANC > 0.5 × 10^9/L for 1–2 days
[b]Platelets > 20–50 × 10^9/L or platelet transfusion independence 1–2 days
[c]NS, not significant

14

better with engraftment than the total number of CD34$^+$ cells. These same PBSC subsets were also shown to be the best predictors of engraftment in a multivariate analysis. Subsequent studies by other groups have yielded mixed results when comparing the CD34$^+$/CD33$^-$ subset with total CD34$^+$ cells. However, all groups have found the CD34$^+$/CD33$^-$ subset dose to correlate well with platelet recovery, and most groups have reported the CD34$^+$/CD33$^-$ cell dose to be a better predictor of platelet engraftment than total CD34$^+$ cell dose *(55–58)*. Although the CD34$^+$/CD33$^-$ cell dose shows a good correlation with platelet engraftment, some groups have not observed a correlation between CD34$^+$/CD33$^-$ cell dose and time to neutrophil engraftment *(55,56)*. Reasons for these discrepancies have not been elucidated, but it is possible that an as-yet-unidentified subpopulation within the CD34$^+$/CD33$^-$ compartment accounts for these differences, and that enrichment levels vary in different patient populations or with the mobilization regimen used. Despite these discrepancies, in general, the minimum CD34$^+$/CD33$^-$ cell dose required for engraftment appears to be approx 1×10^6/kg (range, 0.9–2.8×10^6/kg).

Buscemi et al. *(59)* and Hénon et al. *(60)* have examined the CD34$^+$/CD38$^-$ cell dose infused in patients undergoing autologous PBSCT, and reported that the dose of this CD34$^+$ subset correlates better than both total CD34$^+$ cell numbers or the CD34$^+$/CD33$^-$ cell dose, with respect to the time to either platelet engraftment or trilineage engraftment. The minimum dose of CD34$^+$/CD38$^-$ cells required for engraftment was found to be 0.05×10^6 cells/kg (average dose 0.15×10^6/kg, range 0.011–1.62×10^6/kg) *(60)*, much lower than that reported for either total CD34$^+$ or CD34$^+$/CD33$^-$ cell numbers (Table 3).

4.2.2. PEDIATRIC PBSCT

PBSC collections in children weighing less than 25 kg is complicated by a low blood volume and poor vascular access, which has limited the use of PBSC for autotransplantation in children. However, the safety and efficacy of PBSCT in children has recently been established *(61)*. Data regarding factors affecting engraftment kinetics in children from trials with larger number of patients are beginning to accumulate. Although the number of groups that have analyzed the effects of CD34$^+$ cell dose on engraftment in pediatric patients has been limited, the number of CD34$^+$ cells infused appears to correlate with time to engraftment of neutrophils and, perhaps, platelets. Leibundgut et al. *(62)* reported that the number of both total CD34$^+$ and CD34$^+$/CD33$^-$ cells infused correlated with neutrophil recovery, but that only MK-CFU doses correlated with platelet engraftment. The only threshold observed in this study was for the GM-CFU dose ($>5 \times 10^4$ GM-CFU/kg), although few patients received low doses of CD34$^+$ cells. Investigators in Madrid *(63,64)* have also examined various CD34$^+$ cell subsets. These investigators have reported optimal doses of $>0.5 \times 10^6$ CD34$^+$/CD38$^-$ cells/kg for neutrophil engraftment, $>2 \times 10^6$ CD34$^+$/CD38$^+$ cells/kg for platelet engraftment, and $>5 \times 10^6$ CD34$^+$ cells/kg for engraftment of both lineages. Additional large studies will be required to establish a statistically significant correlation between CD34$^+$ cell dose and engraftment kinetics, and to determine valid threshold values in children undergoing PBSCT.

4.2.3. ALLOGENEIC PBSCT

In the allogeneic setting, PBSCT have not been as extensively studied as in the autologous setting. The safety of hematopoietic growth factor administration for stem cell mobilization in normal individuals has been one concern with utilization of PBSC, instead of BM, for allotransplants. Although the use of G-CSF has not been reported to result in any significant or irreversible toxicities to healthy donors, careful monitoring of donors is still required to assess its long-term safety *(65)*. Another major concern with the use of PBSC for allotransplants has been the potential for an increased risk of GVHD, because of the 10-fold higher concentration of T-lymphocytes in PB than in BM. Studies to date suggest that there is no increased risk of acute GVHD with allogeneic PBSCT, but that chronic GVHD may occur at a higher frequency with transplantation of PBSC than BM cells.

Several groups have investigated parameters that affect the engraftment of allo-PBSC. Körbling et al. *(66)* and Rosenfeld et al. *(67)* have reported no correlation between the CD34+ cell dose and the time to engraftment of neutrophils or platelets, although, in both studies, most patients received relatively high numbers of CD34+ cells (mean or median of $8–10 \times 10^6$/kg). More recently, other groups *(68,69)* have found that the CD34+ cell dose in allo-PBSCT significantly affects the speed of engraftment. Threshold CD34+ cell doses of $>5 \times 10^6$ CD34+ cells/kg and $>4.6 \times 10^6$ CD34+ cells/kg have been reported by Brown et al. *(68)* and Urbano-Ispizua et al. *(69)*, respectively.

4.2.4. Effect of Positive-selection of CD34+ PBSC on Engraftment

Many groups are currently investigating the safety and efficacy of CD34+ cell selection as a means of decreasing the volume of PBSC grafts in order to limit DMSO-associated infusional toxicity, decreasing tumor contamination of autografts, and depleting T-cells to reduce the risk of severe GVHD in allo-PBSCT. While tumor cells have been detected in the circulation, and their levels may even increase in PB following mobilization, tumor cell numbers have been found to be lower in PBSC products than in BM autografts *(70–72)*. Many groups are examining the relevance of contaminating tumor cells to disease-free survival. Currently, it is not clear that positive selection of CD34+ cells will affect disease-free survival rates *(27,73)*. However, CD34+ cell selection does not appear to adversely affect engraftment kinetics. Similar CD34+ cell dose thresholds have been observed in patients receiving positively selected CD34+ PBSC, and historical controls receiving unmanipulated PBSC *(46,74,75)*. Randomized trials addressing this issue need to be performed.

4.3. Predictive Parameters of CD34+ Cell Yields

CD34+ cell enumeration is an attractive choice for making real-time decisions about the timing of apheresis and the assessment of the adequacy of PBSC collections due to intralaboratory precision in CD34+ cell quantitation and relatively rapid result turnaround time. More recently, CD34 analyses have been suggested for use in predicting the likelihood of successful PBSC mobilization in individual patients. PB CD34+ cell counts, taken either during the steady state prior to mobilization or following mobilization on the day of, or day preceding, leukapheresis, have been reported, by several groups *(76–78)*, to correlate with the yield of CD34+ cells in leukapheresis products. Any extrapolation of data from these studies by individual transplant centers must take into account differences in patient characteristics, mobilization protocols, timing for initiation of apheresis, definition of target CD34+ cell yields, and method for CD34+ cell enumeration. However, analysis of steady-state CD34+ PBSC counts may prove useful in identifying those patients who are likely to be poor mobilizers, who might benefit from alternative mobilization strategies, or in identifying patients from whom large numbers of progenitor cells are likely to be collected, who would then be good candidates for ex vivo procedures associated with low CD34$^+$ cell recoveries, such as positive selection of CD34$^+$ cells or tumor purging.

Unfortunately, steady-state CD34$^+$ PBSC counts have not been adequately analyzed to firmly establish their value in predicting hematopoietic reserve. Two studies, using small patient cohorts, found a strong correlation between steady-state PB CD34$^+$ cell numbers and leukapheresis yields after mobilization with G-CSF alone or in combination with CT (76,79). However, a third study (80) has reported no correlation after mobilization with G-CSF alone.

4.4. Use of Growth Factors After PBSC Infusion

The use of myeloid growth factors to accelerate neutrophil recovery after PBSCT is currently a topic of some debate. In a retrospective analysis of 243 patients, Bensinger et al. (52) showed that the use of postinfusion growth factor was associated with a significant delay in platelet recovery only in patients who received $<5 \times 10^6$ CD34$^+$ cell/kg (Table 2). Those authors therefore suggested that, in patients with CD34$^+$ cell yields below 5×10^6 CD34$^+$ cells/kg, and particularly when below 2.5×10^6 CD34$^+$ cells/kg, posttransplant myeloid growth factors should not be used. The results of several randomized trials examining the benefit of G-CSF treatment on outcome after PBSCT have also been reported. Most groups report a significant improvement in neutrophil recovery in the G-CSF group, although all patients in one study received relatively high doses of CD34$^+$ cells ($>5 \times 10^6$ CD34$^+$ cells/kg), and the effect of CD34$^+$ cell dose on G-CSF efficacy was not analyzed in the other studies (81–83). In contrast to the findings reported by Bensinger, Linch et al. (84) examined 90 patients transplanted for lymphoma, and found that postinfusion G-CSF administration did not cause a delay in platelet recovery when low CD34$^+$ cell doses ($<5 \times 10^6$/ CD34$^+$ cells/kg) were received.

Studies in children have led to further controversy regarding the use of post-PBSCT growth factor administration. In a large randomized study, Kawano et al. (85) reported a 10-d delay in median time to platelet recovery in all non-ALL patients who received G-CSF posttransplant, regardless of the CD34$^+$ cell dose infused. In addition, they observed only a 1-d improvement in the median time to neutrophil engraftment in those children receiving growth factor post-PBSCT. Determination of the benefit of growth factors post-PBSCT will require the completion of large randomized trials in which adequate numbers of patients receiving low CD34$^+$ cell doses, with or without post-PBSCT growth factor, are included, and the effects of stem cell dose on growth factor efficacy are analyzed.

4.5. PBSC Viability

Cryopreservation and short-term storage (less than 6 mo) of leukapheresis products does not appear to result in lower recoveries of MNC or CD34$^+$ cells (86,87). However, recovery of in vitro colony-forming activity (GM-CFU and burst-forming units, erythrocytes) appears to decrease dramatically with extended periods of storage, especially beyond 2 yr (88,89). Improved recovery of GM-CFU following long-term storage (2–5 yr) can be achieved by the use of polyolefin bags and storage at −135°C, instead of PVC bags with storage at −80°C (88), or by the inclusion of hydroxyethyl starch (HES) in the cryoprotectant solution and storage at −80°C (90,91).

4.6. Summary

Measurement of the CD34[+] cell content of PBSC collections by flow cytometry is currently the most powerful and practical surrogate for PB progenitor cell content, and has become a routine practice of most transplant centers. Some centers also quantitate CD34[+] cell subsets. PBSC CD34[+] cell doses, but not NC doses, have been shown to correlate with speed of engraftment and overall engraftment. Based on currently available data, a CD34[+] cell dose of $2–5 \times 10^6$/kg is recommended. For CD34[+] cell subsets, minimum doses of 1×10^6 CD34[+]/CD33[-] cells/kg and 0.05×10^6 CD34[+]/CD38[-] cells/kg have been suggested. For patients in whom such doses cannot be reasonably collected, alternative therapies should probably be considered.

5. UMBILICAL CORD BLOOD

Hematopoietic stem and progenitor cells from placental blood, also referred to as CB, have recently been identified as an alternative source of allogeneic HSCs for transplantation (11,15,92–95). Compared to adult HSCs, stem cells from CB have distinct proliferative advantages, including enrichment in the most primitive stem cells producing long-term repopulation in vivo, increased clonogenicity, increased cell cycle rate, autocrine growth factor production, and increased telomere length (13,96–99).

In patients for whom no suitable BM donor is identified, CB stem cells have successfully been used to reconstitute the BM. The first CB transplant (CBT) was performed using CB from an HLA-identical sibling in 1988 (11). In 1994, the first unrelated CBT was reported by Kurtzberg et al. (100). Since then, more than 1000 CBTs have been performed worldwide for the treatment of various malignant and nonmalignant diseases, using both sibling and unrelated donors.

CB as a source of allogeneic stem cells offers the advantages of rapid availability, decreased likelihood of transmission of clinically important viral infections such as cytomegalovirus (CMV) and Epstein-Barr virus due to the low viral infection rate at birth, and a low risk of severe GVHD (92–95,100–102). The decreased risk of both acute and chronic GVHD reported with CBT allows an increase in the permissible degree of histoincompatibility between donor and recipient. CB grafts mismatched for up to two HLA Ags have been used effectively to reconstitute the BM (92–95). Thus, CB will probably provide an appropriate source of HSC for increasing numbers of patients belonging to ethnic groups not well-represented in BM donor registries. The use of CB from unrelated donors may also provide the benefits of a graft-vs-tumor effect, without the associated risks of GVHD and treatment-related mortality.

At the end of 1998, approx 21,000 CB units, nearly 100% of which were typed for HLA-A, -B, and -DR Ags, were available worldwide from 16 CB centers (103). This contrasts with the more than 5 million donors in BM registries worldwide, of which only 50% have been HLA-A-, -B-, and -DR-typed. The ability to collect CB from ethnic groups not well-represented in BM registries, with no risk to the mother or donor, has prompted the collection of CB from these groups. CB searches have recently been integrated into the established search procedures for an unrelated marrow donor through the Bone Marrow Donors Worldwide database. Despite efforts to increase representation of ethnic groups by CB collection centers, the weight of the intended recipient remains a major obstacle to the use of CB cells for transplantation. Although sufficient stem cells for transplantation can generally be collected and stored from BM and mobilized PB, the availability of stem cells in CB is limited. Because the clinical outcome of CBT has been shown to be related to the numbers of NC/kg infused, the use of CB for transplantation has primarily been restricted to children and smaller adults.

5.1. Optimal CB Cell Dose

Analysis of 102 patients who underwent related CBT by the Eurocord group revealed a median time to neutrophil engraftment of 28 d and a median of 48 d for platelet engraftment *(94,104)*. Factors favorably influencing survival were age ≤6 yr, ≤20 kg recipient weight, recipient CMV-negative serology, sex match, and NC dose ≥3.7 × 10^7/kg. Analysis of the outcome in 143 patients undergoing unrelated CBT by the Eurocord group showed the same trends observed in related CBT *(105)*. A relationship between the numbers of cells infused and engraftment was observed. The number of NC/kg infused after thawing was found to be the major factor that predicted for neutrophil and platelet engraftment after CBT. Patients receiving <3.7 × 10^7 NC/kg experienced delayed engraftment, with a median of 34 d required for neutrophil engraftment and 134 d for platelet engraftment compared to 25 and 47 days, respectively, in patients receiving a larger cell dose. Notably, no adult patients who received <1 × 10^7 NC/kg survived. Patients receiving <2 × 10^7 NC/kg had a 69 and 49% probability of achieving neutrophil and platelet engraftment, respectively, by d 60. The results from these studies demonstrate that infusion of low numbers of NC is associated with both an increased risk of nonengraftment and delayed engraftment.

Kurtzberg et al. *(92)* has also reported a correlation between NC dose and the rate of myeloid engraftment in a series of 25 patients undergoing unrelated CBT, who all received G-CSF to accelerate engraftment. Wagner et al. *(106)* has shown in a univariate analysis of 111 patients receiving CBT that the speed of engraftment is associated not only with the number of NC infused but also with the number of CD34+ cells and GM-CFU infused. In their analysis, the only factor predictive for survival was the number of cells infused.

Rubinstein et al. *(95)* recently reported the outcome of 562 patients undergoing unrelated CBT with CB units provided by the Placental Blood Program at the New York Blood Center. A correlation between the numbers of infused CB leukocytes or white blood cells/kg recipient weight (leukocyte count determined prior to cryopreservation) and successful myeloid engraftment was observed. Notably, only 97 (17%) of the 562 patients evaluated in this study were ≥18 yr of age. The median time to neutrophil engraftment was 28 d and 90 d for platelet engraftment. Successful engraftment was reported in 91% of patients receiving ≥1.0 × 10^8 leukocytes/kg; engraftment occurred in only 74% of patients receiving doses of 7–24 × 10^6 leukocytes/kg. In multivariate analyses, only the cell dose correlated with myeloid engraftment, whereas both the number of leukocytes/kg infused and the recipient's age were associated with the incidence of transplant-related events. Conversely, age, but not cell dose, correlated significantly with event-free survival after engraftment. Thus, the leukocyte content of CB grafts may primarily determine the speed and overall success of engraftment, and only secondarily affect transplant-related events and event-free survival.

In contrast to previous studies suggesting delayed platelet reconstitution after CBT compared to allo-BMT, Rubinstein et al. *(95)* reported that the probability and timing of platelet engraftment after CBT were similar to those observed after MUD-BMT. The rate and speed of myeloid engraftment were also found to be associated with the degree of donor–recipient HLA compatibility. This study also found that CMV positivity of the recipient prior to CBT was significantly associated with active CMV disease post-CBT and most strongly correlated with secondary graft failure.

Migliaccio et al. *(96)* have reported an association between the dose of CB CFC infused/kg and time to myeloid engraftment. The CFC dose was shown to directly correlate with the likelihood for engraftment, and inversely correlated with the time to myeloid engraftment after CBT. Engraftment was observed in 80% of patients receiving >4 × 10⁴ CFC/kg. Qualitative analyses of thawed CB cells may help to clarify the lack of engraftment observed in the remaining 20% of recipients who received the same CFC dose.

In vivo administration of G-CSF post-CBT has not been observed to increase the percentage of patients that successfully engraft. Recent studies with cytokine cocktails for ex vivo expansion of CB cells have been particularly exciting, with greater than 80-fold increases in CD34$^+$ cells observed with cultured CB cells (reviewed in ref. *13*). Future studies of CB expansion may permit sufficient stem cell amplification to increase the number of eligible adults for CBT. Additionally, the decreased immunological reactivity of transplanted CB cells may make it possible to combine several CB units from different donors, to increase stem cell numbers for transplantation.

5.2. CB Stem Cell Viability

Factors associated with the timing for processing and cryopreservation of CB are critical to the survival and quality of CB stem cells. Standardized methods for processing and storing CB units have not been universally adopted by collection centers. Following collection, CB units are stored at 4 or 25°C until processing. Processing of CB is generally completed within 24 h after collection *(107,108)*. Until recently, CB was routinely cryopreserved as an unseparated product, because of progenitor cell losses in excess of 30% reported with a variety of cell separation and volume reduction procedures *(95,101,109,110)*. In order to maintain cost-effectiveness and optimal use of space, it has become necessary to store CB as a separated product. Currently, most CB centers routinely volume-reduce CB units to 20–25 mL by removal of excess plasma and red cells with HES sedimentation before cryopreservation in 10% DMSO/dextran40 solution, which has been reported to result in approx 85% recovery of both NC and CD34$^+$ cells *(95,111–113)*.

The viability and yield of stem cells from CB stored at 4°C prior to processing has been reported to be reduced *(108)*. Recently, Shlebak et al. *(114)* also demonstrated that storage of CB at room temperature (25°C) prior to processing also resulted in a significant reduction in progenitor cell numbers. These investigators found a 59% reduction in d 7 GM-CFU when CB was stored at 25°C for 9 h prior to cell separation, and a 77% reduction when processing was further delayed until 24 h. Notably, MNC recovery was not as greatly affected as recovery of GM-CFU, with recovery of 88% MNC after 9 h and 51% after 24 h, implying a selective loss of stem and progenitor cells following prolonged storage. Thus, processing of collected CB should optimally be undertaken within 6 h.

The effects of cryopreservation on recovery of processed MNC and fractionated CD34$^+$ cells have been extensively studied. Broxmeyer et al. *(115)* has reported that computer-controlled freezing results in insignificant losses in stem and progenitor cells, with over 90% recovery of GM-CFU. Cryopreservation has also been reported to affect neither the recovery nor the clonogenic capacity of progenitor cells in frozen, unseparated CB for up to 7 yr *(116–118)*. However, recently, Shlebak et al. *(114)* reported that, although cryopreservation following either controlled-rate freezing or passive cooling did not result in a significant reduction in numbers or viability of MNC and GM-CFU, there was a significant reduction in the ability of GM-CFU to produce secondary colonies on replating after cryopreservation. Thus, functional deterioration in CB stem and progenitor cells following cryopreservation could explain the failure of engraftment observed in up to 20% of patients receiving adequate cell doses for CBT, as reported by Migliaccio et al. *(96)*.

5.3. Summary

The variability in parameters used to monitor cell doses and engraftment, such as NC dose, leukocyte count, number of CD34$^+$ cells, number of GM-CFU, and number of CFC, emphasizes the importance of the universal adoption of standardized methods for assessing the stem cell content of CB units in interpretation of CBT results. Data pre- and postthawing is likely to be most informative and to permit identification of the appropriate indicators for engraftment and speed of engraftment, as well as the determination of minimum and optimum doses. Based on the preponderance of data on NC and leukocyte doses in CBT, and the relative paucity of data regarding CD34$^+$ cell doses, a dose of 2×10^7 NC/kg prior to thawing has been recommended, because of estimated cell losses that occur during thawing *(103)*. Notably, this dose is approx 1 log lower than the cell number infused with a standard allo-BMT or -PBSCT, further supporting the qualitative advantage of stem cells from CB over adult sources. Future studies should address more precisely the numbers of stem cells required for successful CBT by analysis of CD34$^+$ cell doses, as well as CD34$^+$ subpopulations in large numbers of patients.

6. FUTURE PERSPECTIVES

The CD34 Ag is a clinically useful marker for the human HSC, but it should not be considered an absolute boundary for defining the stem cell population. Recent studies in mice indicate the existence of a CD34$^-$ HSC capable of self-renewal and hematopoietic reconstitution. Long-term reconstitution of myeloablated mice has been accomplished with injection of a single murine CD34$^-$ stem cell *(119)*. In addition, transgenic mice lacking CD34 have been found to be viable, with normal hematologic profiles, and to experience normal trilineage recovery following sublethal irradiation *(120)*. The search for the human CD34$^-$ stem cell counterpart will be complicated by the requirement for the use of xenogeneic models, in which negative results will be difficult to interpret. However, there is already evidence that human BM contains cells that can efflux Hoechst 33342 dye in a manner identical to a small, homogenous population of murine CD34$^-$ HSC *(121)*. Although isolation of the true human HSC has remained elusive, it is likely that this will be accomplished in the near future. The potential use of such cells opens exciting prospects as these cells may possess more desirable biological characteristics, such as increased gene transduction frequencies to facilitate gene transfer into human cells or enhanced ex vivo expansion capabilities.

REFERENCES

1. Serke S, Arseniev L, Watts M, Fritsch G, Ingles-Esteve J, Johnson JE, et al. Imprecision of counting CFU-GM colonies and CD34-expressing cells, *Bone Marrow Transplant.*, **20** (1997) 57–61.

2. Andrews RG, Singer JW, and Bernstein ID. Precursors of colony-forming cells in humans can be distinguished from colony-forming cells by expression of the CD33 and CD34 antigens and light scatter properties. *J. Exp. Med.*, **169** (1989) 1721–1731.

3. Bernstein ID, Leary AG, Andrews RG, and Ogawa M. Blast colony-forming cells and precursors of colony-forming cells detectable in long-term marrow culture express the same phenotype (CD33⁻CD34⁺), *Exp. Hematol.*, **19** (1991) 680–682.

4. Sakabe H, Ohmizono Y, Tanimukai S, Kimura T, Mori KJ, Abe T, et al. Functional differences between subpopulations of mobilized peripheral blood-derived CD34⁺ cells expressing different levels of HLA-DR, CD33, CD38 and c-kit antigens. *Stem Cell*, **15** (1997) 73–81.

5. Terstappen LWMM, Huang S, Safford M, Lansdorp PM, and Loken MR. Sequential generations of hematopoietic colonies derived from single nonlineage-committed CD34⁺CD38⁻ progenitor cells. *Blood*, **77** (1991) 1218–1227.

6. Prosper F, Stroncek D, and Verfaillie CM. Phenotypic and functional characterization of long-term culture-initiating cells present in peripheral blood progenitor collections of normal donors treated with granulocyte colony-stimulating factor. *Blood*, **88** (1996) 2033–2042.

7. Van Epps DE, Bender J, Lee W, Schilling M, Smith A, Smith S, et al. Harvesting, characterization, and culture of CD34⁺ cells from human bone marrow, peripheral blood, and cord blood. *Blood Cells*, **20** (1994) 411–423.

8. Kasai M and Masauzi N. Characteristics of umbilical cord blood (UCB) and UCB transplantation. *Semin. Thromb. Hemostasis.*, **24** (1998) 491–495.

9. Huang S, Law P, Young D, Ho AD. Candidate hematopoietic stem cells from fetal tissues, umbilical cord blood vs. adult bone marrow and peripheral blood. *Exp. Hematol.*, **26** (1998) 1162–1171.

10. Theilgaard-Mönch K, Raaschou-Jensen K, Heilmann C, Andersen H, Bock J, Russel CA, et al. A comparative study of CD34⁺ cells, CD34⁺ subsets, colony forming cells, and cobblestone area forming cells in cord blood and bone marrow allografts. *Eur. J. Haematol.*, **62** (1999) 174–183.

11. Gluckman E, Broxmeyer HE, Auerbach AD, et al. Hematopoietic reconstitution in a patient with Fanconi's anemia by means of umbilical cord blood from an HLA-identical sibling. *N. Engl. J. Med.*, **321** (1989) 1174–1178.

12. Timeus F, Crescenzio N, Marranca D, et al. Cell adhesion molecules in cord blood hematopoietic progenitors. *Bone Marrow Transplant.*, **22** (1998) S61–S62.

13. Cairo MS and Wagner JE. Placental and/or umbilical cord blood: An alternative source of hematopoietic stem cells for transplantation. *Blood*, **90** (1997) 4665–4678.

14. Gratama JW, Orfao A, Barnett D, Brando B, Huber A, Janossy G, et al. Flow cytometric enumeration of CD34⁺ hematopoietic stem and progenitor cells. *Cytometry*, **34** (1998) 128–142.

15. Wagner JE, Kernan NA, Steinbuch M, Broxmeyer HE, and Gluckman E. Allogeneic sibling umbilical cord blood transplantation in children with malignant and non-malignant disease. *Lancet.*, **346** (1995) 214–219.

16. Lapidot T, Pflumio F, Doedens M, Murdoch B, Williams DE, and Dick JE. Cytokine stimulation of multilineage hematopoiesis from immature human cell engrafted in SCID mice. *Science*, **255** (1992) 1137–1141.

17. Vormoor J, Lapidot T, Pflumio F, et al. Immature human cord blood progenitors engraft and proliferate to high levels in severe combined immunodeficient mice. *Blood*, **83** (1994) 2489–2497.

18. Pflumio F, Izac B, Katz A, Shultz LD, Vainchenker W, and Coulombel L. Phenotype and function of human hematopoietic cells engrafting immune-deficient CB17-severe combined immunodeficiency mice and nonobese diabetic-severe combined immunodeficiency mice after transplantation of human cord blood mononuclear cells. *Blood*, **88** (1996) 3731.

19. Hogan CJ, Shpall EJ, McNiece I, and Keller G. Multilineage engraftment in NOD/LtSz-scid/scid mice from mobilized human CD34⁺ peripheral blood progenitor cells. *Biol. Blood Marrow Transplant.*, **3** (1997) 236–246.

20. Hogan CJ, Shpall EJ, McNulty O, et al. Engraftment and development of human CD34(+)-enriched cells from umbilical cord blood in NOD/LtSz-scid/scid mice. *Blood*, **90** (1997) 85–96.

21. Noort WA, Willemze R, and Falkenburg JHF. Comparison of repopulating ability of hematopoietic progenitor cells isolated from human umbilical cord blood or bone marrow cells in NOD-SCID mice. *Bone Marrow Transplant.*, **22** (1998) S58–S60.

22. Thomas ED and Storb R. Technique for human marrow grafting. *Blood*, **36** (1970) 507–515.

23. Storb R, Prentice RL, and Thomas ED. Marrow transplantation for treatment of aplastic anemia. An analysis of factors associated with graft rejection. *New Engl. J. Med.*, **296** (1977) 61–66.

24. Al-Fiar F, Prince HM, Imrie K, Stewart AK, Crump M, and Keating A. Bone marrow mononuclear cell count does not predict neutrophil and platelet recovery following autologous bone marrow transplant: value of the colony-forming unit granulocytic-macrophage (CFU-GM) assay. *Cell Transplantation*, **6** (1997) 491–495.

25. Brandwein JM, Callum J, Sutcliffe SB, Scott JG, and Keating A. Analysis of factors affecting hematopoietic recovery after autologous bone marrow transplantation for lymphoma. *Bone Marrow Transplant.*, **6** (1990) 291–294.

26. Douay L, Gorin N, Mary J, Lemarie E, Lopez M, Najman A, et al. Recovery of CFU-GM from cryopreserved marrow and in vivo evaluation after autologous bone marrow transplantation are predictive of engraftment. *Exp. Hematol.*, **14** (1986) 358–365.

27. Sharp JG, Kessinger A, Mann S, Crouse DA, Armitage JO, Bierman P, et al. Outcome of high-dose therapy and autologous transplantation in non-Hodgkin's lymphoma based on the presence of tumor in the marrow or infused hematopoietic harvest. *J. Clin. Oncol.*, **14** (1996) 214–219.

28. Laporte J, Douay L, Lopez M, Labopin M, Jouet JP, Lesage S, et al. One hundred twenty-five adult patients with primary acute leukemia autografted with marrow purged by mafosfamide: a 10-year single institution experience. *Blood*, **84** (1994) 3810–3818.

29. Rowley SD, Piantadosi S, Marcellus, DC, Jones RJ, Davidson NE, Davis JM, et al. Analysis of factors predicting speed of hematologic recovery after transplantation with 4-hydroperoxyclophosphamide-purged autologous bone marrow grafts. *Bone Marrow Transplant.*, **7** (1991) 183–191.

30. Gorin N, Lopez M, Laporte J, Quittet P, Lesage S, Lemoine F, et al. Preparation and successful engraftment of purified CD34$^+$ bone marrow progenitor cells in patients with non-Hodgkin's lymphoma. *Blood*, **85** (1995) 1647–1654.

31. Shpall E, LeMaistre CF, Holland K, Ball E, Jones R, Saral R, et al. A prospective randomized trial of buffy coat versus CD34-selected autologous bone marrow support in high-risk breast cancer patients receiving high dose chemotherapy. *Blood*, **90** (1997) 4313–4320.

32. Attarian H, Feng Z, Buckner CD, MacLeod B, and Rowely SD. Long-term cryopreservation of bone marrow for autologous transplantation. *Bone Marrow Transplant.*, **17** (1996) 425–430.

33. Torres A, Alonso MC, Gomez-Villagran JL, Manzanares MR, Martinez F, Gomez P, et al. No influence of number of donor CFU-GM on granulocyte recovery in bone marrow transplantation for acute leukemia. *BLUT*, **50** (1985) 89–94.

34. Atkinson K, Norrie S, Chan P, Downs K, and Biggs J. Lack of correlation between nucleated bone marrow cell dose, marrow CFU-GM dose or marrow CFU-E dose and the rate of HLA-identical sibling marrow engraftment. *Br. J. of Hematology*, **60** (1985) 245–251.

35. Bacigalupo A, Piaggio G, Podesta M, Figari O, Benvenuto F, Sogno G, et al. Influence of marrow CFU-GM content on engraftment and survival after allogeneic bone marrow transplantation. *Bone Marrow Transplant.*, **15** (1995) 221–226.

36. Gerhartz H, Kolb H, Clemm C, and Wilmanns W. Clonogenic assays and engraftment in allogeneic bone marrow transplantation. *Bone Marrow Transplant.*, **1** (1986) 221–226.

37. Bortin M, Gale R, Kay H, and Rimm A. Bone marrow transplantation for acute myelogenous leukemia. *JAMA*, **249** (1983) 1166–1175.

38. Sierra J, Storer B, Hansen J, Bjerke J, Martin P, Petersdorf E, et al. Transplantation of marrow cells from unrelated donors for treatment of high risk acute leukemia: the effect of leukemic burden, donor HLA-matching and marrow cell dose. *Blood*, **89** (1997) 4226–4235.

39. Mavroudis D, Read E, Cottler-Fox M, Couriel D, Molldrem J, Carter C, et al. CD34$^+$ cell dose predicts survival, posttransplant morbidity, and rate of hematologic recovery after allogeneic marrow transplants for hematologic malignancies. *Blood*, **8** (1996) 3223–3229.

40. Bender JG, To LB, Williams S, and Schwartzberg LS. Defining a therapeutic dose of peripheral blood stem cells. *J. Hematother.*, **1** (1992) 329–341.

41. Schwella N, Siegert W, Beyer J, Rick O, Zingsem J, Eckstein R, et al. Autografting with blood progenitor cells: predictive value of preapheresis blood cell counts on progenitor cell harvest and

correlation of the reinfused cell dose with hematopoietic reconstitution. *Ann. Hematol.*, **71** (1995) 227–234.

42. Smith RJ and Sweetenham JW. A mononuclear cell dose of 3×10^8/kg predicts early multilineage recovery in patients with malignant lymphoma treated with carmustine, etoposide, Ara-C and melphalan (BEAM) and peripheral blood progenitor cell transplantation. *Exp. Hematol.*, **23** (1995) 1581–1588.

43. Watts MJ, Sullivan AM, Jamieson E, Pearce R, Fielding A, Devereux S, et al. Progenitor-cell mobilization after low-dose cyclophosphamide and granulocyte colony-stimulating factor: an analysis of progenitor-cell quantity and quality and factors predicting for these parameters in 101 pretreated patients with malignant lymphoma. *J. Clin. Oncol.*, **15** (1997) 535–546.

44. Haas R, Witt B, Mohle R, Goldschmidt H, Hohaus S, Fruehauf S, et al. Sustained long-term hematopoiesis after myeloablative therapy with peripheral blood progenitor cell support. *Blood*, **85** (1995) 3754–3761.

45. To LB, Haylock DN, Simmons PJ, and Juttner CA. The biology and clinical uses of blood stem cells. *Blood*, **89** (1997) 2233–2238.

46. Hermouet S, Niaussat AE, Briec A, Pineau D, Robillard N, Bataille R, et al. Analysis of platelet recovery after autologous transplantation with G-CSF mobilized CD34$^+$ cells purified from leukapheresis products. *Hematol. Cell Ther.*, **39** (1997) 317–325.

47. Tricot G, Jagannath S, Vesole D, Nelson J, Tindle S, Miller L, et al. Peripheral blood stem cell transplants for multiple myeloma: identification of favorable variables for rapid engraftment in 225 patients. *Blood*, **85** (1995) 588–596.

48. Glaspy JA, Shpall EJ, LeMaistre CF, Briddell RA, Menchaca DM, Turner SA, et al. Peripheral blood progenitor cell mobilization using stem cell factor in combination with filgrastim in breast cancer patients. *Blood*, **90** (1997) 2939–2951.

49. Weaver CH, Hazelton B, Birch R, Palmer P, Allen C, Schwartzberg L, et al. An analysis of engraftment kinetics as a function of the CD34 content of peripheral blood progenitor cell collections in 692 patients after the administration of myeloablative chemotherapy. *Blood*, **86** (1995) 3961–3969.

50. Rossi A, Cortelazzo S, Bellavita P, Viero P, Bassan R, Comotti B, et al. Long-term haematological reconstitution following BEAM and autologous transplantation of circulating progenitor cells in non-Hodgkin's lymphoma. *Brit. J. Haematol.*, **96** (1997) 620–626.

51. Bolwell B, Goormastic M, Andresen S, Koo A, Wise K, Overmoyer B, et al. Variables associated with the platelet count 6 weeks after autologous peripheral blood progenitor cell transplantation. *Bone Marrow Transplant.*, **22** (1998) 547–551.

52. Bensinger W, Appelbaum F, Rowley S, Storb R, Sanders J, Lilleby K, et al. Factors that influence collection and engraftment of autologous peripheral-blood stem cells. *J. Clin. Oncol.*, **13** (1995) 2547–2555.

53. Weaver CH, Potz J, Redmond J, Tauer K, Schwartzberg LS, Kaywin P, et al. Engraftment and outcomes of patients receiving myeloablative therapy followed by autologous peripheral blood stem cells with a low CD34$^+$ cell content. *Bone Marrow Transplant.*, **19** (1997) 1103–1110.

54. Dercksen MW, Rodenhuis S, Dirkson MKA, Schaasberg WP, Baars JW, van der Wall E, et al. Subsets of CD34$^+$ cells and rapid hematopoietic recovery after peripheral-blood stem-cell transplantation. *J. Clin. Oncol.*, **13** (1995) 1922–1932.

55. Copelan EA, Ceselski SK, Ezzone SA, Lasky LC, Penza SL, Bechtel TP, et al. Mobilization of peripheral-blood progenitor cells with high-dose etoposide and granulocyte colony-stimulating factor in patients with breast cancer, non-Hodgkin's lymphoma, and Hodgkin's disease. *J. Clin. Oncol.*, **15** (1997) 759–765.

56. Millar BC, Millar JL, Shepherd V, Blackwell P, Porter H, Cunningham D, et al. The importance of CD34$^+$/CD33$^-$ cells in platelet engraftment after intensive therapy for cancer patients given peripheral blood stem cell rescue. *Bone Marrow Transplant.*, **22** (1998) 469–475.

57. Pecora AL, Preti RA, Gleim GW, Jennis A, Zahos K, Cantwell S, et al. CD34$^+$CD33$^-$ cells influence days to engraftment and transfusion requirements in autologous blood stem-cell recipients. *J. Clin. Oncol.*, **16** (1998) 2093–2104.

58. Sampol Mayol A, Besalduch Vital J, Galmés Llodrá A, Bargay Lleonart J, Matamoros Flori N, Morey Sureda M, et al. CD34$^+$ cell dose and CD33$^-$ subsets: collection and engraftment kinetics in autologous peripheral blood stem cells transplantation. *Haematologica*, **83** (1998) 489–495.

59. Buscemi F, Indovina A, Scimè R, Santoro A, Pampinella M, Fiandaca T, et al. CD34$^+$ cell subsets and platelet recovery after PBSC autograft. *Bone Marrow Transplant.*, **16** (1995) 855–860.

60. Hénon P, Sovalat H, Becker M, Arkam Y, Ojeda-Uribe M, Raidot JP, et al. Primordial role of

CD34$^+$38$^-$ cells in early and late trilineage haemopoietic engraftment after autologous blood cell transplantation. *Brit. J. Haematol.*, **103** (1998) 568–581.

61. Takue Y, Kawano Y, Abe T, Okamoto Y, Suzue T, Shimizu T, et al. Collection and transplantation of peripheral blood stem cells in very small children weighing 20 kg or less. *Blood*, **86** (1995) 372–380.

62. Leibundgut K, von Rohr A, Brülhart K, Hirt A, Ischi E, Jeanneret C, et al. The number of circulating CD34$^+$ blood cells predicts the colony-forming capacity of leukapheresis produces in children. *Bone Marrow Transplant.*, **15** (1995) 25–31.

63. Diaz MA, Alegre A, Villa M, Granda A, de la Vega A, Ramirez M, et al. Pediatric experience with autologous peripheral blood progenitor cell transplantation: influence of CD34$^+$ cell dose in engraftment kinetics. *Bone Marrow Transplant.*, **18** (1996) 699–703.

64. Gonzelez-Requejo A, Madero L, Diaz MA, Villa M, Garcia-Escribano C, Balas A, et al. Progenitor cell subsets and engraftment kinetics in children undergoing autologous peripheral blood stem cell transplantation. *Brit. J. Haematol.*, **101** (1998) 104–110.

65. Anderlini P, Körbling M, Dale D, Gratwohl A, Schmitz N, Stroncek D, et al. Allogeneic blood stem cell transplantation: considerations for donors. *Blood*, **90** (1997) 903–908.

66. Körbling M, Huh YO, Durett A, Mirza N, Miller P, Engel H, et al. Allogeneic blood stem cell transplantation: peripheralization and yield of donor-derived primitive hematopoietic progenitor cells (CD34$^+$ Thy-1^{dim}) and lymphoid subsets, and possible predictors of engraftment and graft-versus-host disease. *Blood*, **86** (1995) 2842–2848.

67. Rosenfeld C, Collins R, Piñeiro L, Agura E, and Nemunaitis J. Allogeneic blood cell transplantation without posttransplant colony-stimulating factors in patients with hematopoietic neoplasm: a phase II study. *J. Clin. Oncol.*, **14** (1996) 1314–1319.

68. Brown RA, Adkins D, Goodnough LT, Haug JS, Todd G, Wehde M, et al. Factors that influence the collection and engraftment of allogeneic peripheral-blood stem cells in patients with hematologic malignancies. *J. Clin. Oncol.*, **15** (1997) 3067–3074.

69. Urbano-Ispizua A, Solano C, Brunet S, de la Rubia J, Odriozola J, Zuazu J, et al. Allogeneic transplantation of selected CD34$^+$ cells from peripheral blood: experience of 62 cases using immunoadsorption or immunomagnetic technique. *Bone Marrow Transplant.*, **22** (1998) 519–525.

70. Brugger W, Bross KJ, Glatt M, Weber F, Mertelsmann R, and Kanz L. Mobilization of tumor cells and hematopoietic progenitor cells into peripheral blood of patients with solid tumors. *Blood*, **83** (1994) 636–640.

71. Vescio RA, Han EJ, Schiller GJ, Lee JC, Wu CH, Cao J, et al. Quantitative comparison of multiple myeloma tumor contamination in bone marrow harvest and leukapheresis autografts. *Bone Marrow Transplant.*, **18** (1996) 103–110.

72. Ross AA, Cooper BW, Lazarus HM, Mackay W, Moss TJ, Ciobanu N, et al. Detection and viability of tumor cells in peripheral blood stem cell collections from breast cancer patients using immunocytochemical and clonogenic assay techniques. *Blood*, **82** (1993) 2605–2610.

73. Cooper BW, Moss TJ, Ross AA, Ybanez J, and Lazarus HM. Occult tumor contamination of hematopoietic stem-cell products does not affect clinical outcome of autologous transplantation in patients with metastatic breast cancer. *J. Clin. Oncol.*, **16** (1998) 3509–3517.

74. Negrin RS, Kusnierz-Glaz CR, Still BJ, Schriber JR, Chao NJ, Long GD, et al. Transplantation of enriched and purged peripheral blood progenitor cells from a single apheresis product in patients with non-Hodgkin's lymphoma. *Blood*, **85** (1995) 3334–3341.

75. Watts MJ, Sullivan AM, Ings SJ, Leverett D, Peniket AJ, Perry AR, et al. Evaluation of clinical scale CD34$^+$ cell purification: experience of 71 immunoaffinity column procedures. *Bone Marrow Transplant.*, **20** (1997) 157–162.

76. Fruehauf S, Haas R, Conradt C, Murea S, Witt B, Möhle R, et al. Peripheral blood progenitor cell (PBPC) counts during steady-state hematopoiesis allow to estimate the yield of mobilized PBPC after filgrastim (R-metHuG-CSF)-supported cytotoxic chemotherapy. *Blood*, **85** (1995) 2619–2626.

77. Elliott C, Samson DM, Armitage S, Lyttelton MP, McGuigan D, Hargreaves R, et al. When to harvest peripheral-blood stem cells after mobilization therapy: prediction of CD34-positive cell yield by preceding day CD34-positive concentration in peripheral blood. *J. Clin. Oncol.*, **14** (1996) 970–973.

78. Chapple P, Prince HM, Quinn M, Bertoncello I, Juneja S, Wolf M, et al. Peripheral blood CD34$^+$ cell count reliably predicts autograft yield. *Bone Marrow Transplant.*, **22** (1998) 125–130.

79. Husson B, Ravoet C, Dehon M, Wallef G, Hougardy N, and Delannoy A. Predictive value of the steady-state peripheral blood progenitor cell (PBPC) counts for the yield of PBPC collected by

leukapheresis after mobilization by granulocyte colony-stimulating factor (G-CSF) alone or chemo-therapy and G-CSF. *Blood*, **87** (1996) 3526–3528.

80. Roberts AW, Begley CG, Grigg AP, and Basser RL. Do steady-state peripheral blood progenitor cell (PBPC) counts predict the yield of PBPC mobilized by filgrastim alone? [letter]. *Blood*, **86** (1995) 2451.

81. Tarella C, Castellino C, Locatelli F, Caracciolo D, Corradini P, Falda M, et al. G-CSF administration following peripheral blood progenitor cell (PBPC) autograft in lymphoid malignancies: evidence for clinical benefits and reduction of treatment costs. *Bone Marrow Transplant.*, **21** (1998) 401–407.

82. Klumpp TR, Mangan KF, Goldberg SL, Pearlman ES, and Macdonald JS. Granulocyte colony-stimulating factor accelerates neutrophil engraftment following peripheral-blood stem-cell transplant-ation: a prospective, randomized trial. *J. Clin. Oncol.*, **13** (1995) 1323–1327.

83. Lee SM, Radford JA, Dogson L, Huq T, Ryder WDJ, Pettengell R, et al. Recombinant human granulocyte colony-stimulating factor (filgrastim) following high-dose chemotherapy and peripheral blood progenitor cell rescue in high-grade non-Hodgkin's lymphoma: clinical benefits at no extra cost. *Brit. J. Cancer*, **77** (1998) 1294–1299.

84. Linch DC, Milligan DW, Winfield DA, Kelsey SM, Johnson SA, Littlewood TJ, et al. G-CSF after peripheral blood stem cell transplantation in lymphoma patients significantly accelerated neutrophil recovery and shortened time in hospital: results of a randomized BNLI trial. *Brit. J. Haematol.*, **99** (1997) 933–938.

85. Kawano Y, Takaue Y, Mimaya J, Horikoshi Y, Watanabe T, Abe T, et al. Marginal benefit/disadvan-tage of granulocyte colony-stimulating factor therapy after autologous blood stem cell transplantation in children: results of a prospective randomized trial. *Blood*, **92** (1998) 4040–4046.

86. Pettengell R, Woll PJ, O'Connor DA, Dexter TM, and Testa NG. Viability of haemopoietic progenitors from whole blood, bone marrow and leukapheresis product: effects of storage media, temperature of time. *Bone Marrow Transplant.*, **14** (1994) 703–709.

87. Humpe A, Riggert J, Vehmeyer K, Troff C, Hiddemann W, Köhler M, et al. Comparison of CD34+ cell numbers and colony growth before and after cryopreservation of peripheral blood progenitor and stem cell harvests: influence of prior chemotherapy. *Transfusion*, **37** (1997) 1050–1057.

88. Valeri CR and Pivacek LE. Effects of the temperature, the duration of frozen storage, and the freezing container on in vitro measurements in human peripheral blood mononuclear cells. *Transfusion*, **36** (1996) 303–308.

89. Galmés A, Besalduch J, Bargay J, Novo A, Morey M, Guerra JM, et al. Long-term storage at −80°C of hematopoietic progenitor cells with 5-percent dimethyl sulfoxide as the sole cryoprotectant. *Transfusion*, **39** (1999) 70–73.

90. Katayama Y, Yano T, Bessho A, Deguchi S, Sunami K, Mahmut N, et al. The effects of a simplified method for cryopreservation and thawing procedures on peripheral blood stem cells. *Bone Marrow Transplant.*, **19** (1997) 283–287.

91. Ayello J, Semidei-Pomales M, Preti R, Hesdorffer C, and Reiss RF. Effects of long-term storage at −90 degrees C of bone marrow and PBPC on cell recovery, viability, and clonogenic potential. *J. Hematother.*, **7** (1998) 385–390.

92. Kurtzberg J, Laughlin M, Graham ML, et al. Placental blood as a source of hematopoietic stem cells for transplantation into unrelated recipients. *N. Engl. J. Med.*, **335** (1996) 157–166.

93. Wagner JE, Rosenthal J, Sweetman R, et al. Successful transplantation of HLA-matched and HLA-mismatched umbilical cord blood from unrelated donors: analysis of engraftment and acute graft-vs-host disease. *Blood*, **88** (1996) 795–802.

94. Gluckman E, Rocha V, Boyer-Chammard A, et al. Outcome of cord blood transplantation from related and unrelated donors. *N. Engl. J. Med.*, **337** (1997) 373–381.

95. Rubinstein P, Carrier C, Scaradavou A, et al. Outcomes among 562 recipients of placental-blood transplants from unrelated donors. *N. Engl. J. Med.*, **339** (1998) 1565–1577.

96. Migliaccio AR, Adamson JW, Rubinstein P, and Stevens C. Correlation between progenitor cell dose, likelihood to engraft and time to myeloid engraftment in 130 unrelated placental/cord blood transplants. 3rd Eurocord Concerted Action Workshop, Annecy, France, 1998 (Abstr.).

97. Morrison SJ, Wandycz AM, Akashi K, et al. The aging of hematopoietic stem cells. *Nature Med.*, **2** (1996) 1011–1016.

98. Morrison SJ, Prowse KR, Ho P, et al. Telomerase activity in hematopoietic cells is associated with self-renewal potential. *Immunity*, **5** (1996) 207–216.

99. Mayani H and Lansdorp PM. Thy-1 expression is linked to functional properties of primitive hematopoietic progenitor cells from human umbilical cord blood. *Blood*, **83** (1994) 2410–2417.

100. Kurtzberg J, Graham M, Casei J, et al. The use of umbilical cord blood in mismatched related and unrelated hemapoietic stem cell transplantation. *Blood*, **20** (1994) 275–284.

101. Rubinstein P, Rosenfield RE, Adamson JW, and Stevens CE. Stored placental blood for unrelated bone marrow reconstitution. *Blood*, **81** (1993) 1679–1690.

102. Rubinstein P. Placental blood-derived hematopoietic stem cells for unrelated bone marrow reconstitution. *J. Hematother.*, **2** (1993) 207–210.

103. Gluckman E, Rocha V, and Chastang CI. Ham-Wasserman Lecture: Cord blood hematopoietic stem cells biology and transplantation. *American Society of Hematology Education Program Book.* (1998) 1–14.

104. Rocha V, Chastang CI, Souillet G, et al. for the Eurocord transplant group. Related cord blood transplants: The Eurocord experience of 78 transplants. *Bone Marrow Transplant.*, **21** (1998) S59.

105. Gluckman E, Rocha V, Chastang CI, on behalf of Eurocord. Cord blood banking and transplant in Europe. *Bone Marrow Transplant.*, **22** (1998) S68–S74.

106. Wagner JE, DeFor T, Rubinstein P, and Kurtzberg J. Transplantation of unrelated donor umbilical cord blood (UCB): Outcomes and analysis of risk factors. *Blood*, **90** (1997) 398a (Abstract).

107. Ademokun JA, Chapman C, Dunn J, et al. Umbilical blood collection and separation for hematopoietic progenitor cell banking. *Bone Marrow Transplant.*, **19** (1997) 1023–1028.

108. Campos L, Roubi N, and Guyotat D. Definition of optimal conditions for collection and cryopreservation of umbilical hematopoietic cells. *Cryobiology*, **32** (1995) 511–513.

109. Broxmeyer HE, Douglas GW, Hangoc G, et al. Human umbilical cord blood as a potential source of transplantable hematopoietic stem/progenitor cells. *Proc. Natl. Acad. Sci.*, **86** (1989) 3828–3832.

110. Jacobs HCJM and Falkenburg JHF. Umbilical cord blood banking in The Netherlands. *Bone Marrow Transplant.*, **22** (1998) S8–S10.

111. Rubinstein P, Drobila L, Rosenfield R, et al. Processing and cryopreservation of placental/umbilical cord blood for unrelated bone marrow reconstitution. *Proc. Natl. Acad. Sci. USA*, **92** (1995) 10,119–10,122.

112. Querol S, Gabarro M, Amat L, et al. The placental blood program of the Barcelona Cord Blood Bank. *Bone Marrow Transplant.*, **22** (1998) S3–S5.

113. Kögler G, Sarnowski A, and Wernet P. Volume reduction of cord blood by Hetastarch for long-term stem cell banking. *Bone Marrow Transplant.*, **22** (1998) S14–A15.

114. Shlebak AA, Marley SB, Roberts IAG, Davidson RJ, Goldman JM, and Gordon MY. Optimal timing for processing and cryopreservation of umbilical cord haematopoietic stem cells for clinical transplantation. *Bone Marrow Transplant.*, **23** (1999) 131–138.

115. Broxmeyer HE, Kurtzberg J, Gluckman E, et al. Umbilical cord blood hematopoietic stem and repopulating cells in human clinical transplantation. *Blood Cells*, **17** (1990) 313–329.

116. Almici C, Carlo-Stella C, and Mangoni L. Density separation and cryopreservation of umbilical cord blood cells: evaluation of recovery in short- and long-term cultures. *Acta. Haematica.*, **95** (1996) 171–175.

117. Turner CW, Luzins J, and Hutcheson C. A modified harvest technique for cord blood haematopoietic stem cells. *Bone Marrow Transplant.*, **10** (1992) 89–91.

118. Emminger W, Emminger-Schmidmeir W, Hocker P, et al. Myeloid progenitor cells (CFU-GM) predict engraftment kinetics in autologous transplantation in children. *Bone Marrow Transplant.*, **4** (1989) 415–420.

119. Osawa M, Hanada K, Hamada H, and Nakauchi H. Long-term lymphohematopoietic reconstitution by a single CD34-low/negative hematopoietic stem cell. *Science*, **273** (1996) 242–245.

120. Cheng J, Baumhueter S, Cacalano G, Carver-Moore K, Thibodeaux H, Thomas R, et al. Hematopoietic defects in mice lacking the sialomucin CD34. *Blood*, **87** (1996) 479–490.

121. Goodell MA, Rosenzweig M, Kim H, Marks DF, DeMaria M, Paradis G, et al. Dye efflux studies suggest that hematopoietic stem cells expressing low or undetectable levels of CD34 antigen exist in multiple species. *Nature Med.*, **3** (1997) 1337–1345.

2 Is Bone Marrow Transplantation Appropriate in Older Patients?

Brian J. Bolwell, MD

CONTENTS

1. INTRODUCTION

Many, if not most, protocols involving allogeneic bone marrow transplant (allo-BMT) have eligibility criteria that include parameters of patient age. Generally, eligibility includes patients less than 55, 60, or 65 yr of age. Many autologous BMT (ABMT) protocols also have age cutoffs restricting patient eligibility. The reason for such an age cutoff is presumably that the transplant procedure itself is prohibitively risky in older patients. Common transplant teachings suggest that the older the patient, the higher the risk of graft-vs-host disease (GVHD), treatment-related mortality (TRM), overall toxicity, and decreased disease-free survival (DFS). However, much of this dogma is based on literature comparing pediatric patients to adult patients. Indeed, few series actually examine the potential toxicity of transplantation comparing older adults to younger adults. Additionally, in the field of autologous transplantation (autotransplantation), the use of primed peripheral blood progenitor cells (PBPCs) has drastically reduced the treatment-related toxicities, at least in part, because of enhanced engraftment rates; therefore, some of the older literature concerning autotransplantation in older adults is dated.

This chapter reviews representative large series of transplant outcome over the past 20 years, with emphasis on the contribution of age to overall survival (OS) and DFS. Next, reports describing the impact of age on the incidence of GVHD are examined. This is followed by an examination of published reports that specifically address the

From: *Current Controversies in Bone Marrow Transplantation*
Edited by: B. Bolwell © Humana Press Inc., Totowa, NJ

Table 1
Influence of Age on Outcome of Allo-BMT for AML

Author (ref.)	Yr published	Comment
Mortimer et al. (1)	1983	156 pts reported to IBMTR; 6-mo survival similar in patients aged ≤23 vs ≥24 yr.
Dinsmore et al. (2)	1984	70 pts; 3-yr DFS in good risk pts better if patients age <20 yr. Age had no influence on outcome of poor risk pts.
Boström et al. (3)	1985	39 pts; Age (<14 vs >14 yr) had no influence on DFS.
McGlave et al. (4)	1988	73 pts in CR1; DFS identical in children and adults. Incidence of relapse the same.
Gellar et al. (5)	1989	99 pts; Age ≤20 yr had greater DFS than <20 yr.
Copelan et al. (6)	1991	127 pts; Age had no influence on DFS.
Snyder et al. (7)	1993	99 CR1 pts; Age had negative influence on OS and DFS as a continuous variable; median AML age 26 yr (range 2–47 yr).
Keating et al. (8)	1996	169 pts in CR1; no difference on DFS or relapse rate by age; TRM higher for pts 36–45 vs <25 (33 vs 18%, $p = 0.02$)

Pts, patients; CR, complete remission; OS, overall survival; IBMTR, International Bone Marrow Transplant Registry; DFS, disease-free survival; TRM, treatment-related mortality.

outcome of transplantation in older adults. The author's own institutional data at the Cleveland Clinic Foundation is summarized, as well.

2. ALLO-BMT OUTCOME DATA

Table 1 summarizes some of the early series reporting the efficacy of allo-BMT for acute myeloid leukemia (AML), as well as selected recent reports. This is not a summary of every published article on this subject, but it represents a cross-section of data, based on large numbers of patients from major transplant centers specifically addressing the impact of age on BMT outcome for AML. The first thing one notices is the inconsistency of the influence of age on outcome. Several series found no association of age with OS or DFS; other series did find that patient age influenced outcome.

A closer examination of the reports that described an association of outcome with age reveals that, in reality, the analyses generally compared adults to pediatric patients. One study found those 3-yr DFS good-risk AML patients was better if patients were <20 yr old, compared to ≥20 yr of age (2); this was confirmed in another study using the same age cutoff criteria (5). One study used age as a continuous variable in the analysis; however, the median age of the entire series was 26 yr, meaning that a large pediatric population was included in the overall analysis (7).

Tables 2 and 3 show similar data concerning the influence of age on outcome of allo-BMT for patients with acute lymphoblastic leukemia (ALL) (Table 2) and chronic myeloid leukemia (CML) (Table 3). The original series reported by Thomas et al. (9) of BMT for ALL was a series of patients <30 yr old: Age did not influence outcome, presumably meaning that younger pediatric patients have a prognosis similar to older pediatric patients. As was the case in the series of AML, some studies found a correlation

Table 2
Influence of Age on Outcome of Allo-BMT for ALL

Author (ref.)	Yr published	Comment
Thomas et al. (9)	1979	22 pts, all aged <30 yr; age did not influence outcome.
Barrett et al. (10)	1989	690 pts reported to IBMTR; age ≥16 yr associated with ↑ treatment failure vs <16 yr.
Wingard et al. (11)	1990	74 pts; EFS not influenced by age.
Doney et al. (12)	1991	192 pts; median age 22 yr; ↑ pt age associated with ↓ DFS and ↓ OS.
Uckun et al. (13)	1993	83 pts; age not associated with risk of relapse.
Sutton et al. (14)	1993	184 pts; age not associated with TRM, LFS, or relapse.
Frassoni et al. (15)	1996	790 all in CR1 reported to EBMT; median age 22 (range 1–51 yr); increased age (continuous variable) associated with ↓ LFS.

Pts, patients; CR, complete remission; OS, overall survival; IBMTR, International Bone Marrow Transplant Registry; DFS, disease-free survival; TRM, treatment-related mortality; LFS, leukemia-free survival; EFS, event-free survival; EBMT, European Bone Marrow Transplant Registry.

Table 3
Influence of Age on Outcome of Allo-BMT for CML

Author (ref.)	Yr published	Comment
Thomas et al. (16)	1986	198 pts; age not associated with OS when interval from diagnosis to transplant included in analysis.
McGlave et al. (17)	1987	57 pts; OS better if age <30 vs >30 yr.
Martin et al. (18)	1988	66 pts with accelerated phase; age not associated with OS.
Goldman et al. (19)	1988	405 pts reported to IBMTR; ↑ age associated with ↓ OS and ↓ LFS.
Biggs et al. (20)	1992	115 pts; age not associated with LFS.
McGlave et al. (21)	1993	196 matched unrelated donor transplant pts; younger age associated with ↑ DFS.
Gratwohl et al. (22)	1993	1480 pts reported to EBMT; Age >20 (vs ≤20 yr) associated with ↓ LFS and ↑ TRM.
Bacigalupo et al. (23)	1993	100 pts; age not associated with OS or leukemic relapse.

Pts, patients; CR, complete remission; OS, overall survival; IBMTR, International Bone Marrow Transplant Registry; DFS, disease-free survival; TRM, treatment-related mortality; LFS, leukemia-free survival; EFS, event-free survival; EBMT, European Bone Marrow Transplant Registry.

of outcome with age; many others did not. Thus, the overall data is inconsistent regarding the influence of age on transplant outcome.

Most of the series that did find a negative association of increasing age on transplant outcome had a median patient population age in the twenties, again implying that a significant proportion of the transplanted patients were pediatric patients, which means that the overall analysis thus was an examination of comparing adults vs pediatric patients, instead of specifically studying outcome based on older age. Of the series that specifically looked at leukemic relapse (13,14,23), none found an association of leukemic relapse with age.

Therefore, in a manner similar to the data of allo-BMT for AML, the data of allo-BMT for ALL and CML reveals that the influence of age on transplant outcome is conflicting, because some reports found negative association, but others did not. Many of the reports that did find an age influence included a heavy pediatric population, making the analysis one of comparing children with adults, rather than comparing older adults with younger adults. Finally, although some reports did suggest age, as a continuous variable, was associated with decreased DFS and/or OS, no report found that increasing age was associated with higher relapse rates, and no series reported an upper age cutoff at which TRM is prohibitively so high as to preclude attempting the transplant.

3. INFLUENCE OF AGE ON GVHD

One reason why some authors postulate that survival is decreased in older patients receiving allo-BMT is that the risk of GVHD is increased in older patients. Table 4 is a summary of series reporting the influence of age on both acute GVHD and chronic GVHD. Again, data are conflicting. Some reports did find a higher incidence of GVHD in older patients, and others did not. The large series reported by Gale et al. *(25)* in 1987, found that increased age is associated with an increase incidence of acute GVHD, but this was biased by a high incidence of female donor to male recipient transplants; when the analysis was reperformed, of 1818 patients who were not female-to-male transplants, there was no age effect on overall outcome. The large series report in 1995 from the European Bone Marrow Transplantation Registry (EBMT) *(28)* did not find an association of age with an increased incidence of any grade of GVHD. Other reports that did find an influence of age, again, tended to compare adult patients with pediatric patients, comparing patients more than 18 *(26)*, 17 *(31)*, or 23 yrs of age *(24)*, with their younger counterparts.

The influence of age on the data of chronic GVHD is somewhat more consistent, because most series report an increased incidence of chronic GVHD with increasing age. However, most of these series again compare adults to pediatric patients, using age cutoffs of 20 or 17 yr to compare patient groups. One study of T-cell-depleted patients *(35)* found that age was not associated with an increased risk of GVHD, although patients greater than 20 yr of age were associated with increased risk of treatment failure.

This data, when examined in aggregate, strongly suggests that the incidence of both acute and chronic GVHD is somewhat higher in adult patients, when compared to pediatric patients. There is little data, however, suggesting that the incidence of GVHD is significantly higher in older adults, compared to younger adults, and there is little data to suggest that there is an age at which the incidence of GVHD is so prohibitively risky as to withhold the potential benefits of allo-BMT.

4. DATA SPECIFICALLY EXAMINING
BMT OUTCOME IN OLDER ADULTS

Many reports have been published over the past decade specifically examining the outcome of both allo- and autotransplantation in older patients. Several early series, based on small numbers of patients, were published *(36–38)*, which suggested that either there was no difference in outcome in older patients greater than 40 yr, compared

Table 4
Influence of Age on Development of GVHD

Author (ref.)	Yr published	Comment
Acute GVHD		
Bross et al. (24)	1984	136 pts; ↑ risk of a GVHD in pts aged >23.7 yr.
Gale et al. (25)	1987	2036 pts reported to IBMTR; median age 21 yr; ↑ age associated with ↑ incidence of AGVHD, but biased by high incidence of female → male transplants; analysis of 1818 pts not female → male found no age effect.
Weisdorf et al. (26)	1991	469 pts; median age 21 yr; Age ≥18 yr associated with ↑ risk of AGVHD.
Nash et al. (27)	1992	446 pts; pt age associated with ↑ a GHVD univariate analysis, but not in multivariate analysis.
Gratwohl et al. (28)	1995	1294 pts with CML report to EBMT; age not associated with ↑ incidence of any grade of AGVHD (≤20 vs >20 yr).
Hagglund et al. (29)	1995	291pts; age (≤17 vs >17 yr). Not associated with ↑ risk of AGVHD.
Chronic GVHD		
Sullivan et al. (30)	1988	164 evaluable pts; median age 23; age >20 (vs ≤20 yr) associated with ↑ mortality from CGVHD.
Boström et al. (31)	1990	466 pts reported to EBMTR; increased risk of CGVHD in pts aged >17 (vs ≤17 yr).
Atkinson et al. (32)	1990	2534 pts reported to IBMTR surviving 90+ d post-BMT, median age 23 yr; age >20 (vs ≤20 yr) associated with ↑ risk of CGVHD.
Loughran et al. (33)	1990	169 pts; age (continuous variable) associated with ↑ risk of CGVHD (univariate), not in a multivariate analysis.
Ochs et al. (34)	1994	469 pts; age ≥18 yr associated with ↑ risk of CGVHD.
Marmount et al. (35)	1991	731 T-cell depleted pts; age not associated with ↑ GVHD, but age ≥20 yr associated with ↑ risk of treatment failure.

Pts, patients; CR, complete remission; OS, overall survival; IBMTR, International Bone Marrow Transplant Registry; DFS, disease-free survival; TRM, treatment-related mortality; LFS, leukemia-free survival; EFS, event-free survival; EBMT, European Bone Marrow Transplant Registry; AGVHD, acute graft-versus-host disease; CGVHD, chronic graft-versus-host-disease.

to younger patients, or reported that, although the risks may be somewhat greater, the curative potential of the transplant outweighed the potential risks in older patients.

Since that time, many series have confirmed these initial findings. Bär et al. (39) compared three patient groups (ages 40–49, 30–39, and less than 30 yr) receiving T-cell-depleted allo-BMT for acute leukemia in remission, or CML in chronic or accelerated phase. They found that event-free survival (EFS) at 3 yr was identical for patients more than 39 yr, compared with those 30–39, and less than 30 yr. Ringdén et al. (40) reported a series of more than 2000 patients reported to the International Bone Marrow Transplant Registry of allo-BMT for leukemia, and compared outcome in four groups: those age 30–39, 40–44, 45–49, and 50 yr and older. Two-yr DFS was identical in

Table 5
Influence of Age on Outcome of ABMT

Author (ref.)	Yr published	Comment
Sweetenham et al. *(45)*	1994	901 adult pts reported to EBMT with NHL; PFS and OS similar in pts < 55 vs ≥ 55 yr.
Cahn et al. *(46)*	1995	111 AML CR1 pts reported to EBMT; no difference in relapse of pts aged ≥ 50 vs those < 50 yr; ↑ TRM in older adults (28 vs 14%), which resulted in ↓ OS (35 vs 48%, $p = 0.004$).
Miller et al. *(47)*	1996	506 pts, 101 age ≥ 50 yr; pts ≥ 50 yr had ↑ risk of TRM, but no ↑ risk of relapse, slight ↓ in EFS.
Kusnierz-Glaz et al. *(48)*	1997	500 adult and pediatric pts; EFS 34% pts aged ≥50 yr vs 46% in younger pts ($p = 0.03$).
Copelan et al. *(49)*	1996	885 pts reported to OBMTC; OS the same for pts aged < 19 vs 20–34 vs 35–49 vs 50–69.
Lazarus et al. *(50)*	1996	3744 pts with NHL or BC reported to ABMTR; TRM and OS the same in pts aged 20–39 vs 40–49 vs 50–59 vs 60–69 yr.

Pts, patients; CR, complete remission; OS, overall survival; IBMTR, International Bone Marrow Transplant Registry; DFS, disease-free survival; TRM, treatment-related mortality; LFS, leukemia-free survival; EFS, event-free survival; EBMT, European Bone Marrow Transplant Registry; OBMTC, Ohio Bone Marrow Transplant Consortium.

the treatment groups. There was no difference in leukemic relapse. There was a slightly increased TRM in patients greater than 45 yr of age.

Rapoport et al. *(41)* compared EFS in patients >40 yr old with those <40 yr old undergoing either allo-BMT or ABMT. Of patients receiving allo-BMT, 3-yr EFS was actually improved among older patients (56 vs 26%, $p = 0.057$). However, this difference chiefly resulted from a higher proportion of patients with CML and early-stage leukemia in the older age group. The outcome of autotransplantation for non-Hodgkin's lymphoma (NHL) and Hodgkin's disease (HD) found no difference in EFS *(41)*.

Cahn et al. *(42)* compared 192 patients over 40 yr with a group of over 1000 patients aged 16–40 yr reported to the EBMT. Leukemia-free survival, transplant-related to mortality, and OS were the same in the two patient populations groups.

Du et al. *(43)* compared the outcome of allo-BMT in patients over the age of 50 yr, vs those age 40–50 yr, vs those age 18–39 yr. OS was the same in the three age cohorts. The incidence of GVHD was also comparable.

Ringdén et al. *(44)* examined the outcome of unrelated allo-BMT in patients above the age of 40 yr, compared with younger patients, median age 23 yr. There was a trend toward a higher TRM in patients >40 yr of age (46 vs 32%, $p = 0.16$). Three-yr patient survival times were similar in the two groups.

Table 5 summarizes other reports addressing the influence of age on the outcome of auto-BMT. Although there was some suggestion that TRM might be higher in older patients, most of these series report that there is no effect of age on transplant outcome. The largest series, presented at the meeting of the American Society of Clinical Oncology in 1996 *(50)*, found no influence of age on OS for patients undergoing autotransplantation. None of the studies, including those finding a slightly decreased OS in older

Table 6
100-D Mortality of Cleveland Clinic Foundation BMT Patients 1992–1997

Type of transplant	Age (yr)	N	100-D mortality (%)		p-Value (Chi-square)
Auto-PBPC					
Breast cancer	0–29	9	0	0	0.56
	30–39	77	0	0	
	40–49	171	4	2	
	50+	86	2	2	
Auto-PBPC					
NHL and HD	0–29	53	3	6	0.59
	30–39	69	4	6	
	40–49	94	8	8	
	50+	102	11	11	
Allo -BMT					
Matched sibling donor	0–29	32	4	13	0.60
	30–39	44	8	18	
	40–49	58	14	24	
	50+	14	3	21	

PBPC, primed peripheral blood progenitor cells; NHL, non-Hodgkin's lymphoma; HD, Hodgkin's Disease.

patients, suggested that transplant should not be offered to patients in the fifth, sixth, or seventh decade of life. All concluded that this potentially curative therapy was appropriate for these age groups, if clinically indicated.

5. CLEVELAND CLINIC BMT OUTCOME DATA BY AGE

Tables 6–8 summarize the patients undergoing BMT at the Cleveland Clinic Foundation from 1992 through 1997. This time frame was chosen in order to ensure that all patients had a minimum of 18 mo follow-up. Table 6 shows 100-d mortality after autologous stem cell transplantation (ASCT) for breast cancer, and of matched sibling donor allo-BMT for any diagnosis. There is no difference in 100-d mortality, in either auto- or allotransplantation, by age cohorts. Because the presumed reason to exclude older patients from transplantation is related to toxicity of the transplant regimen, the fact that the 100-d mortality was not affected by age is compelling evidence not to have exclusionary criteria in BMT protocols, based solely on age.

Tables 7 and 8 show OS and DFS of the same groups of patients, respectively. The stage IV/metastatic breast cancer population showed a trend toward improved survival in young patients, although differences in OS or DFS differences were not statistically significant. There was little difference in transplant outcome of NHL and HD patients, by age, as shown.

Allo-BMT outcome again showed that there was a trend toward improved OS and DFS in the younger patient population, although this was not a statistically significant difference. Patients over 50 yr actually had a greater DFS with allo-BMT than did patients age 40–49 yr, although, again, this was not a statistically significant difference.

The author's own institutional data, therefore, mimics much of the data reviewed

Table 7
OS of BMT Patients at Cleveland Clinic Foundation 1992–1997

Transplant and diagnosis type	Age (yr)	N	Overall survival		p-Value (log-rank)
			1 yr (%)	2 yr (%)	
Auto-PBPC					
Breast cancer	0–39	41	85	63	0.14
Metastatic/stage IV	40–49	100	71	45	
	50+	46	68	37	
NHL and HD	0–29	53	84	77	0.25
	30–39	69	80	75	
	40–49	94	77	68	
	50+	102	72	61	
Allo-BMT					
Matched sibling donor	0–29	32	59	52	0.12
	30–39	44	61	53	
	40–49	58	45	36	
	50+	14	38	36	

PBPC, primed peripheral blood progenitor cells; NHL, non-Hodgkin's lymphoma; HD, Hodgkin's disease; OS, overall survival.

earlier in this chapter. Specifically, 100-d mortality and overall transplant outcomes are similar in older patients, compared with younger patients. Younger patients may have a trend toward improved outcome, but the real issue is that there is no evidence to suggest that the outcome in older patients is so bad as to exclude them from the curative potential of ASCT/ABMT or allo-SCT/BMT.

6. SUMMARY AND COMMENTARY

Allo-BMT clearly has the ability to cure patients with various types of leukemia and other malignancies, who are otherwise incurable with conventional doses of chemotherapy. In a similar manner, ASCT has been shown to be potentially curative in patients with NHL, HD, and other diagnoses, when conventional therapy offers no such chance of cure. The fact that BMT is potentially curative therapy for patients otherwise incurable is, therefore, not a question. The question at hand is, should older patients be denied this potentially curative therapy?

The answer is, quite simply, that they should not. Older patients might have a slightly higher TRM risk; they may have an increased risk of both acute and chronic GVHD; and these risks may or may not have a deleterious impact on OS and DFS. However, there is no data that suggest that these potential risks prohibit an attempt to cure an older patient, who is otherwise healthy, of their underlying malignancy.

The decision to transplant any patient, regardless of age, involves evaluations of the risks of the procedure vs the potential benefits of the procedure. The risks that need to be determined include an assessment of the patient's underlying clinical status from cardiac, hepatic, renal, pulmonary, and other perspectives. If a patient in their fifties,

Table 8
DFS of BMT Patients at Cleveland Clinic Foundation 1992–1997

Transplant type/diagnosis	Age (yr)	N	DFS 1 yr (%)	DFS 2 yr (%)	p-Value (log-rank)
Auto-PBPC					
Breast cancer	0–39	41	58	43	0.10
Metastatic/stage IV	40–49	100	38	19	
	50+	46	42	29	
NHL and HD	0–29	53	64	57	0.17
	30–39	69	76	68	
	40–49	94	70	62	
	50+	102	64	54	
Allo-BMT					
Matched sibling donor	0–29	32	52	49	0.16
	30–39	44	52	46	
	40–49	58	38	26	
	50+	14	36	36	

PBPC, primed peripheral blood progenitor cells; NHL, non-Hodgkin's lymphoma; HD, Hodgkin's disease; DFS, disease-free survival.

sixties, or even older, is physiologically healthy, the data presented in this chapter strongly suggest that there is no reason that such an older patient be denied the potentially curative therapy of BMT. After reviewing this literature, the recommendation of this author is to delete eligibility criteria in BMT protocols that exclude patients solely on the basis of older age. There is no compelling evidence to support such arbitrary exclusions based on age.

REFERENCES

1. Mortimer MB, Gale RP, Humphrey EM, et al. Bone marrow transplantation for acute myelogeneous leukemia: factors associated with early mortality, *JAMA*, **249** (1983) 1166–1175.
2. Dinsmore R, Kirkpatrick D, Flomenberg N, et al. Allogeneic bone marrow transplantation for patients with acute nonlymphocytic leukemia, *Blood*, **63** (1984) 649–656.
3. Boström B, Brunning RD, McGlave R, et al. Bone marrow transplantation for acute nonlymphocytic leukemia in first remission: analysis of prognostic factors, *Blood*, **65** (1985) 1191–1196.
4. McGlave PB, Haake RJ, Boström BC, et al. Allogenic bone marrow transplantation for acute non-lymphocytic leukemia in first remission, *Blood*, **72** (1988) 1512–1517.
5. Geller RB, Saral R, Piantadosi S, et al. Allogeneic bone marrow transplantation after high-dose busulfan and cyclophosphamide in patients with acute nonlymphocytic leukemia, *Blood*, **73** (1989) 2209–2218.
6. Copelan EA, Biggs JC, Thompson JM, et al. Treatment for acute myelocytic leukemia with allogeneic bone marrow transplantation following preparation with BuCy2, *Blood*, **78** (1991) 838–843.
7. Snyder DS, Chao NJ, Amylon MD, et al. Fractionated total body irradiation and high-dose etoposide as a preparatory regimen for bone marrow transplantation for 99 patients with acute leukemia in first complete remission, *Blood*, **82** (1993) 2920–2928.
8. Keating S, Suciu S, deWitte T, et al. Prognostic factors of patients with acute myeloid leukemia (AML) allografted in first complete remission: an analysis of the EROTC-EIMEMA AML 8A trial, *Bone Marrow Transplant.*, **17** (1996) 993–1001.
9. Thomas ED, Sanders JE, Flournoy N, et al. Marrow transplantation for patients with acute lymphoblastic leukemia in remission, *Blood*, **54** (1979) 468–476.

10. Barrett AJ, Horowitz MM, Gale RP, et al. Marrow transplantation for acute lymphoblastic leukemia: factors affecting relapse and survival, *Blood*, **74** (1989) 862–871.

11. Wingard JR, Piantadosi S, Santos GW, et al. *J. Clin. Oncol.*, **8** (1990) 820–830.

12. Doney K, Fisher LD, Appelbaum FR, et al. Treatment of adult acute lymphoblastic leukemia with allogeneic bone marrow transplantation. Multivariate analysis of factors affecting acute graft-versus-host disease, relapse, and relapse-free survival, *Bone Marrow Transplant.*, **7** (1991) 453–459.

13. Uckun FAM, Kersey JH, Haake R, et al. Pretransplantation burden of leukemic progenitor cells as a predictor of relapse after bone marrow transplantation for acute lymphoblastic leukemia, *N. Engl. J. Med.*, **329** (1993) 1296–1301.

14. Sutton L, Kuentz M, Cordonnier C, et al. Allogeneic bone marrow transplantation for adult acute lymphoblastic leukemia in first complete remission: factors predictive of transplant-related mortality and influence of total body irradiation modalities, *Bone Marrow Transplant.*, **12** (1993) 583–589.

15. Frassoni F, Labopin M, Gluckman E, et al. Results of allogeneic bone marrow transplantation for acute lymphoblastic leukemia have improved in europe with time: a report of the acute leukemia working party of the european group for blood and marrow transplantation (EBMT), *Bone Marrow Transplant.*, **17** (1996) 13–18.

16. Thomas ED, Clift RA, Fefer A, et al. Marrow transplantation for the treatment of chronic myelogenous leukemia, *Ann. Intern. Med.* **104** (1986) 155–163.

17. McGlave P, Arthur D, Haake R, et al. Therapy of chronic myelogenous leukemia with allogeneic bone marrow transplantation. *J. Clin. Oncol.*, **5** (1987) 1033–1040.

18. Martin PJ, Clift RA, Fisher LD, et al. HLA-Identical marrow transplantation during accelerated-phase chronic myelogenous leukemia: analysis of survival and remission duration, *Blood*, **72** (1988) 1978–1984.

19. Goldman JM, Gale RP, Horowitz MM, et al. Bone marrow transplantation for chronic myelogenous leukemia in chronic phase, *Ann. Intern. Med.*, **108** (1988) 806–814.

20. Biggs JC, Szer J, Crilley P, et al. Treatment of chronic myelogenous leukemia with allogeneic bone marrow transplantation after preparation with BuCy2, *Blood*, **80** (1992) 1352–1357.

21. McGlave P, Gartsch G, Anasetti C, et al. Unrelated donor marrow transplantation therapy for chronic myelogenous leukemia: initial experience of the national marrow donor program, *Blood*, **81** (1993) 543–550.

22. Gratwhol A, Hermans J, Niederwieser D, et al. Bone marrow transplantation for chronic myelogenous leukemia: long-term results, *Bone Marrow Transplant.*, **12** (1993) 509–516.

23. Bacigalupo A, Gualandi F, Van Lint MT, et al. Multivariate analysis of risk factors for survival and relapse in chronic granulocytic leukemia following allogeneic marrow transplantation: Impact of disease related variables (Sokal score), *Bone Marrow Transplant.*, **12** (1993) 443–448.

24. Bross DS, Tutschka PJ, Farmer ER, et al. Predictive factors for acute graft-versus-host disease in patients transplanted with HLA-identical bone marrow, *Blood*, **63** (1984) 1265–1270.

25. Gale RP, Bortin MM, van Bekkum DW, et al. Risk factors for acute graft-versus-host disease, *Br. J. Haematol.*, **67** (1987) 397–406.

26. Weisdorf D, Hakke R, Blazar B, et al. Risk factors for acute graft-versus-host disease in histocompatible donor bone marrow transplantation, *Transplantation*, **51** (1991) 1197–1203.

27. Nash RA, Pepe SM, Storb R, et al. Acute graft-versus-host disease: Analysis of risk factors after allogeneic bone marrow transplantation and prophylaxis with cyclosporine and methotrexate, *Blood*, **80** (1992) 1838–1845.

28. Gratwoh A, Hermans J, Apperley J, et al. Acute graft-versus-host disease: Grade and outcome in patients with chronic myelogenous leukemia, *Blood*, **86** (1995) 813–818.

29. Hägglund H, Boström L, Remberger M, et al. Risk factors for acute graft-versus-host disease in 291 consecutive HLA-identical bone marrow transplantation recipients, *Bone Marrow Transplant.*, **16** (1995) 747–753.

30. Sullivan KM, Witherspoon RP, Storb R, et al. Prednisone and azathioprine compared with prednisone and placebo for treatment of chronic graft-vs-host disease: Prognostic influence of prolonged thrombocytopenia after allogeneic marrow transplantation, *Blood*, **72** (1988) 546–554.

31. Boström L, Ringdén O, Jacobsen N, et al. A European multicenter study of chronic graft-versus-host disease, *Transplantation*, **49** (1990) 1100–1105.

32. Atkinson K, Horowitz MM, Gale RP, van Bekkum DW, et al. Risk factors for chronic graft-versus-host disease after HLA-identical sibling bone marrow transplantation, *Blood*, **75** (1990) 2459–2464.

33. Loughran TP, Sullivan K, Morton T, et al. Value of day 100 screening studies for predicting the

development of chronic graft-versus-host disease after allogeneic bone marrow transplantation, *Blood*, **76** (1990) 228–234.

34. Ochs LA, Miller WJ, Filipovich AH, et al. Predictive factors for chronic graft-versus-host disease after histocompatible sibling donor bone marrow transplantation, *Bone Marrow Transplant.*, **13** (1994) 455–460.

35. Marmont AM, Horowitz MM, Gale RR, et al. T-cell depletion of HLA-identical transplants in leukemia, *Blood*, **78** (1991) 2120–2130.

36. Klingemann H-G, Storb R, Fefer A, et al. Bone marrow transplantation in patients aged 45 years and older, *Blood*, **67** (1986) 770–776.

37. Blume KG, Forman SJ, Nademanee AP, et al. Bone marrow transplantation for hematologic malignancies in patients aged 30 years or older, *J. Clin. Oncol.*, **4** (1986) 1489–1492.

38. Copelan EA, Kapoor N, Berliner M, and Tutschka PJ. Bone marrow transplantation without total body irradiation in patients aged 40 and older, *Transplantation*, **48** (1989) 65–68.

39. Bär BMAM, DeWitte T, Schattenberg A, et al. Favourable outcome of patients older than 40 years of age after transplantation with marrow grafts depleted of lymphocytes by counterflow centrifugation, *Br. J. Haematol.*, **74** (1990) 53–60.

40. Ringdén O, Horowitz MM, Gale RP, Biggs JC, et al. Outcome after allogeneic bone marrow transplant for leukemia in older adults, *JAMA*, **270** (1993) 57–60.

41. Rapoport AP, DiPersio JF, Martin BA, et al. Patients ≥ age 40 years undergoing autologous or allogeneic BMT have regimen-related mortality rates and event-free survivals comparable to patients < age 40 Years, *Bone Marrow Transplant.*, **15** (1995) 523–530.

42. Cahn J-Y, Labopin M, Schattenberg A, et al. Allogeneic bone marrow transplantation for acute leukemia in patients over the age of 40 years, *Leukemia*, **11** (1997) 416–419.

43. Du W, Dansey R, Abella EM, et al. Successful allogeneic bone marrow transplantation in selected patients over 50 years of age: A single institution's experience, *Bone Marrow Transplant.*, **21** (1998) 1043–1047.

44. Ringdén O, Remberger M, Mattsson J, et al. Transplantation with unrelated bone marrow in leukaemic patients above 40 years of age, *Bone Marrow Transplant.*, **21** (1998) 43–49.

45. Swettenham JR, Pearce R, Philip T, et al. High-dose therapy and autologous bone marrow transplantation for intermediate and high grade non-Hodgkin's lymphoma in patients aged 55 years and over: Results from the European group for bone marrow transplantation, *Bone Marrow Transplant.*, **14** (1994) 981–987.

46. Cahn JY, Laboprin M, Mandelli F, et al. Autologous bone marrow transplantation for first remission acute myeloblastic leukemia in patients older than 50 years: A retrospective analysis of the European bone marrow transplant group, *Blood*, **85** (1995) 575–579.

47. Miller CB, Piantadosi S, Vogelsang GB, et al. Impact of age on outcome of patients with cancer undergoing autologous bone marrow transplant, *J. Clin. Oncol.*, **14** (1996) 1327–1332.

48. Kusierz-Glaz CR, Schlegel PG, Wong RM, et al. Influence of age on the outcome of 500 autologous bone marrow transplant procedures for hematologic malignancies, *J. Clin. Oncol.*, **15** (1997) 18–25.

49. Copelan E, Bolwell B, Harris R, et al. Analysis of age as a predictor of survival following allogeneic and autologous marrow transplantation, *Proc. ASCO*, **15** (1996) 84 (Abstract).

50. Lazarus H, Horowitz M, and Nugent M. Outcome of autotransplants in older adults, *Proc. ASCO*, **15** (1996) 338 (Abstract).

3

What Is an Accurate Risk/Benefit Ratio for Umbilical Cord Cell Transplantation in Children and Adults?

Mary J. Laughlin, MD

CONTENTS

ALLOGENEIC UMBILICAL CORD BLOOD CELL
    TRANSPLANTATION
PRECLINICAL STUDIES AND CLINICAL REPORTS
UMBILICAL CORD CELL TRANSPLANTATION
    Graft Characteristics and Hematopoietic Recovery
    Incidence and Severity of Acute and Chronic GVHD
    Rate and Quality of Immunologic Recovery
    Graft Vs Leukemia/Lymphoma
SUMMARY
REFERENCES

1. ALLOGENEIC UMBILICAL CORD BLOOD CELL TRANSPLANTATION

Allogeneic transplantation (allotransplantation) can cure a significant fraction of patients with high-risk or recurrent hematologic malignancies *(1)*. However, this approach has been limited by the availability of suitable human leukocyte antigen (HLA)-matched related donors, and by the occurrence of severe graft-vs-host disease (GVHD) when bone marrow (BM) from HLA-matched unrelated donor (MUD), or partially HLA-mismatched family member grafts, are utilized *(2–4)*. Attempts to reduce GVHD in recipients undergoing allotransplantation with MUD, or partially HLA-mismatched family member grafts by T-cell depletion (TCD) has been shown to reduce acute GVHD. However, this benefit of reduced GVHD is offset by increases in the rates of graft failure, lymphoproliferative disorders associated with Epstein-Barr virus, and recurrent leukemia *(5,6)*.

Approaches to identify alternative unrelated donors initially focused on the established of volunteer living donor registries, including the National Marrow Donor Pro-

From: *Current Controversies in Bone Marrow Transplantation*
Edited by: B. Bolwell © Humana Press Inc., Totowa, NJ

Table 1
Advantages of UCB vs Bone Marrow as Alternative Source of
HSCs for Allotransplantation

1. Placental or UCB is an abundantly available source of stem cells that can be harvested at no risk to the mother or infant.
2. Ethnic balance in a cord blood repository can be maintained automatically in heterogeneous populations, or can be controlled via collection from birthing centers representing targeted minority populations.
3. Important infectious agents, particularly cytomegalovirus, are much less common in the newborn than in adults, and will be less likely to contaminate UCB.
4. UCB, cryopreserved and banked, could be made available on demand, eliminating delays and uncertainties that now complicate marrow collection from unrelated donors.
5. The intensity of graft-vs-host reactivity of fetal lymphocytes may be less than that of adult cells, suggesting that transplantation of UCB will result in less GVHD than transplantation of BM.
6. Frozen UCB can be easily shipped and thawed for use when needed, compared to freshly donated BM, which has a limited shelf-life, necessitating coordination between harvesting surgeons, transportation, and transplantation teams.
7. There is an undistorted accumulation of HLA types encountered, because, unlike volunteer donors who usually retire from the registry, stored placental blood suffers no attrition, except by clinical use, or by culling and substitution.

gram. Because HLA antigens (Ags) are genetically linked, the likelihood of finding an unrelated identical match is dependent on the ethnic background of the recipient, and, because volunteer donor pools are comprised primarily of Caucasians, the likelihood of a patient of ethnic minority heritage, e.g., Black, Asian, Hispanic, or American Indian, finding a suitable match in volunteer donor registries is small (7). In addition to possible ethnic imbalances in existing donor registries, logistical problems also decrease the probability of actual donation with time from registration. More than 10% of donors listed in each registry are lost per year, because they have become untraceable, or because of age censoring. Further compounding the problem is the cumbersome process of identifying, typing, and harvesting an unrelated donor, with the time interval between initiation of a search and the donation of marrow averaging a minimum of 4–6 mo. This is impractical for some patients whose underlying disease may not stabilize for a long-enough period of time to allow for this process to occur.

Unrelated umbilical cord blood (UCB) offers advantages over the use of matched unrelated BM from adult donors, including ready availability, ease of collection, absence of risk to the donor, and lack of contamination by latent viruses. Table 1 outlines the advantages of UCB as an alternative source of hematopoietic stem cells (HSCs) for allotransplantation.

2. PRECLINICAL STUDIES AND CLINICAL REPORTS

Transplantation of UCB from partially HLA-matched related and unrelated donors has been shown to successfully engraft pediatric patients (and a few reported adult patients) with hematologic malignancies, immunodeficiency syndromes, inborn errors of metabolism, or marrow failure syndromes (8–16,20,21). An unrelated UCB bank, supported by the National Heart Lung and Blood Institute, was established at the New

Table 2
UCB-related and -Unrelated Allotransplantation: Clinical Results

No. patients	Median age (yr)	Grade II–IV acute GVHD (%)	Probability engraftment	ANC > 500/μL (d)	Event-free survival (%)[a]	Ref.
44	4	3	.82	22	62	7
25	7	43	.92	22	48	8
18	2.7	50	1.0	24	48	9
143	6	24	.87	30	29–63	6
562	–	46	.91	28	22–62	17

[a]EFS percentages shown are Kaplan-Meier estimates.

York Blood Center in 1992. Over the past 6 yr, approx 9000 UCBs have been banked at this facility, and this group recently reported outcomes for 562 transplants performed *(16)*.

One would expect improved survival, if the graft-vs-leukemia (GVL) effects of allotransplantation, mediated by T-cell interactions between the donor graft and host leukemia-associated or major histocompatibility complex (MHC)-restricted Ags *(17–19)*, could be elicited, independent of the complications of severe GVHD. The incidence and severity of acute and chronic GVHD observed in UCB recipients, the majority of whom are children, has thus far been lower than that previously reported in recipients of MUD or partially HLA-mismatched family member grafts *(8–13,16)*. The degree and/or type of HLA disparity effects on UCB transplant outcomes is currently not well understood. Initial reports pointed to a lack of correlation between HLA disparity and incidence of GVHD *(13)*. Nevertheless, more recent data points to HLA disparity as an important indicator of UCB transplant outcomes *(16)*. At this point, it is unclear whether the decreased incidence of GVHD associated with UCB grafts also results in a decrease in GVL effects. Clinical reports of allogeneic UCB recipients have not pointed to increased relapse rates, but patient numbers are small, and length of follow-up thus far is of short duration.

Early UCB allotransplantation clinical reports point to significant delays in time to hematopoietic recovery, with median to attained neutrophil recovery of 26 d, and overall probability of engraftment in the range of 90%. GVHD grades II–IV are reported to range 35–40%, with the majority of recipients receiving grafts disparate at two or more loci. Table 2 summarizes published clinical reports of these early trials using UCB grafts for allotransplantation.

Although graft cell dose is a consistent indicator of time to hematopoietic recovery, the number of HSCs required to provide durable engraftment in an ablated adult recipient is not established. Although some reports have included a few adult recipients transplanted with UCB, a critical issue is whether UCB contains sufficient numbers of HSCs to predictably engraft full-stature adults. UCB graft variables, including cell count, CD34, and colony-transforming unit (CFU) content, have been studied to determine those factors with consistent predictive value for time to myeloid engraftment. The author et al. *(20,21)* have reported preliminary experience with using this alternative stem cell source in adult recipients. Preliminary analyses indicate that UCB contains sufficient HSCs to provide long-term engraftment in adult recipients over 40 kg in weight. Although significant delays in time to hematopoietic recovery are observed in these adult recipients, the time to neutrophil, red blood cell (RBC), and platelet recovery does not differ significantly, compared with that observed in children grafted with UCB. Nevertheless, there are further uncertainties concerning UCB grafting from unrelated donors into adult patients: will the reduced incidence and severity of GVHD observed thus far in pediatric recipients hold true for adult recipients; what is the time required for immune reconstitution; and are GVL/lymphoma effects maintained?

3. UMBILICAL CORD CELL TRANSPLANTATION

3.1. Graft Characteristics and Hematopoietic Recovery

Hematopoietic reconstitution is delayed after UCB grafting, compared with conventional allogeneic BM or peripheral stem cell grafts. The cause of delayed hematopoietic recovery in UCB recipients is not clear, but it may result from either reduced HSC dose, or from the fact that UCB contains a higher proportion of immature progenitor cells. Although the durability of these UCB grafts has not been studied extensively, given the limited follow-up in published reports, to date, there have been only four late graft failures observed in patients receiving gancyclovir for cytomegalovirus infections (16). UCB graft analyses that have predictive value for hematopoietic engraftment include reinfused mononuclear cell (MNC) and CFU assays (8–13,16). UCB grafts contain 2–2.5×10^4 granulocyte-macrophage-CFU/mL sample, and can be stored in a cryopreserved state for as long as 10 yr, with no adverse effect on cell viability at the time of thawing (22). CD34 quantification has thus far not been consistently predictive of time to hematopoietic engraftment in UCB recipients. The lack of correlation between CD34 content of infused UCB grafts and time to hematopoietic engraftment may be related to the quantification of CD34 in these UCB grafts postthaw, rather than prior to cryopreservation, and/or to reduced surface epitope density (23,24) of CD34 on UCB progenitor cells. In vitro analyses of UCB CD34 progenitors, compared with adult marrow and peripheral blood stem cells, point to a less-mature phenotype (25).

Because of concern that manipulation of UCB, including centrifugation, MNC fractionation, or RBC depletion, would result in loss of hematopoietic progenitor cells, and because fetal RBCs are larger than adult RBCs, rendering standard density gradient separation techniques inefficient in separating out UCB MNC fractions, the early banking of UCB included cryopreservation without volume reduction, RBC depletion, or MNC isolation. Since the hematocrit of UCB is high (55–70%), a large volume of RBCs are included in the cryopreserved unit, and are subsequently lysed upon thawing, delivering a significant load of free hemoglobin to the recipient during infusion. Subsequently, with the development of efficient methods to fractionate UCB, thereby removing RBCs and decreasing volume for cryopreservation, collected UCB units are routinely fractionated prior to cryopreservation (26–29). Concern within the transplant community prompted an initiative sponsored by the National Heart Lung and Blood Institute in 1995 to focus on all aspects of UCB transplantation, including the development of standard operating procedures for the collection and processing of UCB for grafting (30). This work is currently ongoing to establish three UCB banks, six transplant centers, and one medical coordinating center.

Effects of graft cell dose on the rate of hematopoietic recovery and transplant survival has laid the basis for laboratory and phase I clinical trials focused on ex vivo expansion of UCB grafts. Although early clinical trials reported thus far do not point to more rapid hematopoietic recovery in UCB recipients, laboratory studies reveal that UCB primitive hematopoietic stem and progenitor cells differ from those collected from adult donors *(31)*. UCB contains hematopoietic progenitor cells at a higher frequency, and these UCB progenitors also have a higher proliferative capacity. Laboratory studies reveal that 1-wk liquid cultures of CD34-enriched UCB progenitor cells, in the presence of early-acting cytokines, results generally in a 2–3-fold expansion of progenitors capable of reinitiating long-term stromal cell cultures *(32)*. An important observation in these studies is that CD34 selection may be necessary for optimal expansion of UCB *(33)*.

Obvious concerns are raised in ex vivo expansion of UCB, about whether differentiation of primitive stem cells will increase the risk of late graft failure *(34)*. Preliminary work points to the presence of immature progenitors that have limited proliferative response to cytokines, thereby maintaining the stem cell component in expanded UCB grafts, and, further, that observed cell expansion is derived from committed progenitor cells *(35)*. These preclinical studies identify questions yet to be addressed, including the role of accessory lymphoid populations in ex vivo expanded allogeneic grafts *(36,37)*, as well as the role of stromal elements in maintaining immature stem cells with self-renewal capacity during expansion *(38–40)*. UCB HSCs have also been studied intensively as a possible target for gene transfer in gene therapy trials. Improved retroviral transduction of UCB hematopoietic progenitor cells has been reported *(41,42)*.

3.2. Incidence and Severity of Acute and Chronic GVHD

HLA disparity between the donor and recipient is the most powerful factor governing severity of GVHD *(43)*. Because of the extreme polymorphism of the HLA system, the current probability of finding a MUD via the available large volunteer donor registries is only approx 20%, leaving approx 50% of patients still without a donor. Because histocompatibility is a key determinant in the development of GVHD after allotransplantation, molecular characterization of HLA class I and II Ags assists in the selection of the best available family or unrelated donor graft. Age of both the donor and recipient is another key factor associated with the development of acute GVHD. Graft source is also a key factor influencing the incidence and severity of GVHD after allotransplantation. A high incidence of acute GVHD has been observed with marrow from HLA-MUDs, compared with matched sibling grafts, despite HLA matching at high-resolution molecular tissue typing. This may be attributable to reactivity of donor T-cells, with recipient minor histocompatibility Ags presented within the MHC *(44,45)*. Minor histocompatibility Ag disparity is expectedly greater between unrelated individuals.

Unmodified BM generally contains approx 1×10^{10} MNCs, with up to 10–15% mature T-cells. Almost all clinical reports show a significant reduction in the incidence and severity of acute GVHD when TCD of the graft is performed. However, overall survival is not improved with TCD of the graft, because of associated increases in the rates of graft failure and recurrent leukemia. The cumulative results of these TCD trials thus far *(46–48)* point to the importance of quantifying and characterizing the absolute numbers of residual graft T-cells, T-cell subsets, and progenitor and accessory cells, to reduce GVHD, while preserving engraftment potential and GVL effects.

GVHD is dependent on alloreactivity of T-lymphocytes contained in the donor graft, which proliferate in response to disparate histocompatibility Ags on host tissues. These alloreactive T-lymphocytes directly, or indirectly (via natural killer [NK] cells and/or release of lymphokines), attack recipient cells. Tolerance can be achieved first by elimination (clonal deletion) in the recipient thymus of host reactive immature CD3[+] CD4[+]CD8[+] T-cells directed toward class II MHC (MHC-II) Ags by marrow-derived Ag presenting cells (APCs). Tolerance induction to MHC-I Ags, as well as minor histocompatibility Ags, also occurs peripherally after allotransplantation. Murine studies point to the presence of two sets of APCs in the periphery, to maintain tolerance in mature T-cells: stimulatory APCs (e.g., macrophages and dendritic cells) and deleting APCs (veto cells) *(49)*. Alternatively, the presence of specific suppressor T-cell or deleting APCs (veto cells) in the graft may be of importance in the development of transplantation tolerance in the recipient. Here, host MCH-I restricted cytotoxic T-lymphocytes specific for donor-cell Ags receive negative, deletional signals from donor CD8[+] APCs (veto cells) *(50)*.

Although the exact mechanism underlying the observed decreased incidence of severe GVHD after allogeneic UCB transplantation is unclear, it may be related to fetal immune tolerance to noninherited maternal Ags. Initial in vitro analyses of UCB pointed to a low frequency of alloreactive lymphocytes in UCB, but recent reports *(51)* demonstrate that UCB contains normal frequencies of cytotoxic and helper T-lymphocyte precursors against noninherited maternal and paternal Ags.

Further immunologic features, unique to UCB, to explain this observed reduction in elicited GVHD, include phenotypic analysis of lymphocyte populations contained in UCB grafts, notable for the presence of a predominant population of immature unprimed T-lymphocytes, which may serve to limit the cytokine and cellular cascade necessary to amplify donor alloreactivity to recipient Ags *(52,53)*. Alternatively, this low incidence of GVHD may be related to the extensive immunosuppression from the preparative regimens, provided to ensure donor engraftment, or to the lower dose of UCB graft T-cells infused.

Several in vitro studies of UCB point to the inherent lack of full expression of immunomodulatory cytokines by alloreactive T-cells contained in UCB grafts *(54,55)*. Saito et al. *(56)* reported reduced interleukin 2 receptor (IL-2R) γ-chain expression in UCB early and mature lymphoid cells (T-, B-, NK), in part accounting for their relative unresponsiveness to allogeneic stimuli. IL-2R γ-chain expression in UCB lymphocytes was notably one-third that of adult cells. The IL-2R γ-chain is shared with receptors for IL-4, IL-7, IL-9, and IL-15. In primary mixed leukocyte culture, UCB T-cells demonstrate proliferative responses to allogeneic stimulation, but little generation of cytotoxic effector function. In addition, restimulation of primary UCB cultures results in a state of proliferative unresponsiveness *(57)*. Therefore, the reduced GVHD summarized in clinical reports after UCB may be related to these in vitro observations that immunologically competent cells contained in an UCB graft, although capable of recognizing noninherited Ags, do not elicit the normal cascade of events to expand these alloreactive lymphocytes. Preliminary observations point to reduced expression of nuclear factor of activated T-cells-1 as an important molecular mechanisms underlying this reduced cytokine production by UCB T-cells *(58)*.

3.3. Rate and Quality of Immunologic Recovery

Following allotransplantation, all patients experience a period of profound immuno-deficiency. Immune reconstitution of T- and B-cell compartments following allotransplantation may require as long as 12–24 mo. The slow process of immune reconstitution, together with postengraftment immunosuppression, create an immunologic environment in which the host is susceptible to opportunistic infections *(59)*, as well as to virally induced malignancies *(60)*. Recipients of unrelated donor or HLA-nonidentical transplants appear to have a higher rate of infectious complications than matched sibling allotransplant recipients. Also, GVHD and its treatment also delays immune recovery after allotransplantation.

By reducing the incidence and severity of GVHD, graft TCD would be expected to benefit immune reconstitution. Such a benefit, however, may be counteracted by the removal of functionally mature cells from the treated BM graft. Reported studies have shown variable quantitative and temporal differences in immune recovery following allotransplantation utilizing TCD grafts *(61–65)*. These reports point to immune reconstitution in patients who underwent TCD BM transplantation (BMT) using either closely MUDs or partially matched familial donors marked by depressed circulating total lymphocytes, CD3, and CD4 T-cell counts until 2 yr posttransplant; CD8$^+$ T-cell counts generally normalize by 18 mo, resulting in an inverted CD4:CD8 ratio until 24 mo posttransplant. Analysis of the pattern of immunologic recovery after allotransplantation also may be useful in predicting the onset of GVHD. Soiffer et al. *(63)* observed higher circulating CD8$^+$ T-cells and lower CD56$^+$ NK cells in patients who developed grades 2–4 GVHD, compared with those patients with grades 0–1 GVHD. This report, however, may reflect unique biology of immune reconstitution in patients receiving CD6-depleted grafts.

The author et al.'s preliminary analyses of immune recovery in UCB adult transplant recipients points to immune recovery within the first year posttransplant *(15,66)*. Immune recovery in this series of adult UCB transplant recipients was marked by profound lymphopenia and immunodeficiency during the first 6–12 mo after transplant. However, when immune recovery was attained, generally 9–12 mo after transplant, recovery of both T- and B-cell function was noted. Immune function studies, including enumeration of T-, B-, and NK cells via flow cytometric analyses, and T-lymphocyte proliferative responses to mitogens, performed on these patients after transplantation with UCB, revealed increased proportions of circulating lymphocytes expressing CD56$^+$CD3$^-$ phenotype, indicating an NK rebound effect, as previously reported in BMT recipients *(67,68)*. However, the absolute lymphocyte counts measured in the early posttransplant time period were very low, and the absolute numbers of circulating NK cells did not differ from that of adult controls. Proportions and absolute numbers of B-cells were noted to increase, beginning 6 mo post-UCB transplant, and persisted at 1-yr follow-up, as previously described *(69)*. It is unclear whether this B-cell rebound, observed post-UCB transplant, is related to tapering of immunosuppressive drugs, including cyclosporine, occult viral infections, and/or a recapitulation of normal B-cell ontogeny in the adult transplant recipient. Lymphocyte proliferation responses to plant mitogens ranged 30–50% that of normal controls during the first 6 mo post-UCB transplant.

3.4. Graft Vs Leukemia/Lymphoma

GVL effects after allotransplantation represent graft NK and T-lymphocyte interactions with Ags expressed on malignant cells. The contributions and interplay between NK and effector T-cells in the generation of GVL effects are not well defined. Because leukemic blasts are weakly immunogenic *(70)*, cells using MHC-nonrestrictive effector mechanisms, including NK, lymphokine-activated killer (LAK), and a subset of CD3[+] CD8[-]CD4[-] T-cells, have been the focus of study for their contribution to the development of cytotoxic T-lymphocytes (CTLs) specifically reactive with malignant cells. Graft T-lymphocyte interactions with Ags expressed on leukemic blasts have been shown to elicit GVL effects. Leukemia-reactive MHC-II-restricted CD4[+] CTL cell lines have been generated from allotransplant sibling donors by stimulating their peripheral blood lymphocytes (PBL) with leukemic blasts from the patient *(71,72)*. Mechanisms of presentation of tumor-associated Ags, in association with MHC molecules, moreover, has been further elucidated with evidence of the exclusive presentation by marrow-derived APCs *(73)*.

Currently, the capacity of UCB to mediate GVL in vivo is unknown. The observations of reduced GVHD elicited after UCB transplantation raises the question of concomitant reduction of GVL effects. Current clinical reports utilizing UCB have not pointed to increased relapse rates, but patient numbers are small and length of follow-up is short. NK cells are the first lymphoid cell population emerging from the recovering BM after near-ablative chemoradiotherapy. The role of NK cells in mediating GVL effects has been verified in recent reports of higher relapse rates observed in CML patients *(74)*, with reduced circulating NK cells during the first 9 mo after allotransplantation. In vitro phenotypic analyses of UCB have pointed to differences in lymphocyte subsets, compared with adult PBL. A study reported by Harris et al. *(75)* demonstrated that the proportion of cells expressing CD3, CD20, and CD56 were identical in UCB and PBL. However, CD8 cells are reduced, resulting in an increased CD4:CD8 ratio. Han et al. *(76)* did not verify this inversion of CD4:CD8 ratio in UCB. These authors noted that both the percentage and absolute number of CD4[+]CD8[+] T-cells are significantly increased in UCB, and that, because UCB has a higher lymphocyte count, compared with adult PBL, the absolute NK cell count is higher. Moreover, UCB LAK activity has been shown to be more readily induced in UCB, compared with that seen in adult PBL. These UCB LAK cells are able to lyse fresh leukemia targets from patients with acute lymphoblastic leukemia, acute myeloid leukemia, and CML *(77)*.

4. SUMMARY

Human allotransplantation is limited by a lack of available HLA-matched related donors, as well as by the risk of significant GVHD when alternative HLA-matched unrelated or partially mismatched family member grafts are utilized. These drawbacks have prompted the evaluation of banked unrelated UCB as a substitute allogeneic stem cell source. Thus far, clinical reports regarding UCB transplantation have focused primarily on pediatric or young adult recipients of small stature. Clinical reports thus far point to acceptable rates of hematopoietic engraftment and reduced GVHD, even when HLA-disparate grafts are infused. Mechanisms of reduced GVHD in UCB grafting have yet to be elucidated. Despite reduced acute and chronic GVHD, relapse rates in these UCB recipients is low. Understanding of the mechanisms underlying these observed clinical outcomes in recipients of allogeneic UCB grafts awaits further investigation.

REFERENCES

1. Buchner T. Treatment of adult acute leukemia, *Curr. Opin. Oncol.*, **9** (1997) 18–25.
2. Kernan NA, Bartsch G, Ash RC, et al. Analysis of 462 transplantations from unrelated donors facilitated by the National Marrow Donor Program, *N. Engl. J. Med.*, **328** (1993) 593–602.

3. Davies SM, Wagner JE, Weisdorf DJ, et al. Unrelated donor base marrow transplantation for hematologic malignancies: current status, *Leukemia Lymphoma*, **23** (1996) 221–226.

4. Carlens S, Ringden O, Remberger M, et al. Risk factors for chronic graft-versus-host disease after bone marrow transplantation: a retrospective single centre analysis, *Bone Marrow Transplant.*, **22** (1998) 755–761.

5. Goldman JM, Gale RP, Bortin MM, et al. Bone marrow transplantation for chronic myelogenous leukemia in chronic phase: increased risk of relapse associated with T-cell depletion, *Ann. Intern. Med.*, **108** (1988) 806–814.

6. Champlin RE. T-cell depletion for allogeneic bone marrow transplantation: impact on graft-versus-host disease, engraftment, and graft-versus-leukemia, *J. Hematother.*, **2** (1993) 27–42.

7. Beatty PG, Kollman C, and Howe CW. Unrelated-donor marrow transplants: the experience of the National Marrow Donor Program, *Clin. Transplant.*, (1995) 271–277.

8. Gluckman E, Rocha V, Boyer-Chammard A, et al. Outcome of cord-blood transplantation from related and unrelated donors, *New Eng. J. Med.*, **337** (1997) 373–381.

9. Wagner JE, Kernan NA, Steinbuch M, et al. Allogeneic sibling umbilical-cord-blood transplantation in children with malignant and non-malignant disease, *Lancet*, **346** (1995) 214–219.

10. Kurtzberg J, Laughlin M, Graham ML, et al. Placental blood as a source of hematopoietic stem cells for transplantation into unrelated recipients, *N. Engl. J. Med.*, **335** (1996) 157–166.

11. Wagner JE, Rosenthal J, Sweetman R, et al. Successful transplantation of HLA-matched and HLA-mismatched umbilical cord blood from unrelated donors: analysis of engraftment and acute graft-versus-host disease, *Blood*, **88** (1996) 795–802.

12. Cairo MS and Wagner JE. Placental and/or umbilical cord blood: an alternative source of hematopoietic stem cells for transplantation, *Blood*, **90** (1997) 4665–4678.

13. Wagner JE and Kurtzberg, J. Cord blood stem cells, *Curr. Opin. Hematol.*, **4** (1997) 413–418.

14. Laporte J, Gorin N, Rubinstein P, et al. Cord-blood transplantation from an unrelated donor in an adult with chronic myelogenous leukemia, *N. Engl. J. Med.*, **335** (1996) 167–170.

15. Laughlin MJ, Rizzieri DA, Smith CA, et al. Engraftment and reconstitution of immune function post unrelated cord blood transplant in an adult with Philadelphia chromosome positive acute lymphocytic leukemia, *Leukemia Res.*, **22** (1998) 215–219.

16. Rubinstein P, Carrier C, Scaradavou A, et al. Outcomes among 562 recipients of placental-blood transplants from unrelated donors, *New Eng. J. Med.*, **339** (1998) 1565–1577.

17. Faber LM, van Luxemburg-Heijs SAP, Veenhof WFJ, et al. Generation of CD4[+] cytotoxic T-lymphocyte clones from a patient with severe graft-versus-host disease after allogeneic bone marrow transplantation: implications for graft-versus-leukemia reactivity, *Blood*, **86** (1995) 2821–2828.

18. Jiang YZ, Kanfer EF, Macdonald D, Cullis JO, Goldman JM, and Barrett AJ. Graft-versus-leukaemia following allogeneic bone marrow transplantation: emergence of cytotoxic T lymphocytes reacting to host leukaemia cells, *Bone Marrow Transplant.*, **8** (1991) 253–258.

19. Falkenburg HF, Faber LM, van den Elshout M, et al. Generation of donor-derived antileukemic cytotoxic T-lymphocyte responses for treatment of relapsed leukemia after allogeneic HLA-identical bone marrow transplantation, *J. Immunother.*, **14** (1993) 305.

20. Laughlin MJ, Smith CA, Martin P, et al. Hematopoietic engraftment using placental cord blood (PCB) unrelated donor transplantation in recipients > 40 kg weight, *Blood,* **88 (Suppl 1)** (1996) 266a.

21. Kurtzberg J, Laughlin MJ, Smith CA, et al. Hematopoietic recovery in adult recipients following unrelated umbilical cord blood (UCB) transplantation, *Blood,* **90 (Suppl 1)** (1997) 110a.

22. Broxmeyer HE and Cooper S. High-efficiency recovery of immature haematopoietic progenitor cells with extensive proliferative capacity from human cord blood cryopreserved for 10 years, *Clin. Exp. Immunol.*, **107(Suppl 1)** (1997) 45–53.

23. Almici C, Carlo-Stella C, Wagner JE, et al. Biologic and phenotypic analysis of early hematopoietic progenitor cells in umbilical cord blood, *Leukemia*, **11** (1997) 2143–2149.

24. Bender JG, Unverzagt K, Walker DE, et al. Phenotypic analysis and characterization of CD34[+] cells from normal human bone marrow, cord blood, peripheral blood, and mobilized peripheral blood from patients undergoing autologous stem cell transplantation, *Clin. Immunol. Immunopathol.*, **70** (1994) 10.

25. Gomi S, Hasegawa S, Dan K, and Wakabayashi I. A comparative analysis of the transplant potential of umbilical cord blood versus mobilized peripheral blood stem cells, *Nippon Ika Daigaku Zasshi*, **64** (1997) 307–313.

26. Rubinstein P, Dobrila L, Rosenfield RE, et al. Processing and preservation of placental/umbilical cord blood for unrelated bone marrow reconstitution, *Proc. Natl. Acad. Sci. USA.*, **92** (1995) 10,119–10,122.

27. Almici C, Carlo-Stella C, Wagner JE, and Rizzoli V. Density separation and cryopreservation of umbilical cord blood cells: evaluation of recovery in short- and lon-term cultures, *Acta Haematol.*, **95** (1996) 171–175.

28. Regidor C, Posada M, Monteagudo D, et al. Umbilical cord blood banking for unrelated transplantation: evaluation of cell separation and storage methods, *Exp. Hamatol.*, **27** (1999) 30–35.

29. Denning-Kendall P, Donaldson C, Nicol A, et al. Optimal processing of human umbilical cord blood for clinical banking, *Exp. Hematol.*, **24** (1996) 1394–1401.

30. Fraser JK, Cairo MS, Wagner EL, et al. Cord blood transplantation study (COBLT): cord blood bank standard operating procedures. *J. Hematother.*, **7** (1998) 521–561.

31. Theilgaard-Monch K, Raaschou-Jensen K, Heilmann C, et al. A comparative study of CD34+ cells, CE34+ subsets, colony forming cells and cobblestone area forming cells in cord blood and bone marrow allografts, *Eur. J. Haematol.*, **62** (1999) 174–183.

32. DiGiusto DL, Lee R, Moon J, et al. Hematopoietic potential of cryopreserved and ex vivo manipulated umbilical cord blood progenitor cells evaluated in vitro and in vivo, *Blood*, **87** (1996) 1261–1271.

33. Briddell RA, Kern BP, Zilm KL, Stoney GB, and McNiece IK. Purification of CD34+ cells is essential for optimal ex vivo expansion of umbilical cord blood cells, *J. Hematother*, **6** (1997) 145–150.

34. Genechea G, Segovia JC, Albella B, et al. Delayed engraftment of nonobese diabetic/severe combined immunodeficient mice transplanted with ex vivo-expanded human CD34+ cord blood cells, *Blood*, **93** (1999) 1097–1105.

35. Rice A, Flemming C, Case J, et al. Comparative study of the in vitro behavior of cord blood subpopulations after short-term cytokine exposure, *Bone Marrow Transplant.*, **23** (1999) 211–220.

36. Bonnet D, Bhatia M, Wang JC, Kapp U, and Dick JE. Cytokine treatment or accessory cells are required to initiate engraftment of purified primitive human hematopoietic cells transplanted at limited doses into NOD/SCID mice, *Bone Marrow Transplant.*, **23** (1999) 203–209.

37. Welniak L, Murphy WJ, Iacobucci M, et al. IL-15 increases lymphoid and myeloid engraftment of ex vivo expanded human umbilical cord blood (UCB) in NOD.SCID mice, *Blood,* **92 (Suppl 1)** (1998) 290b.

38. Gauthier L, Fougereau M, and Tonnelle C. Construction of temperature and Zn-dependent human stromal cell lines that amplify hematopoietic precursors from cord blood CD34+ cells, *Exp. Hematol.*, **26** (1998) 534–540.

39. Jazwiec B, Solanilla A, Grosset C, et al. Endothelial cell support of hematopoiesis is differentially altered by IL-1 and glucocorticords, *Leukemia*, **12** (1998) 1210–1220.

40. Piacibello W, Sanavio F, Garetto L, et al. Differential growth factor requirement of primitive cord blood hematopoietic stem cell for self-renewal and amplification vs proliferation and differentiation, *Leukemia*, **12** (1998) 718–727.

41. Flasshove M, Banerjee D, Leonard JP, et al. Retroviral transduction of human CD34+ umbilical cord blood progenitor cells with a mutated dihydrofolate reductase cDNA, *Hum. Gene Ther.*, **9** (1998) 63–71.

42. Chatterjee S, Li W, Wong CA, et al. Transduction of primitive human marrow and cord blood-derived hematopoietic progenitor cells with adeno-associated virus vectors, *Blood*, **93** (1999) 1882–1894.

43. Hansen JA, Anasetti C, Beatty PG, et al. Treatment of leukemia by marrow transplantation from HLA-incompatible donors. Effect of HLA-disparity on GVHD, relapse and survival, *Bone Marrow Transplant.*, **6** 108–111.

44. Goulmy E, Shipper R, Pool J, et al. Mismatches of minor histocompatibility antigens between HLA-identical donors and recipients and the development of graft-versus-host disease after bone marrow transplantation, *N. Engl. J. Med.*, **334** (1996) 281–285.

45. van der Harst D, Coulmy E, Falkenburg JHF, et al. Recognition of minor histocompatibility antigens on lymphocytic and myeloid leukemic cells by cytotoxic T-cell clones, *Blood*, **83** (1994) 1060.

46. Herrera C, Torres A, Garcia-Castellano JM, et al. Prevention of graft-versus-host disease in high risk patients by depletion of CD4+ and reduction of CD8+ lymphocytes in the marrow graft, *Bone Marrow Transplant.*, **23** (1999) 443–450.

47. Sehn LH, Alyea EP, Weller E, et al. Comparative outcomes of T-cell-depleted and non-T-cell-depleted allogeneic bone marrow transplantation for chronic myelogenous leukemia: impact of donor lymphocyte infusion, *J. Clin. Oncol.*, **17** (1999) 561–568.

48. Novitzky N, Thomas V, Hale G, and Waldmann H. Ex vivo depletion of T cells from bone marrow grafts with CAMPATH-1 in acute leukemia: graft-versus-host disease and graft-versus-leukemia effect, *Transplantation*, **67** (1998) 620–626.

49. Zhang L, Martin DR, Fung-Leung WP, et al. Peripheral deletion of mature CD8[+] antigen-specific T cells after in vivo exposure to male antigen, *J. Immunol.*, **148** (1992) 3740–3745.

50. Burlingham WJ, Grailer AP, Fechner JH, et al. Microchimerism linked to cytotoxic T lymphocyte functional unresponsiveness (clonal anergy) in a tolerant renal transplant recipient, *Transplantation*, **59** (1995) 1147–1155.

51. Falkenburg JH, van Luxemburg-Heijs SA, Lim FT, et al. Umbilical cord blood contains normal frequencies of cytotoxic T-lymphocytes precursors (CTLp) and helper T-lymphocyte precursors against noninherited maternal antigens and noninherited paternal antigens, *Ann. Hematol.*, **72** (1996) 260–264.

52. Han P, Hodge G, Story C, et al. Phenotypic analysis of functional T-lymphocyte subtypes and natural killer cells in human cord blood: relevance to umbilical cord blood transplantation, *Br. J. Haematol.*, **89** (1995) 733–740.

53. Risdon G, Gaddy J, Stehman FB, et al. Proliferative and cytotoxic responses of human cord blood T lymphocytes following allogeneic stimulation, *Cell Immunol.*, **154** (1994) 14–24.

54. Chalmers IM, Janossy G, Contreras M, and Navarrete C. Intracellular cytokine profile of cord and adult blood lymphocytes, *Blood*, **92** (1998) 11–18.

55. Andersson U, Andersson J, Lindfors A, Wagner K, Moller G, and Heusser CH. Simultaneous production of interleukin 2, interleukin 4 and interferon-gamma by activated human blood lymphocytes, *Eur. J. Immunol.*, **20** (1990) 1591–1596.

56. Saito S, Morii T, Umekage H, et al. Expression of the interleukin-2 receptor gamma chain on cord blood mononuclear cells, *Blood*, **87** (1996) 3344–3350.

57. Risdon G, Gaddy J, and Broxmeyer HE. Allogeneic responses of human umbilical cord blood, *Blood*, **20** (1994) 566–570.

58. Kadereit S, McKinnon K, Mohammad S, Boss L, Junge G, Zakem-Cloud H, Iacobucci M, and Laughlin MJ. Nuclear factor of activated T-cells (NFAT-1) function in umbilical cord blood (UCB) vs adult peripheral blood, *Blood*, **92 (Suppl 1)** (1998) 292b.

59. Wingard JR. Infections in allogeneic bone marrow transplant recipients, *Semin. Oncol.*, **20** (1993) 80–87.

60. Lucas KG, Small TN, Heller G, et al. The development of cellular immunity to Epstein-Barr virus after allogeneic bone marrow transplantation, *Blood*, **87** (1996) 2594–2603.

61. Keever CA, Small TN, Flomenberg N, et al. Immune reconstitution following bone marrow transplantation: comparison of recipients of T-cell depleted marrow with recipients of conventional marrow grafts, *Blood*, **73** (1989) 1340–1350.

62. Verdonck LF, Dekker AW, de Gast GC, et al. Allogeneic bone marrow transplantation with a fixed low number of T cells in the marrow graft, *Blood*, **83** (1994) 3090.

63. Soiffer RJ, Bosserman L, Murray C, et al. Reconstitution of T-cell function after CD6 depleted allogeneic bone marrow transplantation, *Blood*, **75** (1990) 2076–2084.

64. Roux E, Helg C, Ffurmont-Girard, et al. Analysis of T-cell reproduction after allogeneic bone marrow transplantation: significant differences between recipients of T-cell depleted and unmanipulated grafts, *Blood*, **87** (1996) 3984–3992.

65. Kook H, Goldman F, Giller R, et al. Reconstitution of the immune system after unrelated or partially matched T-cell-depleted bone marrow transplantation in children: functional analyses of lymphocytes and correlation with immunophenotypic recovery following transplantation, *Clin. Diag. Lab. Immunol.*, **4** (1997) 96–103.

66. Laughlin MJ, McKinnon K, Demarest J, et al. Immune recovery post unrelated allogeneic umbilical cord blood (UCB) transplantation in adult recipients, *Blood*, **90 (Suppl 1)** (1997) 420a.

67. Ault KA, Antin JH, Ginsburg D, et al. Phenotype of recovering lymphoid cell populations after marrow transplantation, *J. Exp. Med.*, **161** (1985) 1483–1111.

68. Hercend T, Takvorian T, Nowill A, et al. Characterization of natural killer cells with antileukemia activity following allogeneic bone marrow transplantation, *Blood*, **67** (1986) 722–728.

69. Locatelli F, Maccario R, Comoli P, et al. Hematopoietic and immune recovery after transplantation of cord blood progenitor cells in children, *Bone Marrow Transplant.*, **18** (1996) 1095–1101.

70. Sulitzeanu D. Human cancer-associated antigens: present status and implications for immunodiagnosis, *Adv. Cancer Res.*, **44** (1985) 1–42.

71. Faber LM, va Luxemburg-Heijs SA, Veenhof WF, et al. Generation of CD4[+] cytotoxic T-lymphocyte clones from a patient with severe graft-versus-host disease after allogeneic bone marrow transplantation: implications for graft-versus-leukemia reactivity, *Blood*, **86** (1995) 2821.

72. Falkenburg HF, Faber LM, van den Elshout M, et al. Generation of donor-derived antileukemic cytotoxic T-lymphocyte responses for treatment of relapsed leukemia after allogeneic HLA-identical bone marrow transplantation, *J. Immunother.*, **14** (1993) 305.

73. Huang AY, Golumbek P, Ahmadzadeh M, et al. Role of bone marrow-derived cells in presenting MHC class I-restricted tumor antigens, *Science*, **264** (1994) 961.

74. Jiang YZ, Barrett AJ, Goldman JM, and Mavroudis DA. Association of natural killer cell immune recovery with a graft-versus-leukemia effect independent of graft-versus-host disease following allogeneic bone marrow transplantation, *Ann. Hematol.*, **74** (1997) 1–6.

75. Harris DT, Schumacher MJ, Locascio J, et al. Phenotypic and functional immaturity of human umbilical cord blood T lymphocytes, *Proc. Natl. Acad. Sci. USA.*, **89** (1992) 10,006–10,010.

76. Han P, Hodge G, Story C, et al. Phenotypic analysis of functional T-lymphocyte subtypes and natural killer cells in human cord blood: relevance to umbilical cord blood transplantation, *Br. J. Haematol.*, **89** (1995) 733–740.

77. Keever CA, Abu-Hajir M, Graf W, et al. Characterization of the alloreactivity and anti-leukemia reactivity of cord blood mononuclear cells, *Bone Marrow Transplant.*, **15** (1995) 407–419.

4

Are Busulfan-Based Preparative Regimens Equivalent, Worse, or Better than Total Body Irradiation Regimens?

Edward A. Copelan, MD

CONTENTS

1. INTRODUCTION

There is no simple answer to the question posed in the chapter title. Comparisons of total body irradiation (TBI) and busulfan (Bu) can only be made for the methods and doses of administration that have been studied. The best Bu-based and best TBI-

From: *Current Controversies in Bone Marrow Transplantation*
Edited by: B. Bolwell © Humana Press Inc., Totowa, NJ

based regimens in specific situations have not been established. For Bu, in particular, recent developments offer promise for improved results. Further, the relative effectiveness of TBI and Bu may depend on the underlying disease, on the stage of disease, the compatibility of the donor and recipient, and on other factors, including prior therapy and co-existing medical problems. In many settings, there are advantages and disadvantages for each approach.

The ability to safely and effectively administer either varies among different institutions. The value of experience cannot be overstated. Learning curves exist for various preparative regiments for bone marrow transplantation (BMT), including those using Bu and TBI. In order to better understand the relative virtues and disadvantages of these two agents, it is useful to first examine animal models and early human studies, and then to critically analyze more recent investigations, including randomized studies.

2. ANIMAL MODELS

2.1. For TBI

Animal models of BMT evolved from attempts to protect individuals from lethal radiation toxicity. Single exposure to high doses of TBI have been shown, in animal models and in humans, to cause lethal cutaneous and gastrointestinal toxicities. Lower doses, in the range of 1000 rads, cause sustained marrow aplasia and lead to lethal infection or bleeding. Infusion of syngeneic cells from the marrow or spleen of mice and guinea pigs could rescue these animals from lethal doses of irradiation (1,2), leading to studies in dogs and humans (3–6). Dogs exposed to 4 Gy of TBI die from complications of marrow failure. However, dogs exposed to 4–15 Gy can be rescued by infusion of previously stored autologous marrow (7–9). Protection can also be provided by marrow from allogeneic dog leukocyte antigen-identical littermates. However, engraftment of marrow from littermates requires TBI doses in excess of 9 Gy. Unrelated or mismatched donor marrow engrafts only with TBI doses in excess of 15 Gy (10). When radiation is split into several fractions, such as over 4 d, higher doses of radiation are required to ensure engraftment than when radiation is administered as a single dose (15 Gy, compared to 9 Gy) (11).

The combination of myeloablation with (relative) sparing of other organs, achieved with whole body irradiation, led Thomas (6) to utilize this technique to treat advanced hematologic malignancies. Compared to drug therapy, advantageous features of TBI are speed of delivery, lack of metabolites (which might interfere with the proliferation of transplanted cells), potent immunosuppressive effects, antileukemic effectiveness, lack of crossresistance with chemotherapy, the ability to reach privileged sites (including the central nervous system), effectiveness independent of blood supply, and the potential for shielding or boosting specific body parts.

2.2. For Bu

Santos and Owens (12,13) used cyclophosphamide (Cy) to achieve engraftment of allogeneic marrow in mice and rats. One hundred mg/kg of Cy ensured consistent and permanent engraftment of marrow from Lewis rats into histocompatible August Copenhagen and Irish hooded gene (ACI) donors (14). Rhesus monkeys engrafted following Cy doses of 180 mg/kg administered over 2 d. As with irradiation, a larger dose was needed if the Cy was administered over 4 d (15).

In contrast to irradiation and Cy, the drugs Bu and dimethylbusulfan cause severe granulocytopenia and thrombocytopenia, with minimal immediate affect on lymphocyte levels or humoral antibody responses *(16–19)*. These agents are not sufficiently immunosuppressive to permit allogeneic engraftment. However, they help achieve engraftment when added to agents such as antilymphocyte serum *(20)*. In rats, 200 mg/kg Cy is needed to permit engraftment. However, when combined with 30 mg/kg Bu, 150 mg/kg Cy suffices. Furthermore, the combination results in more rapid and complete engraftment than Cy alone *(14,21,22)*.

3. PILOT STUDIES

3.1. TBI in Humans

When TBI was first used as a single agent in two patients with acute lymphoblastic leukemia (ALL) who were undergoing syngeneic BMT, leukemia recurred *(23)*. Cy was then added to TBI to provide more antileukemic effectiveness. Of 100 patients with advanced leukemia, transplanted from human leukocyte antigen (HLA)-identical siblings following preparation with TBI and Cy, 13 became long-term survivors *(24)*. Initial studies used a single exposure of 10 Gy. The predominant toxicity of single-dose TBI was interstitial pneumonia *(25,26)*. In a subsequent study, patients who underwent transplantation in remission, who received fractionated TBI, achieved better leukemia-free survival (LFS) rates (approx 50%) than did patients who received irradiation in a single fraction *(27,28)*. By administering TBI in multiple fractions, hematopoietic cell toxicity was increased, compared to other organs, because of less efficient repair of DNA damage in hematopoietic cells.

Subsequent studies by the Seattle group analyzed the effect of higher doses of fractionated TBI on the incidence of relapse. Patients with acute myeloid leukemia (AML) in first remission *(29)* and chronic myeloid leukemia (CML) in chronic phase *(30)* were randomized to receive 120 mg/kg Cy with 12 Gy vs 15.75 Gy TBI. Patients receiving higher radiation doses exhibited higher incidences of interstitial pneumonia, hepatic veno-occlusive disease (VOD), and other transplant-related complications. They experienced higher rates of transplant-related mortality (TRM). However, they also had significantly lower incidences of leukemic relapse. Rates of LFS were similar with both irradiation doses. The lower radiation dose regimens were judged superior, in that failure because of relapse of disease is preferable to early death related to complications of transplantation. Although these studies demonstrated the optimal irradiation dose in these good-risk patients, this issue has not been adequately addressed in patients at higher risk of relapse.

3.2. Bu in Humans

Preliminary human studies of high-dose Bu demonstrated that mucositis and veno-occlusive disease were severe and dose-limiting at 20 mg/kg Bu *(31,32)*. Bu (16 mg/kg) and 200 mg/kg Cy (a substantially higher dose of Cy than that was utilized by Thomas, with TBI), were used by Santos et al. *(33)* at Johns Hopkins, as preparation for patients undergoing transplantation for AML. Initial studies demonstrated this busulfan/cyclophosphamide (Bu/Cy) regimen to be effective in AML; however, transplant-related complications, including TRM, were higher than with studies of Cy/TBI *(33)*. Because of the toxicity with 16 mg/kg BU and 200 mg/kg Cy (Bu/Cy$_4$), Tutschka et al. *(34)*, at Ohio State, decreased the dose of Cy to 60 mg/kg (Bu/Cy$_2$) on each of

2 consecutive d in patients with AML. Initial results with this regimen demonstrated success rates in AML similar to those reported with Cy/TBI. Bu/Cy$_2$ was then utilized as a preparative regimen in other hematologic disorders. Results were analyzed in a series of large multi-institutional trials (35–37).

To compare Bu-based regimens to TBI-based regimens, it is essential to define ground rules for such a discussion. Substantial amounts of information are available on various Bu-based and TBI-based regimens. To permit a meaningful comparison of Bu to TBI, this discussion focuses primarily on traditional fractionated TBI regimens with 120 mg/kg Cy vs 16 mg/kg Bu with 120 mg/kg Cy as preparation for allogeneic BMT (allo-BMT). The relevant areas that require comparison are immunosuppressive capacity, acute and delayed toxicities, and effectiveness against the underlying malignancy.

4. IMMUNOSUPPRESSION

TBI is a potent immunosuppressive agent. In contrast to TBI, Bu does not acutely lower the lymphocyte count (17–19). Bu is generally described as not being immunosuppressive, but animal and human studies demonstrate that high-dose Bu eradicates lymphocytes, although much more slowly than irradiation (38,39). Neutrophil counts also decline more slowly following high-dose Bu than following irradiation (35), although the difference is not as dramatic as that for lymphocytes. Lymphoid and hematopoietic reconstitution in animals and humans is similar following busulfan or TBI (38,39). Thus, Bu does exert immunosuppressive activity, but this effect is delayed, compared to that of irradiation.

Bu contributes substantially to the immunosuppressive capacity of the Bu/Cy regimen. Patients undergoing allo-BMT from HLA-identical siblings consistently engraft following preparation with the Bu/Cy regimen (35–37). A single study suggested a high rate of rejection of HLA-identical sibling marrow following Bu/Cy (40), but this finding has not been supported by other studies. A small study of 16 mg/kg Bu and 90 mg/kg Cy demonstrated rapid and sustained engraftment in all recipients of HLA-identical sibling grafts (41). Furthermore, unmanipulated, well-matched unrelated donor marrow recipients also consistently engraft (42,43). There is a low incidence of graft rejection in unrelated transplants, particularly as the degree of mismatch increases. It appears that the rate of nonengraftment in unrelated transplants may be slightly greater following Bu/Cy than with Cy/TBI (43). This is a logical expectation in view of the inferior early immunosuppressive capacity of busulfan.

Slattery et al. (44) demonstrated a correlation between Bu levels and rejection. When steady-state ($\overline{C}_{ss}$) levels of Bu were less than 200 ng/mL, 4/4 patients rejected grafts. When levels were 200-600 ng/mL, 4/11 patients rejected grafts. At levels greater than 600 ng/mL, only 1/23 (a 1-antigen mismatched unrelated donor) patients rejected grafts. This data also demonstrated that partially matched unrelated donors require higher $\overline{C}_{ss}$ levels of Bu than HLA-identical siblings: 600 ng/mL, compared to 200 ng/mL.

Slattery (45) further demonstrated that Cy is cleared more rapidly in patients who have received high-dose Bu. The area-under-the-curve of hydroxycyclophosphamide, the active agent, is greater following Bu than with Cy alone. Thus, Bu results in a greater exposure to hydroxycyclophosphamide, and this exposure correlates with the average steady-state level of Bu (45). Bu's effect on Cy metabolism is, therefore, in part responsible for its immunosuppressive capacity as preparative therapy for transplantation. As previously mentioned, animal studies have demonstrated that, when combined with Bu, lower doses of Cy permit more rapid and complete engraftment than with higher doses of Cy alone *(15,21,22)*.

Bu exerts a potent immunosuppressive effect, but its delay well beyond the period of marrow infusion makes it less helpful than TBI in preventing acute rejection. It does contribute to the immunosuppressive effect of the Bu/Cy regimen, at least in part, through its effect on Cy metabolism. Bu/Cy_2 leads to rapid and consistent engraftment of unmanipulated marrow from well-matched sibling and unrelated donors. Bu/Cy_2 is not recommended for poorly matched related or unrelated transplantation, particularly when accompanied by manipulation, such as T-cell depletion, of hematopoietic progenitor cell grafts.

5. TOXICITY

5.1. Acute Toxicity

Accurate analysis of regimen-related toxicity (RRT) caused by the preparative regimen, independent of other factors (e.g., prior treatment, supportive care following transplant, and the development of graft-vs-host disease [GVHD]), is virtually impossible. However, the system developed by Bearman et al. *(46)* provides a reasonable mechanism for comparing toxicities of different regimens. The most common sites of severe RRT are the liver, kidneys, and lungs.

Bearman et al. *(46)* identified the total dose of irradiation as the most significant risk factor in predicting the development of RRT. Patients undergoing allotransplantation, those with advanced disease, and those receiving methotrexate in addition to cyclosporine, had higher incidences of grade III and IV toxicity, demonstrating that other factors contribute to RRT, and, in addition, emphasizing the complexity of comparing regimens in studies using different patient populations and supportive care techniques.

5.2. Hepatic Toxicity

Nevill et al. *(47)* demonstrated a 44% incidence of grade II or higher hepatic RRT using Bu/Cy, similar to results from the same institution using TBI. In most studies, however, the incidence of clinically detectable hepatic VOD in patients receiving Bu/Cy approaches 50%, higher than is usually reported using fractionated irradiation *(48–50)*. Severe hepatic VOD also appears to occur more frequently following Bu *(49,50)*. A meta-analysis of randomized studies of Bu/Cy vs TBI identified a significantly higher risk of VOD in patients conditioned with Bu/Cy *(51)*. However, a randomized study in CML from Seattle *(52)* was excluded from analysis, because the incidence of VOD was not reported. However, the ratios of maximum bilirubin posttransplant, compared to the pretreatment bilirubin and the incidence of bilirubin >3.0 mg/dL posttransplant, were lower (though not significantly) in the Bu/Cy group in this study. Patients receiving Bu preparative regimens, who previously received Bu *(50)* or nitrosurea *(53)*, or who received methotrexate for prevention of GVHD *(47)* were at significantly greater risk for VOD.

VOD has not been frequently reported as a primary cause of death following transplantation. However, in a study of patients prepared with Bu/Cy, those whose bilirubin

rose to greater than 10 mg/dL within 100 d of transplantation experienced a 91% TRM
(54), compared to TRM for those whose bilirubin did not reach 10 mg/dL of 20%. In
29 patients whose bilirubin reached 10 mg/dL, and who came to autopsy, 18 had
pathologic evidence of VOD, and four had massive hepatic necrosis.

Because of the incidence and significance of VOD following Bu, investigators have
pursued methods to decrease its incidence and severity. Hepatic VOD and severe RRT,
in general, occur more frequently when plasma Bu levels are high *(44,45)*. Only 1/31
patients with $\overline{C}_{ss}$ <900 ng/mL developed grade 3 hepatic VOD, which was the only
severe RRT encountered in patients with Bu levels in this range *(44)*. These data suggest
that adjusting subsequent Bu doses to achieve a targeted plasma level, based on first-
dose pharmacokinetic studies, could achieve less toxicity.

Alternatively, or in conjunction with targeted plasma levels, intravenous forms of
Bu offer the potential for more uniform plasma levels and less toxicity *(56)*. Further,
a recent randomized study has demonstrated a significantly reduced risk of VOD in
patients receiving Bu who were given ursodiol as prophylaxis *(57)*. Another approach
to decrease the incidence and severity of VOD has been to lower the Bu dose to 14
mg/kg, and add high-dose etoposide to 120 mg/kg Cy. This approach has resulted in
significantly lower incidence of RRT, of hepatic VOD, and of severe hepatic VOD in
patients with non-Hodgkin's lymphoma undergoing autotransplantation *(58)*. Similar
results have been present in the allogeneic setting as well (unpublished data). Thus,
although the incidence and severity of VOD appear higher following Bu than following
TBI, numerous techniques for substantially lowering this complication have been
described, and promise to improve further results.

5.3. Pulmonary Toxicity

The incidence of interstitial pneumonia appears to be lower with Bu/Cy than with
Cy/TBI, particularly in individuals at high risk for the development of this complication.
In a study of patients at high risk of interstitial pneumonia because of prior chest
irradiation, 5% of patients with Bu/Cy as preparation developed interstitial pneumoni,
compared to 32% of patients who underwent transplantation with Cy/TBI *(59)*. In most
studies, and in the previously mentioned meta-analysis of randomized trials *(51)*, no
significant difference can be demonstrated.

5.4. Other Toxicities

Mucositis, hemorrhagic cystitis, and renal failure are other toxicities that generally
contribute to morbidity, but less often to mortality. Hemorrhagic cystitis appears to
occur about twice as commonly with Bu-containing regimens as with TBI *(50)*. In the
only study that adequately assessed it *(52)*, renal failure occurred more commonly with
TBI than with Bu. Further, that randomized study demonstrated less-prolonged severe
granulocytopenia, less fevers, and a lower incidence of positive bacterial or fungal
blood cultures. These observations were supported by numerous nonrandomized trials
(34–37).

The overall incidence of RRT and severe RRT caused by Bu, compared to irradiation,
appear roughly similar in most studies. In patients with minimal risk factors for toxicity
(e.g., patients with chronic-phase CML undergoing allotransplant from HLA-identical
sibling donors within 1 yr of diagnosis), single-institution experience with either regimen
have similar and low risks of death from transplant-related complications *(52,60)*. The

capacity to lower the incidence of severe hepatic VOD, using the previously described methods, offer the potential to reduce toxicity with Bu to a level beneath that with TBI.

6. GRAFT VS HOST DISEASE

The incidence of acute GVHD appears similar in most studies using Bu and Cy, compared to that reported for Cy/TBI, when using similar techniques for prevention. A study from Seattle *(52)*, randomizing CML patients between Bu/Cy and Cy/TBI, found a lower incidence of acute GVHD in patients receiving Bu/Cy, but this has not been noted by other studies.

7. DELAYED TOXICITY

The well-documented significant delayed effects of conditioning with TBI *(71)*, including endocrine dysfunction, growth abnormalities, and second malignancies, provided a prime motive for the development of radiation-free preparative therapy. Some delayed complications, e.g., chronic GVHD, have been reported in similar incidences following Bu/Cy or Cy/TBI *(61,62)*. Similarly, deficiency of immunoglobulin subclasses 2 (Ig2) and Ig4 following transplantation has been reported in nonirradiated, as well as irradiated recipients *(63,64)*.

Endocrine dysfunction may be more severe following TBI than following Bu. Hypothyroidism occurs frequently in patients receiving single-dose TBI, and can occur in approx 15% of those receiving fractionated TBI, but its frequency appears to be much less common following By/Cy *(65–68)*. Impaired growth because of deficiency of growth hormone production, and direct affects of radiation on bone, are common following TBI, especially when combined with cranial radiation, where it occurs in approx 90% of individuals *(66,67,69)*. However, Bu also impairs growth velocity. Studies in thalassemia demonstrate decreased growth velocity in children aged 10–11 prepared for transplantation with Bu/Cy, but not in younger children *(67)*. One recent analysis did not find significantly impaired growth following Bu-containing regimens in young children, as long as they did not develop GVHD or receive high-dose corticosteroids *(70)*.

TBI consistently causes primary gonadal failure in both men and women, and reports of pregnancy and fathering of children are rare. Occasional patients have recovered sperm function 6–8 yr following transplantation regimens utilizing TBI. One study of 323 men, evaluated for 12 yr following TBI, demonstrated return of spermatogenesis in five *(69)*. Though infertility is common following Bu, it occurs less frequently. No formal studies have been carried out, but it appears that over 30% of patients with minimal therapy prior to transplant have either demonstrable functioning sperm or have fathered children *(71,72)*.

The risk of lymphoproliferative disorders following allotransplantation appears predominantly related to the extent of immunosuppressive treatment *(73,74)*. However, a lower incidence of lymphoproliferative disorders has been reported with regimens that do not use TBI *(73)*. A recent analysis *(75)* of solid cancers following transplant demonstrated that the TBI dose was critical in determining the risk of solid cancer, and that irradiation-free regimens were associated with a lower incidence of malignancies. Solid tumors occurred most frequently in patients who were transplanted prior to the age of 10 yr. Melanoma and cancer of the buccal cavity, brain, liver, thyroid, and connective tissue occurred with increased frequency following transplantation. Tumors occurred at an incidence 4 × as high in patients receiving high doses of irradiation, compared to those who received no irradiation. Although the delayed effects of Bu have been less thoroughly studied than for TBI, they appear to occur less frequently.

8. EFFECTIVENESS IN SPECIFIC DISEASES

Conventional treatments of specific hematologic malignancies are different, i.e., different malignancies are treated with different regimens. It is increasingly apparent that subgroups of patients with a specific hematologic malignancy, e.g., ALL, benefit from treatment tailored for that specific subgroup (76). A single preparative regimen may not prove optimal for the treatment of all hematologic disorders requiring transplantation. Bu-based regimens may be more effective than TBI in some disorders, and less effective in others.

8.1. Acute Myeloid Leukemia

Generally, 55–60% of patients with AML who undergo allotransplantation from HLA-identical siblings while in first remission achieve sustained disease-free survival (DFS), but DFS rates in excess of 70% have been reported (77–83). Patients treated with more advanced disease have poorer rates of long-term survival. Patients in second remission, or untreated first relapse, have LFS of approx 30%; those with primary refractory or relapsed refractory disease have rates of 10–20%. Results have been reported in patients undergoing transplant with Bu/Cy (35,82) that are roughly similar to those for Cy/TBI. However, only one prospective randomized study (81), comparing Bu/Cy to Cy/TBI, solely in patients with AML in first remission, has been published. This study, from the Groupe d'Etude de la Greffe de Moelle Osseuse, reported a significantly poorer outcome in patients given Bu/Cy. It reported a 72% rate of DFS with Cy/TBI, which is higher than that generally reported. The 47% LFS with Bu/Cy was lower than that reported from other studies, including a large multi-institutional study (35), and retrospective analyses of registry data (72,82). Further, there was no consideration of important risk factors, e.g., cytogenetic abnormalities, which significantly effect transplant outcome (83). In marked contrast to this study, a randomized study in patients with AML, ALL, or CML, by the Nordic Bone Marrow Transplant Group, using the same Bu protocol, achieved an 83% DFS rate in AML patients in first complete remission, compared to 58%, using TBI (84). These conflicting results emphasize the commonly ignored limitations of randomized studies, and the importance, as emphasized by Hellman, of incorporating prior knowledge into one's scrutiny of a trial's design, execution, and results, before formulating an opinion (85).

For more advanced disease, similar results have been reported with Bu/Cy and Cy/TBI. One study suggested that results in patients with advanced disease might be better with Bu/Cy than with etoposide (VP-16)/TBI (86); the previously mentioned Nordic study reported worse results in advanced patients receiving Bu/Cy (84).

In autotransplantation of AML, when the absence of a graft-vs-leukemia effect places an increased burden on the preparative regimen, Bu/Cy is widely utilized, but little meaningful data exists as to its relative effectiveness. A retrospective analysis by the European Group for Blood and Marrow Transplantation (EBMT) compared patients with AML undergoing allo- or autotransplant for AML prepared with Bu/Cy_2 to an equal number prepared with Cy/TBI, matched for various risk factors. Results, including TRM, relapse rate, and LFS, were virtually identical, whether patients received Bu/Cy or Cy/TBI *(82)*.

8.2. Acute Lymphoblastic Leukemia

Limited studies of Bu have been performed in ALL *(87,88)*. The results of nonrandomized studies in ALL indicate that Cy/TBI and Bu/Cy yield comparable results. However, an extensive and well-performed retrospective analysis of children transplanted with Cy/TBI or Bu/Cy, by the IBMTR, reported similar rates of relapse, but a higher transplant-related mortality (TRM) and treatment failure in the Bu/Cy group *(89)*. Review of the EBMT data indicated similar results in transplantation of first remission and more advanced patients who underwent allografts, and in autografts of first remission patients using Bu/Cy or Cy/TBI. Results in more advanced ALL patients undergoing autografting, a technique of unproven effectiveness, were superior with Cy/TBI *(82)*.

8.3. Chronic Myeloid Leukemia

Two randomized studies of Bu/Cy vs Cy/TBI have been performed in chronic-phase CML: one by the Seattle group *(52)* and one by the French *(40)*. Both studies demonstrated similar results using each regimen. In the Seattle study, complications, including renal failure and GVHD, occurred in a lower proportion of patients receiving Bu/Cy. In the French study, a significantly lower rate of relapse was experienced in patients receiving Bu/Cy, compared to Cy/TBI. This low relapse rate with Bu/Cy is supported by a multi-institutional trial *(36)*, and by long-term follow-up data from Ohio State *(60)*, in which a low incidence of molecular and hematologic relapse occurred in CML patients prepared for allotransplant with Bu/Cy. It appears that Bu/Cy is at least comparable, and perhaps superior, in the treatment of chronic-phase CML. Similarly, results, which compare favorably to those reported with Cy/TBI, have been published for patients with advanced stages of CML. However, patient selection and other factors complicate meaningful interpretation of these data *(90)*.

8.4. Myelodysplasia

A substantial proportion of patients undergoing allotransplantation for myelodysplastic syndrome (MDS) have therapy-related disorders following combined modality treatment for malignancies. Radiation-free preparative regimens avoid the risk of additional radiation dosages to previously irradiated sites. Large studies have reported similar results with Bu-based regimens, compared to TBI-based regimens in patients undergoing allo-BMT for MDS *(91,92)*.

Seattle performed a prospective study of Bu/Cy in 30 patients with MDS undergoing related or unrelated donor BMT, and compared results with those achieved in 38 historical controls treated with Cy and TBI *(93)*. No significant difference in outcome, based on preparative regimens, was detected.

The European Working Group on Myelodysplastic Syndrome in Children reported a better event-free survival in children with chronic myelomonocytic leukemia, who received Bu, than with those given TBI prior to allo-BMT from HLA-identical siblings or 1 antigen-disparate relatives, primarily because of a lower probability of relapse *(94)*.

8.5. Nonmalignant Disorders

Busulfan is widely and successfully used in preparative regimens for the treatment of nonmalignant conditions, such as inborn errors of metabolism, Wiskott-Aldrich syndrome, and thalassemia. Such transplants are usually performed in young children, in whom avoidance of known delayed effects of radiation, including growth retardation and secondary malignancy, provided the chief motivating factor for the use of Bu.

Lucarelli and the Pesaro team established the effectiveness of Bu (14 mg/kg) and Cy in children and adults with thalassemia (95,96). Patients who had received adequate chelation therapy, or who lacked substantial hepatomegaly or portal fibrosis of the liver, achieved DFS rates in excess of 80%. Children with all three high-risk factors (Class III) have DFS rates of 53%, largely because of nonrelapse mortality. Class III patients were found to have significantly lower mortality rates when they received less than 200 mg/kg of Cy (97).

9. CONCLUSIONS

This chapter compares Bu/Cy and Cy/TBI as preparative regimens for allogeneic progenitor cell transplantation. Regarding immunosuppression, only one study identified a significant incidence of graft rejection among HLA-identical siblings. Yet, in this study, 4/65 patients undergoing allotransplant with Bu/Cy$_2$ for chronic-phase CML rejected grafts (40). It is difficult to reconcile this result with other randomized studies (52,81,84,86), and with the multitude of single and multi-institutional studies published, in which the rate of graft rejection is as low for Bu/Cy as that reported for regimens containing TBI (35–37,82). Furthermore, similar or only slightly higher rates of rejection occur with Bu/Cy in the well-matched, unmanipulated, unrelated setting (42,43,60,93).

Less acute toxicity was experienced in patients receiving Bu/Cy in the Seattle CML study (52), and in advanced patients in the Southwest Oncology Group study comparing Bu/Cy to VP-16/TBI (86), but significantly greater toxicity was seen using Bu/Cy in the Nordic study (84) in advanced, but not early, patients. Again, it is difficult to reconcile the differences between these studies. In studies of chronic-phase CML, hepatotoxicity with Bu/Cy is not greater than that with Cy/TBI (40,52); in acute leukemias, the incidence appears higher (82). This may be attributable, as pointed out by Clift (52), to substantial pretransplant exposure to chemotherapy in the acute leukemia patients. Exposure to specific agents might be especially dangerous in conjunction with Bu (47,50,53).

The bulk of data does not support a meaningful difference in the incidence or severity of GVHD. The incidence of acute GVHD was less in the Bu/Cy group in the Seattle CML study (52), but grade III acute GVHD was greater in the Bu/Cy group in the Nordic study (84). These conflicts emphasize the need to carefully analyze results from these randomized studies, and to balance the results of individual studies with results achieved in large nonrandomized studies, and with registry data.

Personal experience has demonstrated that different institutions have based dosing of both Bu and Cy on different measures of body size, e.g., ideal body wt, real body wt, or a variety of formulas for determining an adjusted ideal body wt. Policies regarding redosing following emesis, administration of other drugs, e.g., phenytoin, which effect Bu metabolism, and frequency of dosing of Bu (e.g., every 6 h vs qid), vary considerably from institution to institution. Inclusion of patients, e.g., those with abnormal liver function tests (LFTs), also differs considerably between institutions. Last, institutions that have substantially greater experience with TBI than with Bu have participated in trials of Bu, often entering small numbers of patients, and lack of expertise may effect results. Such discrepancies may, in part, account for differences in results achieved in different trials.

Insufficient information is available to fully answer the question posed in the chapter title. The greater ease of administration, lesser expense, and lower incidence and severity of delayed complications favor the use of Bu when results are otherwise equivalent. However, the effectiveness of treatment is the most critical issue in choosing a preparative regimen.

In AML, the bulk of evidence supports the equivalence of Bu/Cy and Cy/TBI. A single randomized study favors Cy/TBI (81). A reasonable argument can be made for either regimen in early or advanced AML. In ALL, for which less data exists, doubt remains as to whether Bu/Cy is as effective as Cy/TBI. Modification of Bu/Cy, e.g., the addition of VP-16 may improve results, but Bu/Cy has not been proven as effective as Cy/TBI. In myelodysplasia, CML, and thalassemia and other nonmalignant marrow disorders, Bu/Cy appears to be at least as effective than Cy/TBI, and its use should be favored.

In the unrelated setting, substantially more data exists, and increasingly favorable results have been obtained with Cy/TBI. Sufficient data does exist, however, in the well-matched unrelated setting to support the use of Bu/Cy$_2$ (42,43,60,92). In mismatched family and unrelated transplants, and following marrow manipulation, e.g., T-cell depletion, there is insufficient data to recommend the use of Bu/Cy. Although larger doses of Cy, e.g., 200 mg/kg, result in greater immunosuppression, much more data exists to support TBI-based regimens in these settings. Studies in thalassemia (97) demonstrate less toxicity, and studies in leukemia demonstrate no increase in relapse with Bu/Cy$_2$, compared to Bu/Cy$_4$ (82).

Bu has been less extensively utilized and less well studied than TBI. Advances in its use promise to further improve results. The availability of iv formulations, improved definition of optimal plasma levels for dose-targeting, the use of ursodiol or other agents to decrease hepatic VOD, and further study of combinations with other agents, e.g., etoposide, or radionuclide-labeled monoclonal antibodies, suggest that, in many settings, the question posed in the title may soon be more simply answered.

REFERENCES

1. Jacobson L, Marks E, Robson M, et al. Effect of spleen protection on mortality following x-irradiation, *J. Lab. Clin. Med.*, **34** (1949) 1538.
2. Lorenz E, Uphoff D, Reid T, et al. Modification of irradiation injury in mice and guinea pigs by bone marrow infections, *J. Natl. Cancer Inst.*, **12** (1951) 197.
3. Thomas E, Lochte H Jr, Lu W, et al. Intravenous infusion of bone marrow in patients receiving radiation and chemotherapy, *N. Engl. J. Med.*, **257** (1957) 491.
4. Ferrebee J, Lochte H Jr, Jarezki A III, et al. Successful marrow homograft in the dog after radiation, *Surgery*, **43** (1958) 516.
5. Epstein R, Storb R, Ragde H, et al. Cytotoxic typing antisera for marrow grafting in littermate dogs, *Transplantation*, **6** (1968) 45–58.
6. Thomas E. The role of marrow transplantation in the eradication of malignant disease. *Cancer* **49** (1982) 1963.
7. Thomas E, LeBlond R, Graham T, et al. Marrow infusions in dogs given midlethal or lethal irradiation. *Radiat. Res.* **41** (1970) 113–124.

8. Mannick J, Lochte H Jr, Ashley C, et al. Autografts of bone marrow in dogs after lethal total-body radiation. *Blood* **15** (1960) 255.

9. Cavins J, Kasakura S, Thomas E, et al. Recovery of lethally irradiated dogs following infusion of autologous marrow stored at low temperatures in dimethyl-sulphoxide. *Blood* **20** (1962) 730.

10. Storb R and Deeg H. Failure of allogeneic canine marrow grafts after total body irradiation; allogeneic "resistance" vs transfusion induced sensitization. *Transplantation* **42** (1986) 571–580.

11. Storb R, Raff R, and Appelbaum F. Comparison of fractionated to single-dose total body irradiation in conditioning canine littermates for DLA-identical marrow grafts. *Blood* **74** (1991) 1139–1143.

12. Santos G and Owens A Jr. Syngeneic and allogeneic marrow transfusion on cyclophosphamide-induced lethality in the rat. *Exp. Hematol.* **10** (1966) 8–13.

13. Santos G and Owens A Jr. Allogeneic marrow transplantation in cyclophosphamide treated mice. *Transplant Proc.* **1** (1969) 44–46.

14. Santos G and Owens A Jr. Syngeneic and allogeneic marrow transplants in the cyclophosphamide pretreated rat. In Dausset I, Hamgerger I, Mathe G (eds.), *Advance in Transplantation.* Proceedings of the First International Congress of the Transplantation Society, Paris, France, June 27–30, 1976. Munksgaard, Copenhagen, Denmark, 1968, p. 431–438.

15. Storb R, Buckner C, Dillingham L, et al. Cyclophosphamide regimens in Rhesus monkeys with and without marrow infusion. *Cancer Res.* **30** (1970) 2195–2203.

16. Ford C, Micklem H, Evans P, et al. The inflow of bone marrow cells to the thymus: Studies with part body irradiated mice injected with chromosome marked bone marrow and subjected to antigenic stimulation. *Ann. N.Y. Acad. Sci.* **129** (1966) 283–287.

17. Josvasen N and Boyum A. Hematopoiesis in busulfan treated mice. *Scand. J. Hematol.* **11** (1973) 78–86.

18. Santos G and Tutschka P. The effect of busulfan on antibody production and skin allograft survival in the rat. *J. Natl. Cancer Inst.* **53** (1974) 1775–1780.

19. Buckner C, Dillingham L, Giddens W Jr, et al. Toxicologic and marrow transplantation studies in rhesus monkeys given dimethylmyeran. *Exp. Hematol.* **3** (1975) 275–288.

20. Floersheim G and Ruszkiewicz M. Bone marrow transplantation after antilymphocytic serum and lethal chemotherapy. *Nature* **333** (1969) 854–857.

21. Tutschka P and Santos G. G-B incompatible bone marrow transplantation in the rat after treatment with cyclophosphamide and busulfan. *Fed. Proc.* **32** (1973) 226–232.

22. Tutschka P and Santos G. Bone marrow transplantation in the busulfan treated rat. III. Relationship between myelosuppression and immunosuppression for conditioning bone marrow recipients. *Transplantation* **24** (1977) 52–61.

23. Thomas E, Lochte H Jr., Cannon J, et al. Supralethal whole body irradiation and isologous marrow transplantation in man. *J. Clin. Invest.* **38** (1959) 1709–1714.

24. Thomas E, Buckner C, Banaji M, et al. One hundred patients with acute leukemia treated by chemotherapy, total body irradiation and allogeneic marrow transplantation. *Blood* **49** (1977) 511–533.

25. Bortin M. Pathogenesis of interstitial pneumonitis following allogeneic bone marrow transplantation for acute leukemia. In Gale RP (ed.), *Recent Advances in Bone Marrow Transplantation.* Liss, New York, 1978, pp. 445–452.

26. Fryer C, Fitzpatrick P, Rider W, et al. Radiation pneumonitis: experience following a large single dose of radiation. *Intl. J. Rad. Oncol. Biol. Phys.* **4** (1978) 931–936.

27. Thomas E, Buckner C, Clift R, et al. Marrow transplantation for acute nonlymphoblastic leukemia in first remission. *N. Engl. J. Med.* **301** (1979) 597–599.

28. Thomas E, Clift R, Hersman J, et al. Marrow transplantation for acute nonlymphoblastic leukemia in first remission using fractionated or single-dose irradiation. *Intl. J. Radiat. Oncol. Biol. Phys.* **8** (1982) 817–821.

29. Clift R, Buckner C, Appelbaum F, et al. Allogeneic marrow transplantation in patients with acute myeloid leukemia in first remission: a randomized trial of two irradiation regimens. *Blood* **76** (1990) 1867–1871.

30. Clift R, Buckner C, Frederick R, et al. Allogeneic transplantation in patients with chronic myeloid leukemia in the chronic phase: a randomized trial of two irradiation regimens. *Blood* **77** (1991) 1660–1665.

31. Tutschka P, Santos G, and Elfenbein G. Marrow transplantation in acute leukemia following busulfan and cyclophosphamide. *Blut.* **25** (1980) 375–380.

32. Peters W, Henner W, Grochow L, et al. Clinical and pharmacologic effects of high dose single agent busulfan with autologous bone marrow support in the treatment of solid tumors. *Cancer Res.* **47** (1987) 6402–6406.

33. Santos G, Tutschka P, Brookmeyer R, et al. Marrow transplantation for acute nonlymphocytic leukemia after treatment with busulfan and cyclophosphamide. *N. Engl. J. Med.* **309** (1983) 1347–1353.

34. Tutschka P, Copelan E, and Klein J. Bone marrow transplantation for leukemia following a new busulfan and cyclophosphamide regimen. *Blood* **70** (1987) 1382–1388.

35. Copelan E, Biggs J, Thompson J, et al. Treatment for acute myelocytic leukemia with allogeneic bone marrow transplantation following preparation with BuCy$_2$. *Blood* **78** (1991) 838–843.

36. Biggs J, Szer J, Crilley P, et al. Treatment of chronic myeloid leukemia with allogeneic bone marrow transplantation following preparation with BuCy$_2$. *Blood* **80** (1992) 1352–1357.

37. Copelan E, Biggs J, Avalos B, et al. Radiation-free preparation for allogeneic bone marrow transplantation in adults with acute lymphoblastic leukemia. *J. Clin. Oncol.* **10** (1992) 237–242.

38. Yeager A, Shinn C, Pardoll D, et al. Lymphoid reconstitution after transplantation of congenic hematopoietic cells in busulfan-treated mice. *Blood* **78** (1991) 3312–3316.

39. Fishleder A, Bolwell B, and Lichtin A. Incidence of mixed chimerism using busulfan/cyclophosphamide containing regimens in allogeneic bone marrow transplantation. *Bone Marrow Transplant.* **9** (1992) 293–297.

40. Devergie A, Blaise D, Attal M, et al. Allogeneic bone marrow transplantation for chronic myeloid leukemia in first chronic phase: a randomized trial of busulfan-cytoxan versus cytoxin-total body irradiation as preparative regimen: a report from The French Society of Bone Marrow Graft (SFGM). *Blood* **85** (1995) 2263–2268.

41. Avalos B, Klein J, Kapoor N, et al. Allogeneic bone marrow transplantation following busulfan and 90 mg/kg of cyclophosphamide. *Bone Marrow Transplant.* **12** (1993) 655–658.

42. Klein J, Avalos B, Belt P, et al. Bone marrow engraftment following unrelated donor transplantation utilizing busulfan and cyclophosphamide preparatory chemotherapy. *Bone Marrow Transplant.* **17** (1996) 479–483.

43. Sahebi F, Copelan E, Crilley P, et al. Unrelated allogeneic bone marrow transplantation using high dose busulfan and cyclophosphamide (Bu-Cy) for the preparative regimen. *Bone Marrow Transplant.* **17** (1996) 685–689.

44. Slattery J, Clift R, Buckner C, et al. Marrow transplantation for chronic myeloid leukemia: The influence of plasma busulfan levels on the outcome of transplantation. *Blood* **89** (1997) 3055–3060.

45. Slattery J, Kalhorn T, McDonald G, et al. Conditioning regimen-dependent disposition of cyclophosphamide and hydroxycyclophosphamide in human marrow transplantation patients. *J. Clin. Oncol.* **14** (1996) 1484–1494.

46. Bearman S, Appelbaum F, Buckner C, et al. Regimen-related toxicity in patients undergoing bone marrow transplantation. *J. Clin. Oncol.* **6** (1988) 1562–1568.

47. Nevill T, Barnett M, Klingemann H, et al. Regimen-related toxicity of a busulfan–cyclophosphamide conditioning regimen in 70 patients undergoing allogeneic bone marrow transplantation. *J. Clin. Oncol.* **9** (1991) 1224–1232.

48. McDonald G, Hinds M, Fisher L, et al. Veno-occlusive disease of the liver and multiorgan failure after bone marrow transplantation: a cohort study of 355 patients. *Ann. Intern. Med.* **118** (1993) 255–267.

49. Jones R, Lee K, Beshorner W, et al. Venocclusive disease of the liver following bone marrow transplantation. *Transplantation.* **44** (1987) 778–783.

50. Morgan M, Dodds A, Atkinson K, et al. The toxicity of busulfan and cyclophosphamide as the preparative regimen for bone marrow transplantation. *Br. J. Haematol.* **77** (1991) 529–534.

51. Hartman A-R, Williams SF, and Dillon JJ. Survival, disease-free survival and adverse effects of conditioning for allogeneic bone marrow transplantation with busulfan/cyclophosphamide vs total body irradiation: a meta-analysis. *Bone Marrow Transplant.* **22** (1998) 439–443.

52. Clift RA, Buckner CD, Thomas ED, et al. Marrow transplantation for chronic myeloid leukemia: a randomized study comparing cyclophosphamide and total body irradiation with busulfan and cyclophosphamide. *Blood* **84** (1994) 2036–2043.

53. Stiff P, McKenzie R, Sosman J, et al. High-dose busulfan and cyclophosphamide with bone marrow rescue for refractory Hodgkin's disease: a tolerable and effective regimen in patients without prior nitrosourea exposure. *Blood* **76** (1990) 567a(Abstract).

54. Cunningham I, Marmaduke D, Copelan E, et al. Hyperbilirubinemia as a predictor of post-BMT mortality. *Blood* **78** (1991) 240a(Abstract).

55. Grochow L, Jones R, Brundett R, et al. Pharmacokinetics of busulfan: correlation with veno-occlusive in patients undergoing bone marrow transplantation. *Cancer Chemother. Pharmacol.* **25** (1989) 55–61.

56. Schuler US, Ehrsam M, Schneider A, et al. Pharmacokinetics of intravenous busulfan and evaluation of the bioavailability of the oral formulation in conditioning for haematopoietic stem cell transplantation. *Bone Marrow Transplant.* **22** (1998) 241–244.

57. Essell JH, Schroeder MT, Harman GS, et al. Ursodiol prophylaxis against hepatic complications of allogeneic bone marrow transplantation: a randomized, double-blind, placebo-controlled trial. *Ann. Intern. Med.* **128** (1998) 975–981.

58. Copelan E, Penza S, Pohlman B, et al. A novel Bu/Cy/VP-16 regimen in non-Hodgkin's lymphoma. *Blood* **92** (1998) S1:664a(Abstract).

59. Van Der Jagt RHC, Appelbaum F, et al. Busulfan and cyclophosphamide as a preparative regimen for bone marrow transplantation in patients with prior chest radiotherapy. *Bone Marrow Transplant.* **8** (1991) 211–215.

60. Copelan E, Penza S, Theil K, et al. Allogeneic marrow transplantation with BuCy$_2$ in patients with chronic myelogenous leukemia. *Blood* **92 S1** (1998) 285a(Abstract).

61. Sullivan K, Witherspoon R, Storb R, et al. Chronic graft versus host disease: pathogenesis, diagnosis, treatment and prognostic factors. In Baum SJ, Santos GW, and Takaku F (eds.), *Recent Advances and Future Directions in Bone Marrow Transplantation,* Experimental Hematology Today (1987) p. 150–157.

62. Bross D, Tutschka P, Farmer E, et al. Predictive factors for acute graft-versus-host disease in patients transplanted with HLA-identical bone marrow. *Blood* **63** (1984) 1265–1270.

63. Aucouturier P, Barra A, Intator L, et al. Long-lasting IgG subclass and antibacterial polysaccharide antibody deficiency after allogeneic bone marrow transplantation. *Blood* **70** (1987) 779–785.

64. Sheridan J, Tutschka P, Sedmak D, et al. Immunoglobulin G subclass deficiency and pneumocele infection after allogeneic bone marrow transplantation. *Blood* **75** (1990) 1583–1586.

65. Sklar C, Kim T, and Ramsay N. Thyroid function among long-term survivors of bone marrow transplantation. *Am. J. Med.* **73** (1982) 688–694.

66. Sanders J, Buckner C, Sullivan, et al. Growth and development in children after bone marrow transplantation. *Horm. Res.* **30** (1988) 92–97.

67. Manenti F, Galimberti M, Lucarelli G, et al. Growth and endocrine function after bone marrow transplantation for thalassemia. In Buckner C, Gale R, Lucarelli G (eds.), *Advances and Controversies in Thalassemia Therapy: Bone Marrow Transplantation and Other Approaches,* Liss, New York, (1989) pp. 273–280.

68. Sanders J, and the Long-Term Follow-Up Team. Endocrine problems in children after bone marrow transplant for hematologic malignancies. *Bone Marrow Transplant.* **8** (1991) 2–4.

69. Sanders J, and the Seattle Marrow Transplant Team. The impact of marrow transplant preparative regimens on subsequent growth and development. *Semin. Hematol.* **28** (1991) 244–249.

70. Adan L, de Lanversin M-L, Thalassinos C, et al. Growth after bone marrow transplantation in young children conditioned with chemotherapy alone. *Bone Marrow Transplant.* **19** (1997) 253–256.

71. Wingard J, Miller D, and Santos G. Testicular function after busulfan plus cyclophosphamide. *J. Cell Biochem.* **16A** (1992) 216–225.

72. Copelan EA and Deeg HJ. Conditioning for allogeneic marrow transplantation in patients with lympho-hematopoietic malignancies without the use of total body irradiation. *Blood* **80(7)** (1992) 1648–1658.

73. Witherspoon R, Fisher L, and Schoh G. Secondary cancers after bone marrow transplantation for leukemia or aplastic anemia. *N. Engl. J. Med.* **321** (1989) 784–789.

74. Bhatia S, Ramsay N, Steinbuch M, et al. Malignant neoplasms following bone marrow transplantation. *Blood* **87** (1996) 3633–3639.

75. Curtis R, Rowlings P, Deeg H, et al. Solid cancers after bone marrow transplantation. *N. Engl. J. Med.* **336** (1997) 897–904.

76. Copelan EA and McGuire EA. The biology and treatment of ALL in adults. *Blood* **85** (1995) 1151–1168.

77. Clift R, Buckner C, and Thomas E. The treatment of acute non-lymphoblastic leukemia by allogeneic marrow transplantation. *Bone Marrow Transplant.* **2** (1987) 243–258.

78. Report from the Working Party of Leukemia, European Group for Bone Marrow Transplantation. Allogeneic bone marrow transplantation for leukemia in Europe. *Lancet.* **18** (1988) 1379–1382.

79. McGlave P, Haake R, and Bostrom B. Allogeneic bone marrow transplantation for acute nonlymphocytic leukemia in first remission. *Blood* **72** (1988) 1512–1517.

80. Geller R, Saral R, Piantadosi S, et al. Allogeneic bone marrow transplantation after high-dose busulfan and cyclophosphamide in patients with acute nonlymphocytic leukemia. *Blood* **73** (1989) 2209–2218.

81. Blaise D, Maraninchi D, Archimbaud E, et al., for the Groupe d'Etude de la Greffe de Moelle Osseuse. Allogeneic bone marrow transplantation for acute myeloid leukemia in first remission: a randomized trial of busulfan-cytoxan versus cytoxan-total body irradiation as preparative regimen. A report from the Groupe d'Etude de la Greffe de Moelle Osseuse. *Blood* **79** (1992) 2578–2582.

82. Ringdén O, Labopin M, Tura S, et al., for the Acute Leukaemia Working Party of the European Group for Blood and Marrow Transplantation (EBMT). A comparison of busulfan versus total body irradiation combined with cyclophosphamide as conditioning for autograft or allograft bone marrow transplantation in patients with acute leukaemia. *Brit. J. Hematol.* **93** (1996) 637–645.

83. Gale RP, Horowitz MM, Weiner RS, et al. Impact of cytogenetic abnormalities on outcome of bone marrow transplants in acute myelogenous leukemia in first remission. *Bone Marrow Transplant.* **16** (1995) 203–208.

84. Ringdén O, Ruutu T, Remberger M, et al. A randomized trial comparing busulfan with total body irradiation as conditioning in allogeneic marrow transplant recipients with leukemia: a report from the Nordic Bone Marrow Transplant Group. *Blood* **83** (1994) 2723–2730.

85. Emanuel EJ and Patterson WB. Ethics of randomized clinical trials. *J. Clin. Oncol.* **16** (1998) 365–366.

86. Blume K, Kenneth J, Kopecky J, et al. A prospective randomized comparison of total body irradiation-etoposide versus busulfan-cyclophosphamide as preparatory regimens for bone marrow transplantation in patients with leukemia who were not in first remission: a Southwest Oncology Group Study. *Blood* **81** (1993) 2187–2193.

87. Copelan E, Biggs J, Avalos B, et al. Radiation-free preparation for allogeneic bone marrow transplantation in adults with acute lymphoblastic leukemia. *J. Clin. Oncol.* **10** (1992) 237–242.

88. von Bueltzingsloewen A, Esperou-Courdeau H, Souillet G, et al. Allogeneic bone marrow transplantation following busulfan-based conditioning regimen in young children with acute lymphoblastic leukemia: a cooperative study of the Societe Francaise de Greffe de Moelle. *Bone Marrow Transplant.* **16** (1995) 521–527.

89. Davis SM, Ramsay NKC, Klein JP, et al. Comparison of preparative regimens in transplants for children with acute lymphoblastic leukemia. *J. Clin. Oncol.* (1999) in press.

90. Copelan EA, Grever MR, Kapoor N, et al. Marrow transplantation following busulfan and cyclophosphamide for CML in accelerated or blastic phase. *Br. J. Haematol.* **71** (1989) 487–491.

91. Ratanatharathorn V, Karanes C, Uberti J, et al. Busulfan-based regimens and allogeneic bone marrow transplantation in patients with myelodysplastic syndromes. *Blood* **81** (1993) 2194–2199.

92. O'Donnell MR, Long GD, Parker PM, et al. Busulfan/cyclophosphamide as conditioning regimen for allogeneic bone marrow transplantation for myelodysplasia. *J. Clin. Oncol.* **13** (1995) 2973–2979.

93. Anderson JE, Appelbaum FR, Schoch G, et al. Allogeneic marrow transplantation for refractory anemia: a comparison of two preparative regimen and analysis of prognostic factors. *Blood* **87** (1996) 51–58.

94. Locatelli F, Niemeyer C, Angelucci E, et al., for the European Working Group on Myelodysplastic Syndrome in Childhood. Allogeneic bone marrow transplantation for chronic myelomonocytic leukemia in childhood: a report from the European Working Group on Myelodysplastic Syndrome in Childhood. *J. Clin. Oncol.* **15** (1997) 566–571.

95. Lucarelli G, Polchi P, Galimberti M, et al. Bone marrow transplantation in patients with thalessemia. *N. Engl. J. Med.* **322** (1990) 417–421.

96. Lucarelli G, Galimberti M, Polchi P, et al. Bone marrow transplantation in adult thalessemia. *Blood* **80** (1992) 1603–1607.

97. Lucarelli G, Clift RA, Galimberti M, et al. Marrow transplantation for patients with thalessemia: results in Class 3 patients. *Blood* **87** (1996) 2082–2088.

5

Is Total Body Irradiation Necessary in Bone Marrow Transplantation for Pediatric ALL?

Susan R. Wiersma, MD,
and Susan B. Shurin, MD

CONTENTS

1. INTRODUCTION

Allogenic bone marrow transplantation (allo-BMT) for nonmalignant disease requires ablation of the immune system to permit hematopoietic and lymphoid engraftment unless the donor is syngeneic or the recipient is profoundly immunoincompetent. When BMT is performed for malignant disease, treatment of the recipient to permit engraftment is also used to eliminate residual malignancy. The ultimate success of allo-BMT for leukemia clearly depends upon immunomodulation and graft vs tumor effect in addition to the direct antileukemic effect of the preparative regimen. Nonetheless, the importance of an effective preparative regimen is crucial. Optimal regimens remain a topic of uncertainty in transplantation for acute leukemia.

The first reported BMTs for acute leukemia in 1959 *(1)* were performed following preparative regimens of single-dose 850 cGy and 1140 cGy total body irradiation (TBI). This approach resulted in enough immunosuppression to allow engraftment of isologous marrow, and also produced complete, albeit temporary, remission of the leukemia. Several years later, Santos et al. *(2)* reported that the use of high-dose cyclophosphamide (Cy) as a preparative regimen permitted engraftment, but, again, failed to control leukemia for any significant period of time. Not until the early 1970s did reports begin

From: *Current Controversies in Bone Marrow Transplantation*
Edited by: B. Bolwell © Humana Press Inc., Totowa, NJ

to emerge of successful BMTs for acute leukemia, i.e., sustained engraftment and eradication of leukemia *(3)*. These favorable results reflected enhanced knowledge of many factors influencing allogeneic transplantation (allotransplantation), including histocompatibility and donor selection, antimicrobial therapy, transfusion support, and also the use of a better preparative regimen: Cy with TBI (Cy/TBI).

Numerous advances in the field of stem cell transplantation (SCT) have been made in the past quarter century. However, two major issues related to preparative regimens remain: adequacy of antileukemic activity, and acceptable acute and late toxicities. These two issues are of critical importance in the transplantation of children with acute lymphoblastic leukemia (ALL), because some of the toxicities of SCT are most pronounced in the pediatric population, and leukemic relapse still accounts for the majority of SCT failures. Based on the data currently available, what is the best preparative regimen for this group of patients? Should it include TBI?

2. RATIONALE FOR TBI

TBI serves two critical purposes in SCT for ALL: immunosuppression (in the allogeneic setting), and leukemic cell kill. TBI is attractive as a systemic treatment, because it is all-pervasive, eliminating the problem of sanctuary sites, and is cytotoxic by mechanisms of action different than chemotherapy (CT) agents. Doses may also be delivered with precise accuracy *(4)*.

Radiation at low doses is very toxic to normal lymphocytes. Both in vitro and in vivo, lymphocytes appear to have minimal capacity to repair radiation-induced DNA damage. When lymphocyte subsets have been analyzed separately, no differences in radiation sensitivity have been found *(5)*. Many studies have examined the effects of total dose, dose rate, and fractionation on engraftment of allogeneic marrow *(6)*. As expected, greater total dose, higher dose rate, and less fractionation produce increased cell kill. For example, a fractionated schedule of 1.25 cGy 3 ×/d, at 0.25 cGy/min, to a total dose of 7.5 cGy, had the same effect on the hematopoietic system as 7.5 cGy at 0.04 cGy/min in a single dose *(6)*. In non-T-cell-depleted transplants, all TBI regimens allow full engraftment of allogeneic stem cells. In the T-depleted setting, however, problems with sustained engraftment have occurred with lower doses of TBI *(7)*. Because of concerns about the higher potential for graft rejection in this setting, TBI has been routinely employed when using marrow from an unrelated or mismatched donor *(8)*. In general, the potent immunosuppressive properties of TBI make its use advantageous as preparation for transplants in which engraftment may be difficult.

The second goal of TBI in preparation for SCT is eradication of malignant cells, in this case, leukemic lymphoblasts. Historically, leukemias have been considered exquisitely radiation-sensitive, based on the known radiation sensitivity of normal lymphohematopoietic cells. In vitro evidence, however, suggests a broad spectrum of radiosensitivity of leukemic cell lines. This variation is observed between different ALL cell lines, as well as between different acute myeloid leukemia (AML) cell lines *(9)*. Although cell culture conditions do not always predict the in vivo experience, the significant rate of leukemic relapse post-SCT is certainly consistent with these data.

Uckun et al. *(10)* reported results from clonogenic assays of radiosensitivity of childhood ALL cells, and found substantial variation in the cells' ability to repair sublethal radiation damage. Leukemic progenitor cells from patients with high initial white blood cell counts (WBC >100,000 × 10⁹/L) or younger age (<5 yr) had superior ability to repair sublethal radiation damage. High initial WBC and young age are high-risk prognostic features in childhood ALL, both with respect to initial therapy, and also with risk of relapse post-SCT. Uckun et al. *(10)* also examined the effect of dose fractionation on leukemic cell kill. They compared the antileukemic efficacy of fractionated irradiation (2 × 2 cGy) to that of a single dose (1 × 4 cGy). In 71% of cases, a ≥20% increase in leukemic progenitor cell survival was seen with the fraction-ated schedule, compared to the single dose *(10)*. Several mechanisms have been postu-lated to explain the differences in the radiation survival curves with different fraction-ation schedules, any or all of which may be involved in the resistance of ALL cells to radiation *(9,10)*.

The in vitro data, combined with clinical experience, suggest significant variation in radiosensitivity between leukemias. Even for leukemias that are radiation-sensitive, variable doses and schedules of TBI could be needed for optimal cell kill of individual leukemic clones.

3. TOXICITIES OF TBI

In addition to the desirable properties of immunosuppression and leukemic cell kill, TBI also produces numerous deleterious side effects, both acute and late (Table 1). For children with ALL, these effects may be especially severe, as a consequence of both their young age and their prior therapy for ALL.

Acute toxicities of TBI include nausea, vomiting, diarrhea, mucositis, parotitis, alopecia, rash, hepatic enzyme elevation, and veno-occlusive disease (VOD) of the liver. Improved supportive care has resulted in significant amelioration of many of these effects.

The incidence of VOD in children with leukemia receiving a TBI-containing prepara-tive regimen varies between 1 and 27% *(6,11–14)* depending on the criteria used to diagnose VOD, the underlying disease, the amount and type of prior therapy, pre-existing liver disease, the chemotherapeutic agent(s) used in the preparative regimen, the source of allogeneic stem cells, and the dose and fractionation schedule of the TBI.

The late toxicities of TBI have been of utmost concern regarding its use in children. Although any organ may sustain damage from TBI, the major issues are its potentially irreversible effects on pulmonary, endocrine, and neurocognitive function, and the increased risk of second malignancy.

The pulmonary toxicity (both acute and late) of TBI has long ben recognized, serving as the impetus to alter the administration of TBI from its original single-dose schedule and rate. Fractionation, decreased dose rate, and lung-shielding are now commonly used in the delivery of TBI to adults and children. Numerous variables impact the development and extent of the pulmonary toxicity of TBI, including pre-SCT pulmonary function, infectious pneumonitis, graft-vs-host disease (GVHD), and use of certain CT agents (busulfan [Bu], carmustine [BCNU], and Cy). TBI is a major contributing factor to the pulmonary toxicity of SCT. Even with maximum precautions, approx 20% of children will develop chronic interstitial lung disease *(6,12–18)*.

Administration of cytotoxic therapy and TBI to young children is known to impact both growth and endocrine function *(6,19–24)*. The impact on growth plates in bones depends on the age of the child, the dose of irradiation, and whether the epiphyses are

Table 1

Toxicities Experienced by Patients Undergoing BMT for Leukemia

Ref.	Total no. pts	No. pts Bu/Cy	No. pts Cy/TBI	Disease indications	No. pts ALL	VOD (% of pts)		Cystitis (% of pts)		Pulmonary (% of pts)	
						Bu/Cy	Cy/TBI	Bu/Cy	Cy/TBI	Bu/Cy	Cy/TBI
Morgan et al. (36)	233	67	166	AML, ALL, CML	65	19	1.3[a]	30	14[a]	21	28
Ringden et al. (37) (EBMTR)	782	391	391	AML, ALL, CML	246	7.2	3.3[a]	6.6	2[a]	5.6	12.5[a]
Ringden et al. (46) (Nordic BMT)	167	88	79	AML, ALL, CML	38	12	1[a]	32	10[a]	24	5[a]

[a]Statistically significant ($p < .05$).

VOD = veno-occlusive disease; Cystitis = hemorrhagic cystitis; Pulmonary = pulmonary toxicity; Bu/Cy = busulfan and cyclophosphamide; Cy/TBI = cyclophosphamide and total body irradiation; EBMT = European Bone Marrow Transplantation Group; AML = acute myeloid leukemia; CML = chronic myelogenous leukemia; ALL = acute lymphoblastic leukemia.

open or closed. Most of these data derive from administration of higher doses of irradiation to more localized areas for treatment of solid tumors. The impact of irradiation on pituitary production of growth hormone has long been appreciated, from experience with treatment of brain tumors and prophylactic cranial irradiation for ALL. Thus, the evidence to support significant impact of irradiation on these organs is not limited to the transplant experience. Both alkylating agents and irradiation impact gonadal function. The sensitivity of gonads to irradiation-induced damage depends in part on whether a child is pre- or postpubertal, with perhaps greatest sensitivity during puberty. Infertility is virtually assured with administration of TBI, and is common with high-dose alkylator therapy as well. Endogenous production of sex hormones is variable, and may survive both high-dose CT and irradiation. However, failure of production of estrogen and androgen hormones is common with high-dose therapy, with or without irradiation. These are major issues for patients and families, and have a significant impact on both quality of life and development of other medical complications, such as osteoporosis. Endocrine organs are sensitive to damage by virtually all preparative regimens.

The neurocognitive effects of SCT, and specifically of TBI, are not well understood. It is clear that increasing radiation dose and younger age are associated with more significant deficits *(12,25)*. Long-term, detailed neuropsychometric testing on sufficient numbers of patients, treated at multiple institutions, is not available. When compared to a similar group of children who received standard-risk ALL therapy without cranial irradiation, patients who underwent BMT demonstrated lower verbal IQ scores *(25)*. Chronic illness, nutritional problems, high-dose corticosteroids, and the neuropsychologic impact of drugs, such as cyclosporin, are all likely to differentially affect the children receiving SCT. It was not possible to separately address the impact of TBI in this study. Irradiation-induced damage to the central nervous system (CNS) is known to be a significant problem for children with ALL and brain tumors. Despite the lack of prospective or quantitative data in SCT, the deleterious neurocognitive effects of TBI are of major concern in choice of preparative regimen for children with ALL *(12)*.

The risk of secondary malignancy following SCT is related to the original diagnosis, prior therapy, age of the patient, and the dose and fields of irradiation. Curtis et al. *(26)* reported that the risk of development of a solid tumor following BMT, for children under 10 yr of age at the time of BMT, was 36.6× higher than expected. The risk was 4.6 for those aged 10–29 yr at the time of BMT. Identifying the unique contribution of TBI to the increased risk of malignancy in these children will first require reliable data regarding the risk of second malignancy in children with ALL who receive standard therapy. The risk has been reported as low as 0.5% *(27)*, and as high as 4.8% *(28)*. This issue is currently being addressed with national long-term follow-up studies of children who survive ALL, with attention to the multiple factors that may influence the development of malignancy in these patients.

4. RATIONALE FOR BU IN PLACE OF TBI

The substitution of Bu for TBI in the preparative regimen for SCT was initially investigated in patients whose prior therapy precluded the use of TBI *(29)*. Although various combinations of CTs have been employed in preparation for SCT, the greatest experience has been with regimens combining Bu with Cy (Bu/Cy). "Bu/Cy$_2$" refers to 16 mg/kg Bu with 120 mg/kg Cy, and "Bu/Cy$_4$" refers to 16 mg/kg Bu and 200 mg/kg Cy. Both Bu/Cy$_2$ and Bu/Cy$_4$ provide enough immunosuppression to allow engraftment of non-T-depleted marrow, including matched unrelated donors *(30,31)*. Even in the non-T-depleted setting, however, mixed chimerism frequently results when TBI is omitted from the preparative regimen. Ramirez et al. *(32)* reported results of chimerism studies in children undergoing SCT for ALL. Complete donor engraftment was detected only in patients who received TBI; mixed chimerism occurred predominantly in patients receiving only CT, and in some patients who received TBI.

Interpretation of both efficacy and toxicity of Bu is complicated by the fact that the pharmacology of Bu has only recently been employed to optimize its use. The suggestion that dosing needed to be individualized arose from two observations: the rate of relapse in younger patients prepared with Bu-containing regimens appears to be higher than the rate of relapse in older patients transplanted for chronic myelogenous leukemia (CML); and heavily pretreated patients have a significantly higher rate of development of VOD than do less heavily pretreated patients *(33)*. These observations have led to several studies that identified considerable variability in the pharmacokinetics of Bu. Pharmacologically guided dosing has been in use at a few institutions in the United States and Europe, but only recently has this approach been used to adjust and control the area-under-the-curve (AUC) for individual patients at multiple institutions *(34)*. New formulations, including liposomal oral and intravenous preparations of Bu, may significantly impact rational dosing of this drug *(35)*. The changing use of Bu makes its comparison to TBI as part of a preparative regimen difficult, because optimal use may affect both toxicity and efficacy of the drug.

5. TOXICITIES OF BU/CY

Acute toxicities of Bu/Cy include nausea, mucositis, alopecia, seizures, VOD, and hemorrhagic cystitis (Table 1). The incidence of hemorrhagic cystitis following Bu/Cy is generally reported to be at least double the incidence following Cy/TBI, when the two regimens have been compared *(36,37)*. Likewise, VOD is significantly more common and more severe in patients who receive Bu/Cy, compared to those who receive Cy/TBI *(36–38)*.

Many of the late complications of TBI are also encountered with Bu/Cy, including pulmonary and endocrine dysfunction, and increased risk of secondary malignancy.

Earlier studies reported a higher incidence of interstitial pneumonitis in patients who received Cy/TBI, compared to those who received Bu/Cy, and it was more often associated with cytomegalovirus *(36,37)*. However, the case mortality rate from pulmonary complications is higher in patients following Bu/Cy, as reported in two recent studies *(38,39)*. This is a reflection of the incidence and severity of obstructive bronchiolitis, a later complication with limited therapeutic options. Ringden et al. *(39)* found a statistically significant difference in their randomized study, with a 24% incidence of pulmonary toxicity in the Bu/Cy group, compared to 5% in the Cy/TBI patients. Davies et al. *(38)* reviewed the International Bone Marrow Transplantation Register (IBMTR) data for 627 pediatric ALL patients, and found that deaths from pulmonary toxicity were higher in the Bu/Cy group than in the Cy/TBI patients. Although this was not a prospective randomized trial, it addresses an issue raised by BMT studies that include adult patients: their risk factors for pulmonary toxicity (e.g., prior busulfan therapy for CML and smoking history) are higher than for children, and, therefore, historically it

Table 2
Outcome: Percentage of ALL Patients Experiencing each Outcome

| | Preparative Regimen Used in BMT | | | | | |
| | TRM | | Relapse | | EFS | |
Ref.	Bu/Cy	Cy/TBI	Bu/Cy	Cy/TBI	Bu/Cy	Cy/TBI
Ringden et al. (37) (EBMT)	20.3	21.8	30.0	28	55	57
Ringden et al. (46) (Nordic BMT)	34	14[a]	29	29	51	62
Davies et al. (38) (IBMTR)	18.8	5.5[a]	29	24	47	61[a]

[a]Statistically significant ($p < .05$).

TRM = treatment-related mortality; EFS = event-free survival; Bu/Cy = busulfan and cyclophosphamide; Cy/TBI = cyclophosphamide and total body irradiation.

was postulated that pulmonary toxicity might be expected to be of lesser concern in pediatric patients.

No increased risk of thyroid abnormality has been described following Bu/Cy, but growth abnormalities and gonadal dysfunction are encountered. Although not as well-studied, the degree of abnormality is less following Bu/Cy than following TBI (19–24).

The risk of development of a secondary solid malignancy is related to the dose of radiation, so that recipients of Bu/Cy should be spared (26). However, a significant risk of development of secondary myelodysplasia and/or leukemia is associated with the administration of high-dose alkylating agents, including Bu. No published information is available about this risk in children receiving Bu/Cy for SCT for ALL.

A major theoretical advantage of Bu/Cy is avoidance of the neurocognitive effects of TBI, which is greatest in younger children and infants, and in those who have previously received cranial irradiation (25).

6. RESULTS OF CLINICAL TRIALS

The critical question is whether leukemia-free survival (LFS) is significantly better following Cy/TBI, compared to Bu/Cy. A prospective, randomized trial of Bu/Cy vs Cy/TBI in children with ALL has not been published, so the information must be extrapolated from meta-analysis of the results of trials to data, bearing in mind that many reports are from single-institution studies with limited numbers of patients and multiple variables. Data reported include patients with AML and CML, as well as ALL. Toxicity data for all diagnoses are abstracted in Table 1, and the survival data for ALL in Table 2.

Studies through the 1980s generally used a preparative regimen of 120 mg/kg Cy, followed by fractionated TBI for children transplanted for ALL. This resulted in a 3-yr LFS of approx 40%, depending on remission status, prior therapy, age, and other known risk factors in ALL. In 1987, Borchstein et al. (40) reported a 5-yr event-free survival (EFS) of 64% for children who received TBI prior to the Cy.

Gordon et al. (11) reported the results of their experience using high-dose cytosine arabinoside (ara-C) followed by fractionated TBI. They initially published their data in 1988, and Coccia et al. (41) updated the results in 1997. Twenty-seven children with ALL in second complete remission (CR2) were prepared with this regimen prior to allo-BMT. Twenty-three patients received marrow from a matched sibling, two from 5- of 6-antigen-matched sibling or parent, and one from a matched unrelated donor. Fifteen of these children are alive without leukemia 21–160 mo post-BMT, for 5- and 10-yr EFS rates of 59 ± 9% and 51 ± 11%, respectively. Only two patients had relapse of leukemia. The other deaths were related to toxicities: four GVHD, two infection, two interstitial pneumonitis, and one each from multiorgan failure and a second malignancy. Six patients were transplanted in third CR, two of whom are alive and leukemia-free at 24 and 162 mo posttransplant.

Deconinck et al. (42) reported results for matched sibling donor BMT for adult and pediatric patients with high-risk ALL in first remission, using a preparative regimen of TBI (some single-dose, others fractionated), ara-C, and melphalan. The relapse rate was low (31%); however, the toxicities were severe, with 38% of patients experiencing nonleukemia deaths.

Moussalem et al. (43) analyzed 42 pediatric patients who received an allo-BMT in second remission of ALL. Thirty-eight children received marrow from a matched sibling; two from a matched unrelated donor; one, a haploidentical graft from his father; and one, a syngeneic transplant. Ten patients were prepared with Cy (120 mg/kg) and TBI (10 Gy single dose). The relapse rate was 40%, and the EFS was 50%. Eleven patients received Cy, TBI, etoposide (30 mg/kg), and ara-C (1 g/m^2). The relapse rate was 9%, and EFS was 45%. Twenty patients received TBI (12 Gy in six fractions, or 10 Gy single fraction), ara-C (24 g/m^2), and melphalan (140 mg/m^2). No relapses occurred in this group, with EFS of 65% at a median follow-up of 34 mo. They found no difference in transplant-related toxicity between any of the regimens.

Von Bueltzingsloven (44) reported an experience with non-TBI preparative regimens for young children with high-risk or relapsed ALL. Twenty-one children under 4 yr of age received a Bu-based regimen with Cy or melphalan, with or without ara-C, followed by a matched-sibling BMT. Sixteen patients were in CR1, four in CR2, and one in relapse at the time of BMT. Retrospective analysis at a median follow-up time of 47 mo showed a 4-yr disease-free survival of 61.1%, with relapse accounting for all failures. No transplant-related mortality (TRM) occurred. Toxicities included two patients with growth retardation, both of whom had previously received cranial radiation therapy; two patients had thyroid dysfunction; and one patient had impaired hair regrowth. No neuropsychologic assessments were performed.

The Italian Association of Pediatric Hematology-Oncology BMT Study Group experience was reported by Favre et al. (45). From 1983 to 1996, 416 children with ALL were transplanted, 294 of whom received a TBI-containing preparative regimen, and 122 of whom received Bu/Cy. Kaplan-Meier estimates of EFS for various subgroups of patients were calculated. For patients who received an allo-BMT in CR1 (50 patients), EFS was 63.4 ± 9% for the TBI group, and 58.3 ± 14.2% for the CT group (p = .51). For 144 patients in ≥CR2 who received an allo-BMT, EFS was 51.6 ± 5% for the TBI group, and 34.8 ± 9.9% for the CT group (p = .12). One hundred fifty-seven patients received an autologous BMT (ABMT) for acute leukemia in ≥CR2. Overall, their EFS was 44.4 ± 5.6% for the TBI group, and 7.5 ± 4.0% for the CT group (p = .0003). For patients with ALL, the relapse rate was 31.6% for the allo-TBI group, 50% for the allo-CT group, 44% for the auto-TBI group, and 76.2% for the auto-CT group. Combining the results of the allo-BMT and ABMTs for children with ALL and AML (700 patients), there was no difference in 100-d mortality, TRM, VOD, or interstitial pneumonitis between the TBI group and the CT group. Second malignancy developed in two patients in the CT group, and one in the TBI group.

Ringden et al. *(46)* reported a randomized study conducted by the Nordic Bone Marrow Transplantation Group, comparing Bu/Cy to Cy/TBI for patients (adult and pediatric) with leukemia. This data was initially published in 1994, and updated in 1999 *(39)*. For 38 patients with ALL, the 7-yr EFS was 28% for the Bu/Cy group and 45% for the Cy/TBI group ($p = .36$). The patients who received Bu/Cy had significantly more VOD, hemorrhagic cystitis, and acute GVHD than those who received TBI. Relapse rates were not reported for the subgroup of patients with ALL; however, for the group as a whole (ALL, AML, CML), relapse rates were similar in the Bu/Cy and Cy/TBI groups.

Ringden et al. *(37)* retrospectively analyzed the European Cooperative Group for Blood and Marrow Transplantation, to examine the outcome of patients transplanted for acute leukemia using Bu/Cy vs those who received Cy/TBI. Patients were matched for type of transplant, diagnosis, remission status, age, and GVHD prophylaxis. For recipients of matched-sibling allotransplants, there was no significant difference in any of the subgroups in TRM, relapse rate, and LFS between the Bu/Cy and the Cy/TBI patients. There was, however, a significantly higher rate of VOD and hemorrhagic cystitis in the Bu/Cy group, compared to the Cy/TBI group.

A comprehensive analysis of the IBMTR data regarding the issue of preparative regimens for children with ALL has recently been performed by Davies et al. *(38)*. Although not a prospective randomized trial, this analysis provides the best information to date, comparing the toxicities and outcome of Bu/Cy and Cy/TBI in children undergoing allotransplant for ALL. The IBMTR includes data from 144 centers, with a median follow-up of 37 mo, actuarial 3 yr, on 627 children who received a matched sibling transplant between 1988 and 1995. 451 patients received Cy/TBI and 176 received Bu/Cy. No significant difference was found between the Cy/TBI and Bu/Cy groups with regard to any of the following factors: gender, performance status, immunophenotype, reported presence of chromosomal abnormalities, WBC at diagnosis, CNS involvement at diagnosis, time interval from diagnosis to first CR, remission status pretransplant, length of first CR, or interval from most recent CR or relapse to transplant or year of transplant. The Bu/Cy group had a higher proportion of children ≤5 yr old, and the Cy/TBI group had more children with prior CNS radiation therapy and more children with T-cell-depleted transplants. Overall survival and LFS were 55 ± 5% and 50 ± 5%, respectively, in the Cy/TBI group, and 40 ± 8% and 35 ± 7% in the Bu/Cy group ($p < .01$). The use of Bu/Cy was associated with a significantly higher risk of TRM overall mortality and treatment failure. Although relapse accounted for the majority of deaths in both groups, there were relatively more deaths from infection, interstitial pneumonitis, and VOD in the Bu/Cy group, and more multiorgan system failure in the Cy/TBI group.

7. CONCLUSION

Allo-BMT from a matched-sibling donor offers the best chance for LFS for many pediatric patients with relapsed ALL *(47)*. Leukemic relapse following BMT is responsible for the majority of BMT failures, regardless of the preparative regimen used for BMT. Non-TBI-containing preparative regimens, predominantly Bu/Cy, have been used in an effort to avoid the toxicity associated with TBI. Ironically, analysis of multiple studies shows that TRM is higher with Bu/Cy, compared to Cy/TBI. This difference results in a statistically significant inferior LFS in patients treated with Bu/Cy. These patients received a standard dose of Bu (16 mg/kg), and were not, in general, dosed according to Bu pharmacokinetics (AUC), as is the more recent practice. This raises additional concern, however, as the adjusted dose of Bu is usually higher than 16 mg/kg in children, and higher dosing may result in even greater toxicity.

Search for better preparative regimens should continue, because Cy/TBI and Bu/Cy both result in significant toxicity and less-than-optimal leukemia control. In the meantime, present data support the use of Cy/TBI over Bu/Cy in pediatric patients being transplanted for relapsed ALL.

REFERENCES

1. Thomas ED, Lochte HL Jr, Cannon JH, Sahler OD, and Ferrebee JW. Supralethal whole body irradiation and isologous marrow transplantation in man, *J. Clin. Invest.*, **38** (1959) 1709–1716.
2. Santos GW, Sensenbrenner LL, Burke PJ, et al. Marrow transplantation in man following cyclophosphamide, *Transplant. Proc.*, **3** (1971) 400–404.
3. Buckner CD, Clift RA, Fefer A, et al. Marrow transplantation for the treatment of acute leukemia using HLA-identical siblings, *Transplant. Proc.*, **6** (1974) 365–366.
4. Gilson D and Taylor RE. Total body irradiation: report on a meeting organized by the BIR oncology committee, *Br. J. Radiol.*, **70** (1997) 1201–1203.
5. Dutreix J, Girinski T, Cosset JM, et al. Blood cell kinetics and total body irradiation, *Radiother. Oncol.*, **9** (1987) 119–129.
6. Shank B. Radiotherapeutic principles of bone marrow transplantation. In Forman SJ, Blume KJ, Thomas ED (eds.), *Bone Marrow Transplantation*, Blackwell, Boston, (1995), pp. 96–113.
7. Burnett AK, Robertson AG, Hann IM, et al. In vitro T-depletion of allogeneic bone marrow: prevention of rejection in HLA-matched transplants by increased TBI, *Bone Marrow Transplant.*, **1(Suppl 1)** (1986) 121.
8. Casper J, Camitta B, Truitt R, et al. Unrelated bone marrow donor transplants for children with leukemia or myelodysplasia, *Blood*, **85** (1995) 2354–2363.
9. Wheldon TE. Radiobiological basis of total body irradiation, *Int. J. Radiat. Oncol. Biol. Phys.*, **70** (1997) 1204–1207.
10. Uckun FM, Chandan-Langlie M, Jaszcz W, et al. Radiation damage repair capacity of primary clonogenic blasts in acute lymphoblastic leukemia, *Cancer Res.*, **53** (1993) 1431–1436.
11. Gordon BG, Warkentin PL, Strandjord SE, et al. Allogeneic bone marrow transplantation for children with acute leukemia: long-term follow-up of patients prepared with high-dose cytosine arabinoside and fractionated total body irradiation, *Bone Marrow Transplant.*, **20** (1997) 5–10.
12. Chou RH, Wong GB, Kramer JH, et al. Toxicities of total body irradiation for pediatric bone marrow transplantation, *Int. J. Radiat. Oncol. Biol. Phys.*, **34** (1996) 843–851.
13. Deeg HJ. Acute and delayed toxicities of total body irradiation, *Int. J. Radiat. Oncol. Biol. Phys.*, **9** (1983) 1933–1939.
14. Demierer T, Petersen FB, Appelbaum FR, et al. Allogeneic marrow transplantation following cyclophosphamide and escalating doses of hyperfractionated total body irradiation in patients with advanced lymphoid malignancies: a phase I/II trial, *Int. J. Radiat. Oncol. Biol. Phys.*, **32** (1995) 1103–1109.
15. Belkacemi Y, Pene F, Touboul E, et al. Total body irradiation before bone marrow transplantation for acute leukemia in first or second complete remission, *Strahlenther Onkol.* **174** (1998) 92–104.
16. Gore EM, Lawton CA, Ash RC, et al. Pulmonary function changes in long-term survivors of bone marrow transplantation, *Int. J. Radiat. Oncol. Biol. Phys.*, **36** (1996) 67–75.
17. Bradley J, Rett C, Goldman S, et al. High energy total body irradiation as preparation for bone marrow transplantation in leukemia patients: treatment technique and related complications, *J. Pediatr.*, **40** (1998) 391–396.
18. Nysom K, Holm K, Hesse B, et al. Lung function after allogeneic bone marrow transplantation for leukemia or lymphoma, *J. Pediatr.*, **74** (1996) 432–436.
19. Huma Z, Boulad F, Black P, et al. Growth in children after bone marrow transplantation for acute leukemia, *Blood*, **86** (1995) 819–824.

20. Sanders JE, et al. Endocrine problems in children after bone marrow transplant for hematologic malignancies, *Bone Marrow Transplant.*, **8** (1991) 2–4.
21. Holm K, Nysom K, Rasmussen MH, et al. Growth, growth hormone and final height after BMT. Possible recovery of irradiation-induced growth hormone insufficiency, *Bone Marrow Transplant.*, **18** (1996) 163–170.
22. Clement-DeBoers A, Oostdijk W, Van Weel-Sipman MH, et al. Final height and hormonal function after bone marrow transplantation in children, *J. Pediatr.*, **129** (1996) 544–550.
23. Alter CA, Thornton PS, Willi SM, et al. Growth in children after bone marrow transplantation for acute myelogenous leukemia as compared to acute lymphocytic leukemia, *J. Ped. Endocrinol. Metabol.*, **9** (1996) 51–57.
24. Sarafoglov K, Bouvlad F, Gillio A, et al. Gonadal function after bone marrow transplantation for acute leukemia during childhood, *J. Pediatr.*, **130** (1997) 210–216.
25. Cool VA. Long-term neuropsychological risks in pediatric bone marrow transplant: what do we know? *Bone Marrow Transplant.*, **18** (1996) 545–549.
26. Curtis RE, Rawlings PA, Deeg HJ, et al. Solid cancers after bone marrow transplantation, *N. Engl. J. Med.*, **336** (1997) 897–904.
27. Neglia JP, Meadows AT, Robison LL, et al. Second neoplasms after acute lymphoblastic leukemia in childhood, *N. Engl. J. Med.*, **325** (1991) 1330–1336.
28. Kubuta M, Akiyama Y, Koishi S, et al. Second malignancy following treatment of acute lymphoblastic leukemia in children, *Int. J. Hematol.*, **57** (1998) 397–401.
29. Santos GW, Tutschka PJ, Brookmeyer R, et al. Marrow transplantation for acute nonlymphocytic leukemia after treatment with busulfan and cyclophosphamide, *N. Engl. J. Med.*, **309** (1983) 1347–1352.
30. Klein J, Avalos B, Belt P, et al. Bone marrow engraftment following unrelated donor transplantation utilizing busulfan and cyclophosphamide preparatory chemotherapy, *Bone Marrow Transplant.*, **17** (1997) 479–483.
31. Ratanatharathorn V, Uberti JP, Sensenbrenner LL, et al. Preparative regimens without total body irradiation in the recipients of unrelated donor marrow, *Blood*, (1994) 342a.
32. Ramirez M, Diaz MA, Garcia-Sanchez F, et al. Chimerism after allogeneic hematopoietic cell transplantation in childhood acute lymphoblastic leukemia, *Bone Marrow Transplant.*, **18** (1996) 1161–1165.
33. Slattery JD and Risler JL. Therapeutic monitoring of busulfan in hematopoietic stem cell transplantation, *Therapeut. Drug Monitor*, **20** (1998) 543–549.
34. Vassal G, Koscielny S, Challine D, et al. Busulfan disposition and hepatic veno-occlusive disease in children undergoing bone marrow transplantation, *Cancer Chemother. Pharmacol.*, **37** (1996) 247–253.
35. Schuler US, Ehrsam M, Schneider A, et al. Pharmacokinetics of intravenous busulfan and evaluation of the bioavailability of the oral formulation in conditioning for haematopoietic stem cell transplantation, *Bone Marrow Transplant.*, **20** (1998) 241–244.
36. Morgan M, Dodds A, Atkinson K, et al. The toxicity of busulfan and cyclophosphamide as the preparative regimen for bone marrow transplantation, *Br. J. Hematol.*, **77** (1991) 529–534.
37. Ringden O, Labopin M, Tura S, et al. A comparison of busulfan versus total body irradiation combined with cyclopshosphamide as conditioning for autograft or allograft bone marrow transplantation in patients with acute leukemia, *Br. J. Hematol.*, **93** (1996) 637–645.
38. Davies SM, Ramsay NK, Klein JP, et al. Comparison of preparative regimens in transplants for children with acute lymphoblastic leukemia, submitted for publication.
39. Ringden O, Remberger M, Ruutu T, et al. Increased risk of chronic graft-versus-host disease, obstructive bronchiolitis, and alopecia with busulfan versus total body irradiation: long-term results of a randomized trial in allogenic marrow recipients with leukemia, *Blood*, **93** (1999) 2196–2201.
40. Brochstein J, Keman N, Groshen S, et al. Allogeneic bone marrow transplantation after hyperfractionated total body irradiation and cychophosphamide in children with acute leukemia, *N. Engl. J. Med.*, **217** (1977) 1618–1624.
41. Coccia P, Strandjord S, Warkentin P, et al. High-dose cytosine arabinoside and fractionated total body irradiation: an improved preparative regimen for bone marrow transplantation of children with acute lymphoblastic leukemia in remission, *Blood*, **71** (1988) 888–893.
42. Deconinck E, Cahn JY, Milpied N, et al. Allogeneic bone marrow transplantation for high-risk acute lymphoblastic leukemia in first remission: long-term results for 42 patients conditioned with an intensified regimen (TBI, high-dose Ara-C and melphalan), *Bone Marrow Transplant.*, **20** (1997) 731–735.

43. Moussalem M, Esperov Bovrdeau H, Devergie A, et al. Allogeneic bone marrow transplantation for childhood acute lymphoblastic leukemia in second remission: factors predictive of survival relapse and graft versus host disease, *Bone Marrow Transplant.*, **15** (1995) 943–947.

44. Von Bueltzingloeuen A, Esperov-Bourdeau H, Souillet G, et al. Allogeneic bone marrow transplantation following a busulfan-based conditioning regimen in young children with acute lymphoblastic leukemia: a cooperative study of the societe Francaise de Greffede Moelle, *Bone Marrow Transplant.*, **16** (1995) 521–527.

45. Favre C, Nardi M, Dini G, et al. The role of total body irradiation (TBI). The Italian Association of Pediatric Hematology (AIEOP) BMT Study Group, *Bone Marrow Transplant.*, **18(Suppl 2)** (1996) 71–74.

46. Ringden O, Ruutu T, Remberger M, et al. A randomized trial comparing busulfan with total body irradiation as conditioning in allogeneic marrow transplant recipients with leukemia: a report from the Nordic Bone Marrow Transplantation Group, *Blood*, **83** (1994) 2723–2730.

47. Feig SA, Harris RE, and Sather HN. Bone marrow transplantation versus chemotherapy for maintenance of second remission of childhood acute lymphoblastic leukemia: a study of the Children's Cancer Group (CCG-1884), *Med. Pediatr. Oncol.*, **29** (1997) 534–540.

II TRANSPLANTATION FOR HEMATOLOGIC MALIGNANCIES

6

Stem Cell Transplantation for Chronic Myeloid Leukemia

Indications and Timing

Michael R. Bishop, MD

CONTENTS

1. BACKGROUND AND NATURAL HISTORY

Chronic myeloid leukemia (CML) is a hematopoietic stem cell disorder that accounts for approx 20% of all cases of leukemia *(1)*. The death rate attributed to CML is 1.5/100,000/yr *(2)*. CML is characterized by a specific chromosomal abnormality referred to as the Philadelphia chromosome (Ph[1]) *(3,4)*. The Ph[1] results from the reciprocal translocation of the c-*abl* proto-oncogene on the long arm of chromosome 9 (q34.1) to the 5.8 kb breakpoint cluster region (bcr) on the long arm of chromosome 22 (q11.21). The resulting *bcr-abl* oncogene produces an 8.5-kb messenger ribonuclease (mRNA), which encodes for a 210-kDa fusion protein (p210) *(5)*. Depending on whether c-*abl* is between exon 2 or exon 3 of bcr, two different mRNAs may be formed: b2/a2 or b3/a2 *(6)*. The two different mRNAs encode for an identical fusion protein, p210 *(7)*, which has increased tyrosine kinase activity, compared to the normal c-abl protein *(8)*. Cells transfected with *bcr-abl* cDNA have a demonstrated growth advantage over normal hematopoietic cells *(9)*, which may be very important to the development and maintenance of CML.

From: *Current Controversies in Bone Marrow Transplantation*
Edited by: B. Bolwell © Humana Press Inc., Totowa, NJ

CML has been described in terms of phases. The overwhelming percentage of patients present clinically in an indolent or chronic phase, characterized by a significantly elevated white blood count, with varying degrees of myeloid maturation seen on the peripheral smear. Patients are often asymptomatic, but, when patients do experience symptoms, they are often mild; common symptoms include fatigue, headache, low-grade temperatures, nocturnal sweats, and early satiety. The average duration of the chronic phase is 4–5 yr *(10)*. The chronic phase is followed by a gradual progression into an accelerated phase. Exact definitions for the accelerated phase are controversial, but they include an increased number of immature myeloid precursors, basophilia and eosinophilia, both thrombocytosis and thrombocytopenia, and the development of new cytogenetic abnormalities *(11)*. The most consistent feature of the accelerated phase is probably the decreased ability to control the disease with conventional agents. The median duration of the accelerated phase is 12–18 mo, and this is followed by a progression into the blast or acute phase. The blast phase is defined as the evolution of CML into an acute leukemia, defined as greater than 30% blasts in the marrow. Approximately one-third of patients in the blast phase develop acute lymphocytic leukemia (ALL) and the other two-thirds develop acute myeloid leukemia (AML). The median duration of the blast phase is less than 12 mo. The median survival for patients who present with CML in the chronic phase is approx 5–6 yr.

2. TREATMENT

There are a number of treatment options available for CML. They include myelosuppressive agents, biologic response modifiers, allogeneic stem cell transplantation (allo-SCT), and autologous stem cell transplantation (ASCT). The only known curative treatment for CML is allo-SCT, which has a 5-yr disease-free survival (DFS) approaching 50%, when performed in chronic phase, using stem cells from an human leukocyte antigen (HLA)-matched sibling donor *(12)*. However, because of age restrictions and limited donor availability, even when using unrelated bone marrow donors from international registries, this form of treatment is an option for less than 35% of CML patients *(13)*. As such, when considering treatment options for patients with CML, the primary focus are age and donor availability.

2.1. Conventional Therapy

The most common treatments for CML include myelosuppressive agents (e.g., busulfan and hydroxyurea) and biologic response modifiers (e.g., interferon-α [IFN-α]). IFN-α suppresses growth and differentiation of CML, as well as normal myeloid progenitors, in vitro *(14)*. There have now been several randomized trials *(14–19)* that have demonstrated a survival advantage of IFN-α over hydroxyurea and busulfan in the treatment of CML. In a prospective trial by the Italian Cooperative Group on Chronic Myeloid Leukemia *(15)*, 322 patients were randomized to receive hydroxyurea or IFN-α. Hematologic and cytogenetic responses (CytoR) were superior in the IFN-α arm. However, permanent discontinuation of IFN-α was required in 10% of patients, and an additional 21% required transient discontinuation of IFN-α because of side effects. Median survival with IFN-α treatment was 60–65 mo. This survival advantage was observed only in patients who achieve a significant CytoR, which occurred in approx 25% of all cases (16). The survival of patients who did not achieve a significant CytoR with IFN-α was similar to patients randomized to receive hydroxyurea. Similar results were observed in the German CML Study (17), in which patients were randomized to receive either IFN-α or hydroxyurea or busulfan. However, in this trial, patients who achieved a CytoR with IFN-α did not have a significant survival advantage over patients who did not achieve a CytoR. More recently, the French Cooperative Group (19) has demonstrated that the combination of IFN with cytarabine is superior to IFN alone, relative to both the percentage of patients achieving a CytoR and survival.

2.2. Allogeneic Stem Cell Transplantation

Allo-SCT is the only known curative therapy for patients with CML. For patients with a HLA-identical sibling, who are under the age of 50 yr, allo-SCT is considered the treatment of choice (12,20). There has been increasing evidence that allo-SCT should be performed as early in the disease process as possible (21–23). Retrospective analyses have demonstrated superior DFS and overall survival rates for patients transplanted within 12–24 mo of diagnosis (22). These superior results have been attributed to such factors as younger age, and decreasing treatment-related mortality (TRM) (in particular, graft-vs-host disease [GVHD]), and because the disease has not the opportunity to naturally progress, and the patient has not been exposed to potentially toxic agents, such as busulfan or IFN-α. The latter factor is relatively controversial. A retrospective analysis by the International Bone Marrow Transplant Registry (IBMTR) failed to demonstrate any effect of prior IFN-α exposure on survival following allo-SCT (24). When CML patients under the age of 50 yr are transplanted with HLA-matched siblings, within 1 yr of diagnosis, the 3-yr DFS is in excess of 70% (25). The DFS is approx 50–60% for all patients transplanted in chronic phase, and declines to 35–40% and 10–15% for patients in accelerated and blast phases, respectively. These decreased rates primarily result from increased relapse rates, which are as high as 75% for patients transplanted in blast phase.

Unfortunately, only a minority of patients have a fully HLA-matched sibling. A family member mismatched at a single HLA locus may be successfully used as a donor, with results similar to those obtained with a fully matched family member (26). Still, this increases donor availability for only 5–10% of patients (27). For CML patients who lack a suitable HLA-matched related donor, there are alternative sources of allogeneic stems cells, including HLA-matched unrelated donors, partially matched related donors (PMRD), and placental-derived (umbilical cord) blood cells.

There are sufficient data to demonstrate that allogeneic bone marrow transplantation (allo-BMT) from an unrelated donor can be beneficial, relative to survival (28–33). Potential donors may be identified through international marrow registries, such as the National Marrow Donor Program (NMDP). More than 2 million donors were listed in the NMDP, and over 7000 BMTs have been performed using unrelated donors provided by the NMDP. With the current number of donors currently listed in the registry, over 70% of patients are able to have a potential HLA-A, -B, -DR phenotypic match identified for them at their initial search (34). However, because of the reduction in suitable donors after molecular matching and age restrictions, donor availability is still limited to less than 35% of eligible patients. Patients with CML are relatively fortunate, compared to patients with acute leukemia, because the median duration of the chronic phase is 4 yr, permitting adequate time to identify a potential donor: The average time to identify an unrelated donor is approx 3 mo.

An analysis of the first 462 patients to receive unrelated transplants facilitated by the NMDP demonstrated DFS rates at 2 yr to be approx 40% in low-risk patients, which included patients with CML in chronic phase, and 20% in high-risk patients, which included CML patients in accelerated and blast phases (30). The Chronic Leukemia Working Party of the European Group for Blood and Marrow Transplantation (EBMT) retrospectively analyzed the impact of prognostic factors on the outcome of serologically HLA-matched unrelated transplants for CML, in a cohort of 366 patients transplanted in Europe (35). The overall survival was 37% at 2 yr, and leukemia-free survival was 31%. In univariate analysis, transplantation in first chronic phase, short time interval from diagnosis to transplant, GVHD prophylaxis without T-cell depletion (TCD), acute GVHD, and HLA-DRβ1 D/R matching all had favorable statistical significance. Multivariate analysis confirmed that HLA-DRβ1 matching was the most significant factor influencing survival and TRM.

There have recently been two important analyses supporting the use of unrelated transplants earlier in the course of CML. Results from the Fred Hutchinson Cancer Research Center (33) suggest outcomes similar to related donors when the donors are well matched, the recipients are young, and the recipient is transplanted relatively close to their original diagnosis. A retrospective analysis performed through the IBMTR (32) indicates that unrelated transplants provide a survival advantage over conventional chemotherapy including patients receiving IFN.

Another alternative source of allogeneic stem cells, for CML patients who lack a fully matched related allogeneic donor, are cells from PMRDs (36–39), who, potentially, can be identified for greater than 90% of eligible patients (27). The time to identify a potential PMRD is relatively much shorter than the time required to identify and secure an unrelated donor. This shorter time to identify a donor may be particularly advantageous for patients at high risk of disease progression, such as patients with CML in accelerated phases or blast crisis. However, because of major HLA disparity, the use of a PMRD is associated with an increased risk of graft failure, severe acute and chronic GVHD, and delayed immune reconstitution (37–39).

Transplantations from PMRD in patients with advanced CML have been complicated by a relatively high incidence of graft failure, but they have resulted in sustained long-term survival (37). The largest series on PMRD transplantations, which included 72 patients, was reported by the University of South Carolina (38). The engraftment rate for this patient group was 88%, and the incidence of grade II or higher acute GVHD was 16%. The overall incidence of chronic GVHD was 35%. At a median follow-up of 24 mo, the 2-yr probability of survival was 35%.

Following the discovery that placental blood was rich in hematopoietic progenitor and stem cells, a large research interest developed to use this waste product of normal deliveries for allo-SCT (40). Since the first successful placental blood transplant, there has been increasing evidence that transplantation using placental blood can result in prolonged survival in patients with advanced hematologic diseases and malignancies (41–44). Placental blood registries have been established in the United States and Europe. In addition to the advantage of being a readily available stem cell source, particularly for minorities, placental blood has the potential additional benefit of decreased GVHD, because the T-cells in cord blood are relatively immature (45).

Data on 65 patients who received unrelated placental blood transplants were reported by the Eurocord Transplant Group and the EBMT. Engraftment, defined by neutrophil recovery, was observed in 87% of patients, but platelet recovery was significantly delayed (44). The incidence of acute GVHD was approx 40%, and, among the 23 patients who survived beyond 100 d, none were observed to develop chronic GVHD. The overall survival was 29% at a median follow-up of 10 mo.

The difficulty with these results is that they were primarily performed in children, and there is relatively little information on adults in general, and CML in particular (46,47). Weight and age seem to play a significant role relative to survival following placental blood transplantation. In the report by the Eurocord Group (44) only 16% of patients over the age of 15 yr (*n* = 20) were alive at 1 yr after transplantation. There appears to be a correlation between cell dose with hematopoietic recovery, and possibly survival. The Duke Placental Blood Transplant Program reported their results (47) for patients weighing over 40 kg (*n* = 9), including several adults. At the time of this report, five patients were alive, with durable engraftment 4–18 mo following cord blood transplantation.

Outcomes of BMTs performed using different stem cell sources were retrospectively analyzed by the IBMTR (31). The analysis included a total of 2055 patients with chronic CML, AML, and ALL, who received allo-BMTs between 1985 and 1991, from HLA-identical siblings, haploidentical HLA-mismatched relatives, and HLA-matched and mismatched unrelated donors. Donors were HLA-identical siblings (*n* = 1224), haploidentical relatives mismatched for one or two HLA-A, -B, or -DR antigens (*n* = 340), or unrelated donors who were HLA-matched (*n* = 383) or mismatched for one HLA-A, -B, or -DR antigen (*n* = 108). TRM was significantly higher after alternative donor transplants than after HLA-identical sibling transplants. Among patients with low-risk disease, which included CML patients in chronic phase, the 3-yr TRM was 21% after HLA-identical sibling transplants, and greater than 50% after all types of alternative donor transplants studied. For patients with more advanced leukemia, differences in TRM were less striking.

2.3. Autologous Stem Cell Transplantation

Despite numerous sources of stem cells, allo-SCT is a viable option for less than 50% of patients with CML. An alternative in this situation is ASCT. The use of auto-SCT following high-dose chemotherapy (CT) for CML has been limited, compared to other hematologic malignancies (48,49). The first transplantation of autologous peripheral blood stem cells (PBSCs) to a patient with CML was performed in the 1970s (50). Reiffers et al. (51) treated 47 patients with CML in transformation to accelerated and blast phases with high-dose therapy and PBSCs collected in chronic phase. Forty-three patients were restored to the chronic phase for periods of 2–43 mo after transplantation: 48% of evaluable patients achieved a significant CytoR. These encouraging results led investigators to perform ASCT during chronic phase, which resulted in a complete or partial CytoR in approx 60% of patients (52,53).

Both bone marrow and peripheral blood have been used as source of autologous stem cells, but they share the problem of potential contamination with cells expressing *bcr-abl*. Attempts to eradicate residual leukemic cells in the autograft have included incubation with IFN-γ, long-term culture of CML marrow, and ex vivo treatment with 4-hydroperoxycyclophosphamide or oligonucleotides (52,54–56). The most effective method to obtain large numbers of Ph^1-negative progenitors is by collection by apheresis during early hematopoietic recovery following myelosuppressive CT. Cytotoxic CT and hematopoietic cytokines have been used for the mobilization of stem cells and progenitors for ASCT in early chronic-phase CML. Patients mobilized in this manner have normal hematopoietic cells predominantly in the early recovery phase from myelosuppressive therapy. In some situations, the autografts are Ph^1-negative by both cytogenetic analysis and polymerase chain reaction, and contain sufficient numbers of progenitors for transplantation. Carella et al. *(57)* treated 15 patients with CML in chronic phase, with a CT regimen consisting of idarubicin, arabinosylcytosine, and etoposide. The majority of these patients had either primary or secondary resistance to IFN-α. PBSCs were collected from these patients during hematopoietic recovery following combination CT. Collection of adequate numbers of progenitor cells was more difficult in patients who had received prior treatment with IFN-α. In nine of 15 cases, the expression of Ph^1-positive metaphases in the peripheral blood was completely negative, and, in an additional four patients, a reduction of Ph^1-positive metaphases, to less than 35%, was observed. Eight of these patients have subsequently received high-dose therapy and PBSC transplantation. Seven of eight engrafted, and five were alive and Ph^1-negative at 2, 3, 6, 10, and 18 mo after transplantation.

ASCT, although promising, is still under clinical investigation, and is still considered investigational throughout the medical and transplantation community *(58–60)*. However, to date, there has not been any clear evidence that these results are superior to conventional therapy, especially in patients who have had a major CytoR to IFN *(15,59–62)*. The patients who appear to benefit the most from this procedure have been transplanted early (x < 2 yr) after their initial diagnosis *(57,59)*. ASCT appears to be less beneficial in patients with advanced disease *(59)*. Most of the trials addressing the role of ASCT in AML are in phase II and III. This question is actually being addressed in an international cooperative group trial between the Medical Research Council in the United Kingdom and the Eastern Cooperative Oncology Group in the United States, in which patients who lack an HLA-matched sibling are randomized between IFN-α and an ASCT.

3. SPECIAL CLINICAL SITUATIONS IN CML

3.1. Age

The median age at diagnosis of CML of approx 55 yr limits the application of allo-SCT to approx 50% of patients, even if they had a suitable donor *(61)*. Allo-SCT with related donors has been extended to patients up to the age of 60 yr, if the potential candidate has an adequate performance status and normal major organ function, with relatively good results *(21,63)*. Still, there is an increased chance of TRM primarily in the form of GVHD. Age restrictions have been even more stringent for patients utilizing an unrelated donor, because morbidity and mortality rises even higher with age in this patient group. In an attempt to reduce TRM, new nonmyeloablative preparative regimens have been developed *(64)*. These so-called "mini-transplants" may have limited applicability in CML, because they appear to require the achievement of a minimal residual disease state, in order to benefit from the graft-vs-leukemia effect associated with allo-SCT. These regimens do not appear sufficiently cytotoxic to reduce the leukemic load seen in patients with CML. Prior treatment with cytotoxic agents may be required, in order to achieve a minimal residual disease state for this treatment strategy to be effective *(65)*.

The other alternative for older patients is use of ASCT, which has been applied up to age 70 yr. As described in Subheading 2.3., this treatment is limited by the ability to obtain an adequate (i.e., Ph^1-negative) autograft, which is best obtained early in the disease course, prior to IFN exposure *(57,59)*. One practical approach is to mobilize, collect, and store autologous cells at diagnosis, in older patients and patients who lack a suitable allogeneic donor. Patients could then be started on IFN-α, and, if they failed to achieve a significant CytoR, they could be taken to ASCT. This strategy is now being addressed in randomized trials.

3.2. IFN Vs Unrelated BMT

There is still a significant degree of controversy for patients who are potentially eligible for an unrelated BMT relative to timing and use of IFN-α *(32,61)*. Proponents of initial IFN-α use argue that it is documented to extend life, that unrelated transplants are associated with significant morbidity and mortality, especially for older patients, and that, if one fails to respond to IFN-α, the patient could still proceed to an unrelated transplant. Proponents of early unrelated transplant argue that, similar to results with related allo-SCT, the earlier a patient proceeds to transplant, the better the results, and that long-term administration of IFN is also associated with significant morbidity *(66)*. This issue was addressed in a retrospective analysis using the database of the IBMTR *(32)*. This analysis was modeled on a 35-yr-old patient with an intermediate prognosis *(67)*. The analysis demonstrated an increased early mortality for patients who went to transplant early. However, based upon observations that over 50% of patients will fail to achieve a CytoR to IFN-α, it was estimated that 2 yr of life would be lost by these patients by not proceeding directly to transplant *(68)*. Analyses were also performed for 25- and 45-yr-old patients, and also demonstrated a longer predicted life expectancy for patients who went to transplant early. These results are further supported by similar data from the Fred Hutchinson Cancer Research Center *(33)*. It appears reasonable to offer patients under the age of 40 yr the option of an unrelated transplant as initial therapy. For patients over the age of 40 yr, the risks of transplant need to be carefully considered relative to the benefits and potential side effects of initial treatment with IFN-α.

3.3. Advanced Disease

The prognosis for CML patients with advanced disease, either accelerated or blast phases, is poor; the average life expectancy is less than 6 mo, once patients progress into the blast phase *(69)*. Following allo-SCT, long-term survival rates of 35–40% and 10–15% can be expected for patients in accelerated and blast phases, respectively *(25,70,71)*. Allo-SCT may be successfully performed for patients in accelerated phase. There is usually an adequate amount of time to identify an unrelated donor. However, this is not necessarily the case for patients with blast phase. Attempts may be made to induce a remission in patients in the blast phase with conventional agents used to treat acute leukemias, but the chances of obtaining a remission or a second complete chronic phase are less than 50%. In addition, the duration of the remissions tend to be relatively short *(72)*. ASCT is not an option for these patients, unless they are able to achieve a complete remission, because relapse rates are extremely high *(59)*.

3.4. T-Cell Depletion

It has been well documented that TCD of allografts from related donors results in increased relapse rates for patients transplanted for CML. However, this has not been the case for patients receiving a TCD allograft from an unrelated donor *(74)*. With the introduction of donor leukocyte infusions (DLI), there is continued interest among investigators favoring TCD *(75)*. These investigators, wishing to reduce the incidence and risks of GVHD, are willing to accept the risks of higher relapse rates, knowing that they can potentially salvage a significant number of patients with a DLI *(76)*.

4. SUMMARY

There are now a number of treatment options for patients with CML. Allo-SCT has become a viable option for an increasing number of patients, because of the increased sources of allogeneic stem cells from unrelated bone marrow donors, PMRD, and stored placental blood collections. However, all these transplants are not without significant complications, which may be chronic and debilitating, if not fatal. The clinical results of allo-SCT from alternative donors are favorable for younger patients with good prognostic features. Timing of the transplant early in the course of the disease, before malignant clones become resistant to therapy, and while the patient remains in good clinical condition, is a critical variable for transplant success. Further investigation is necessary to determine the appropriate role of ASCT for CML, especially in relation to treatment with IFN-α. However, the results are encouraging enough to move forward with phase III trials, and it provides a viable treatment option for older patients and patients who fail IFN-α.

REFERENCES

1. Fialkow PJ, Jacobson RJ, and Papayannopoulou T. Chronic myelocytic leukemia: clonal origin in a stem cell common to the granulocyte, erythrocyte, platelet, and macrophage, *Am. J. Med.*, **63** (1977) 125–130.
2. Gunz FW. The epidemiology and genetics of chronic leukemias, *Clin. Haematol.*, **6** (1977) 3–20.
3. Rowley JD. A new consistent abnormality in chronic myelogenous leukemia identified by quinicrine fluorescence and Giemsa staining, *Nature*, **243** (1973) 290.
4. Nowell PC and Hungerford DA. A minute chromosome in human chronic granulocytic leukemia, *Science*, **132** (1960) 1497.
5. Davis RL, Konopka JB, and Witte ON. Activation of the c-abl oncogene by viral transduction or chromosomal translocation generates altered c-abl proteins with similar in vitro kinase properties, *Mol. Cell Biol.*, **5** (1985) 204–213.
6. Schaefer-Rego K, Dudek H, Popenoe D, et al. CML patients in blast crisis have breakpoints localized to a specific region of the BCR, *Blood*, **70** (1987) 448–455.
7. Mills KI, MacKenzie ED, and Birnie GD. The site of breakpoint within the bcr is a prognostic factor in Philadelphia-positive CML patients, *Blood*, **72** (1988) 1237–1241.
8. Konopka JP and Witte ON. Detection of c-abl tyrosine kinase activity in vitro permits direct comparison of normal and altered abl gene products, *Mol. Cell Biol.*, **5** (1985) 3116.
9. Cannistra SA. Chronic myelogenous leukemia as a model for the genetic basis of cancer, *Hematol. Oncol. Clin. North Am.*, **4** (1990) 337–357.
10. Wareham NJ, Johnson SA, and Goldman JM. Relationship of the duration of the chronic phase in chronic granulocytic leukemia to the need of treatment during the first year after diagnosis, *Cancer Chemother. Pharmacol.*, **8** (1982) 205–210.
11. Kantarjian HM, Dixon D, Keating MJ, et al. Characteristics of accelerated disease in chronic myelogenous leukemia, *Cancer*, **61** (1988) 1441–1446.

12. Thomas ED, Clift RA, Fefer A, et al. Marrow transplantation for the treatment of chronic myelogenous leukemia, *Ann. Intern. Med.*, **104** (1986) 155–163.

13. Beatty PG and Anasetti C. Marrow transplantation from donors other than HLA identical siblings, *Hem. Oncol. Clin. N. Am.*, **4** (1990) 677–686.

14. Talpaz M, Chernajovsky Y, Troutman-Worden K, et al. Interferon-stimulated genes in interferon-sensitive and -resistant chronic myelogenous leukemia patients, *Cancer Res.*, **52** (1992) 1087–1090.

15. Tura S, Baccarani M, Zuffa E, for the Italian Cooperative Study Group on Chronic Myeloid Leukemia. Interferon alfa-2a as compared to conventional chemotherapy for the treatment of chronic myeloid leukemia. *N. Engl. J. Med.*, **330** (1994) 820–825.

16. Rosti G, DeVivo A, Zuffa A, Baccarani M. Interferon-alpha in the treatment of chronic myeloid leukemia. A summary and an update of the Italian studies. *Bone Marrow Transplant.*, **17**(suppl.) (1996), 511–513.

17. Hehlmann R, Heimpel H, Hasford J, et al. Randomized comparison of interferon-a with busulfan and hydroxyurea in chronic myelogenous leukemia, *Blood*, **84** (1994) 4064–4077.

18. Allan N, Richards S, Shepard P, et al. UK-Medical Research Council randomized, multicenter trial of interferon-α n 1 for chronic myeloid leukemia: improved survival irrespective of cytogenetic response, *Lancet*, **345** (1995) 1392–1397.

19. Guilhot F, Chastang C, Michallet M, et al. Interferon alfa-2b combined with cytarabine versus interferon alone in chronic myelogenous leukemia, *N. Engl. J. Med.*, **337** (1997) 223–229.

20. Armitage JO. Bone marrow transplantation, *N. Engl. J. Med.*, **330** (1994) 827–838.

21. Clift RA, Appelbaum FR, and Thomas ED. Treatment of chronic myeloid leukemia by marrow transplantation, *Blood*, **82** (1993) 1954–1956.

22. Goldman JM, Szydio R, Horowitz MM, et al. Choice of pre-transplant treatment and timing of transplants for chronic myelogenous leukemia, *Blood*, **82** (1993) 2235–2238.

23. Bacigalupo A, Gualaandi F, Van Lint MT, et al. Multivariate analysis of risk factors for survival and relapse in chronic granulocytic leukemia following allogeneic marrow transplantation: impact of disease related variables (Sokal score), *Bone Marrow Transplant.*, **12** (1993) 443–448.

24. Giralt S, Szydlo R, Goldman JM, et al. Effect of prior interferon therapy on the outcome of HLA-identical sibling bone marrow transplantation for chronic myelogenous leukemia: an analysis from the International Bone Marrow Transplant Registry, *Blood*, (1999) in press.

25. Rizzo JD. New summary slides show current trends in BMT, *ABMTR Newsletter*, **5** (1998) 4–12.

26. Anasetti C, Amos D, Beatty PG, et al. Effect of HLA compatibility on engraftment of bone marrow transplants in patients with leukemia or lymphoma, *N. Engl. J. Med.*, **320** (1989) 197–204.

27. Henslee-Downey PJ. Mismatched bone marrow transplantation, *Curr. Opin. Oncol.*, **7** (1995) 115–121.

28. Hows JM, Yin JL, Marsh J, et al. Histocompatible unrelated donors compared with HLA nonidentical family donors in marrow transplantation for aplastic anemia and leukemia, *Blood*, **68** (1986) 1322–1328.

29. McGlave P, Bartsch G, Anasetti C, et al. Unrelated donor marrow transplantation for chronic myelogenous leukemia: initial experience of the National Marrow Donor Program, *Blood*, **81** (1993) 543–550.

30. Kernan NA, Bartsch G, Ash RC, et al. Analysis of 462 transplantations from unrelated donors facilitated by the National Marrow Donor Program, *N. Engl. J. Med.*, **328** (1993) 593–602.

31. Szydlo R, Goldman JM, Klein JP, et al. Results of allogeneic bone marrow transplants for leukemia using donors other than HLA-identical siblings, *J. Clin. Oncol.*, **15** (1997) 1767–1777.

32. Lee SJ, Kuntz KM, Horowitz MM, et al. Unrelated donor bone marrow transplantation for chronic myelogenous leukemia: a decision analysis, *Ann. Intern. Med.*, **127** (1997) 1080–1088.

33. Hansen JA, Gooley TA, Martin PJ, et al. Bone marrow transplants from unrelated donors for patients with chronic myeloid leukemia, *N. Engl. J. Med.*, **338** (1998) 962–968.

34. Beatty PG, Dahlberg S, Mickelson EM, et al. Probability of finding HLA-matched unrelated marrow donors, *Transplantation*, **45** (1988) 714–718.

35. Devergie A, Apperley JF, Labopin M, et al. European results of matched unrelated donor bone marrow transplantation for chronic myeloid leukemia. Impact of HLA class II matching. Chronic Leukemia Working Party of the European Group for Blood and Marrow Transplantation, *Bone Marrow Transplant.*, **20** (1997) 11–19.

36. Beatty PG, Clift RA, Mickelson EM, et al. Marrow transplantation from related donors other than HLA-identical siblings, *N. Engl. J. Med.*, **313** (1985) 765–771.

37. Bishop MR, Henslee-Downey PJ, Anderson JR, et al. Long-term survival in advanced chronic myelogenous leukemia following bone marrow transplantation from haplo-identical donors, *Bone Marrow Transplant.*, **18** (1996) 747–753.

38. Henslee-Downey P, Abhyankar SH, Parrish RS, et al. Use of partially related donors extends access to allogeneic marrow transplant, *Blood*, **89** (1997) 3864–3872.

39. Aversa F, Tabilio A, Velardi A, et al. Treatment of high-risk acute leukemia with T-cell-depleted stem cells from related donors with one fully mismatched HLA haplotype, *N. Engl. J. Med.*, **339** (1998) 1186–1193.

40. Broxmeyer HE, Douglas GW, Hangoc G, et al. Human umbilical cord blood as a potential source of transplantable hematopoietic stem/progenitor cells, *Proc. Natl. Acad. Sci. USA.*, **86** (1989) 3828.

41. Gluckman E, Broxmeyer HE, Auerbach AD, et al. Hematopoietic reconstitution in a patient with Fanconi's anemia by means of umbilical-cord blood from a HLA-identical sibling, *N. Engl. J. Med.*, **321** (1989) 1174–1178.

42. Wagner JE, Kernan NA, Steinbuch M, et al. Allogeneic sibling umbilical-cord-blood transplantation in children with malignant and non-malignant disease, *Lancet*, **346** (1995) 214–219.

43. Kurtzberg J, Laughlin M, Graham ML, et al. Placental blood as a source of hematopoietic stem cells for transplantation into unrelated recipients, *N. Engl. J. Med.*, **335** (1996) 157–166.

44. Gluckman E, Rocha V, Boyer-Chammard A, et al. Outcome of cord-blood transplantation from related and unrelated donors, *N. Engl. J. Med.*, **337** (1997) 373–381.

45. Harris DT, Schumacher MJ, Locascio J, et al. Phenotypic and functional immaturity of human umbilical cord blood T lymphocytes, *Proc. Natl. Acad. Sci. USA*, **89** (1992) 10,006–10,010.

46. Laporte JP, Gorin NC, Rubinstein P, et al. Cord-blood transplantation from an unrelated donor in an adult with chronic myelogenous leukemia, *N. Engl. J. Med.*, **335** (1996) 167–170.

47. Laughlin MJ, Smith CA, Martin P, et al. Hematopoietic engraftment using placental cord blood unrelated donor transplantation in recipients > 40 kg, *Blood*, **88(Suppl 1)** (1996) 266a.

48. Cheson BD, Lacerna L, Leyland-Jones B, et al. Autologous bone marrow transplantation, *Ann. Intern. Med.*, **110** (1989) 51–65.

49. Butturini A, Keating A, Goldman J, and Gale RP. Autotransplants in chronic myelogenous leukemia: strategies and results, *Lancet*, **335** (1990) 1255–1258.

50. McCarthy DM and Goldman JM. Transfusion of circulating stem cells, *CRC Crit. Rev. Clin. Lab. Sci.*, **20** (1984) 1–24.

51. Reiffers J, Trouette R, Marit G et al. Autologous blood stem cell transplantation for chronic myelogenous leukemia in transformation: a report of 47 cases, *Br. J. Haematol.*, **77** (1991) 339–345.

52. Barnett MJ, Eaves CJ, Phillips GL, et al. Successful autografting in chronic myeloid leukemia after maintenance chemotherapy in culture, *Bone Marrow Transplant.*, **4** (1989) 345–351.

53. DeFabritiis P, Meloni G, Alimena G, et al. High-dose chemotherapy and autologous stem cell reinfusion for patients chronic myelogenous leukemia in chronic phase, *Bone Marrow Transplant.*, **4(Suppl 2)** (1989) 62.

54. McGlave PB, Arthur D, Miller WJ, Lasky L, and Kersey J. Autologous transplantation for CML using marrow treated ex vivo with recombinant human interferon gamma, *Bone Marrow Transplant.*, **6** (1990) 115–120.

55. Carlo-Stella C, Mangoni L, Piovani O, et al. Chronic myelogenous leukemia: in vitro marrow purging with mafosfamide and recombinant granulocyte-macrophage colony-stimulating factor. In Dicke KA, Armitage JO, Dicke-Evinger MJ (eds.), *Autologous Bone Marrow Transplantation: Proceedings of the Fifth International Symposium*, Omaha, NB, 1991, pp. 241.

56. Gewirtz AM. Bone marrow purging with antisense oligodeoxynucleotides. *Prog Clin. Biol. Res.*, **377** (1992), 215–224.

57. Carella AM, Podesta M, Frassoni F, et al. Collection of "normal" blood repopulating cells during early hemopoietic recovery after intensive conventional chemotherapy in chronic myelogenous leukemia, *Bone Marrow Transplant.*, **12** (1993) 267–271.

58. Kantarjian HM, O'Brien S, Anderlini P, and Talpaz M. Treatment of chronic myelogenous leukemia: current status and investigational options, *Blood*, **87** (1995) 3069.

59. McGlave PB, De Fabritis P, Deisseroth A, et al. Autologous transplants for chronic myelogenous leukemia: results from eight transplant groups, *Lancet*, **343** (1994) 1486.

60. Carella AM, Frassoni F, Melo J, et al. New insights in biology and current therapeutic options for patients with chronic myelogenous leukemia, *Haematologica*, **82** (1997) 478.

61. Kantarjian HM, O'Brien S, Anderlini P, and Talpaz M. Treatment of chronic myelogenous leukemia: current status and investigational options, *Blood*, **87** (1995) 3069–3081.

62. Sacchi K, Kantarjian HM, Smith TL, et al. Early treatment decisions with interferon-alfa therapy in early chronic-phase chronic myelogenous leukemia, *J. Clin. Oncol.*, **16** (1998) 882–889.

63. Soiffer RJ, Fairclough D, Robertson M, et al. CD6-depleted allogeneic bone marrow transplantation for acute leukemia in first complete remission, *Blood*, **89** (1997) 3039–3047.

64. Giralt S, Estey E, Albitar M, et al. Engraftment of allogeneic hematopoietic progenitor cells with purine analog-containing chemotherapy: harnessing graft-versus-leukemia without myeloablative therapy, *Blood*, **89** (1997) 4531–4536.

65. Cunningham I, Gee T, Dowling M, et al. Results of treatment of Ph′ chronic myelogenous leukemia with an intensive treatment regimen (L-5 protocol), *Blood*, **53** (1979) 375–395.

66. Talpaz M, Kantarjian HM, Kurzrock R, and Gutterman J. Therapy of chronic myelogenous leukemia: chemotherapy and interferons, *Semin. Hematol.*, **25** (1988) 62–73.

67. Sokal JE, Baccarani M, Tura S, et al. Prognostic discrimination among younger patients with chronic granulocytic leukemia: relevance to bone marrow transplantation, *Blood*, **66** (1985) 1352–1357.

68. Kantarjian H, Smith TL, O'Brien S, et al. Prolonged survival in chronic leukemia after cytogenetic response to interferon-α therapy. The Leukemia Service, *Ann. Intern. Med.*, **122** (1995) 254–261.

69. Kantarjian HM, Deisseroth A, Kurzrock R, Estrov Z, and Talpaz M. Chronic myelogenous leukemia: a concise update, *Blood*, **82** (1993) 691–703.

70. McGlave PB, Arthur DC, Kim TH, Ramsay NKC, Hurd DD, and Kersey J. Successful allogeneic bone marrow transplantation for patients in the accelerated phase of chronic myelogenous leukemia, *Lancet*, **ii** (1982) 625–627.

71. Clift RA, Buckner CD, Thomas ED, et al. Marrow transplantation for patients in the accelerated phase of chronic myelogenous leukemia, *Blood*, **84** (1994) 4368–4373.

72. Kantarjian HM, Talpaz M, LeMaistre CF, et al. Diploid hematopoiesis in patients with advanced phases of chronic myelogenous leukemia following high-dose cyclophosphamide, etoposide, and BCNU (CBV) chemotherapy and autologous bone marrow transplantation, *Cancer*, **68** (1991) 1201–1207.

73. Ash RC, Horowitz MM, Gale RP, et al. Bone marrow transplantation from related donors other than HLA-identical siblings: effect of T cell depletion, *Bone Marrow Transplant.*, **7** (1991) 443–452.

74. Hessner MJ, Endean DJ, Casper JT, et al. Use of unrelated marrow grafts compensates for reduced graft-versus-leukemia reactivity after T-cell-depleted allogeneic marrow transplantation for chronic myelogenous leukemia, *Blood*, **86** (1995) 3987–3996.

75. Collins RH Jr, Shpilberg O, Drobyski WR, et al. Donor leukocyte infusions in 140 patients with relapsed malignancy after allogeneic bone marrow transplantation, *J. Clin. Oncol.*, **15** (1997) 433–444.

76. Alyea EP, Soiffer RJ, Canning C, et al. Toxicity and efficacy of defined doses of CD4+ donor lymphocytes for treatment or relapse after allogeneic bone marrow transplant, *Blood*, **91** (1998) 3671–3680.

7

Should All Adult Patients with Acute Lymphoblastic Leukemia in First Remission Undergo Allogeneic Bone Marrow Transplantation?

Sam L. Penza, MD, and
Edward A. Copelan, MD

CONTENTS

1. INTRODUCTION

Rapid clonal proliferation and accumulation of immature lymphocytes characterize acute lymphoblastic leukemia (ALL). Substantial progress in the cure rate achieved with chemotherapy (CT) has occurred in children with ALL, but results in adults remain poor *(1)*. Significant progress in understanding the biology and heterogeneity of this disease has not yet led to significant improvement in outcome *(2)*. This chapter critically reviews present treatment results in ALL, and presents a rationale for an aggressive treatment strategy.

2. CLASSIFICATION AND PROGNOSTIC FEATURES OF ALL

The French–American–British classification of ALL, based on blast morphology, is useful only in the identification of patients with L_3 morphology. This subtype, which accounts for approx 5% of patients, is characterized by a mature B-cell phenotype and translocation (8;14) *(3)*.

Immunophenotypic analysis demonstrates the heterogeneity of ALL; the lymphoblasts are descended from a single transformed progenitor B- or T-cell arrested at a specific level of maturation. Approximately 75% of adults have ALL of B-cell lineage,

From: *Current Controversies in Bone Marrow Transplantation*
Edited by: B. Bolwell © Humana Press Inc., Totowa, NJ

for which three levels of maturation are generally recognized: early pre-B-ALL; pre-B-ALL; and (mature) B-cell ALL. B-lineage ALL is human leukocyte antigen (HLA) DR-positive, with at least one B-cell antigen (CD19, -20, -22) present. Pre-B-ALL is generally common ALL antigen (CALLA) (CD10)-positive; early pre-B-ALL is CD10-negative. Early pre-B-cells lack cytoplasmic and surface immunoglobulin (Ig) expression; pre-B-ALL has cytoplasmic Ig only. B-cell-ALL has surface Ig, and occasionally cytoplasmic Ig *(1)*. Early pre-B-cell is the most common immunophenotype in children, but is less frequent in adults *(4–6)*.

CD7 is the most commonly expressed T-cell antigen in T-cell ALL, distinguishing it from B-cell or myeloid malignancy. The characterization of T-cell ALL is also based on the level of maturation. Seven percent of adult ALL cases are precursor T-cell ALL. Mature T-cell ALL makes up 16% of adult cases of ALL *(1,7–9)*. Myeloid antigens, most commonly CD13 or CD33, are detected in approx 20% of adult cases of ALL. Previous studies have indicated that myeloid expression (CD13,33) on the ALL blasts had some prognostic influence *(1)*, but recent studies have suggested this may not be prognostically significant *(10)*.

Cytogenetic analysis is the most important prognostic test in ALL *(11,12)*. Cytogenetic analysis detects clonal chromosomal aberrations in 50–70% of patients *(11–14)*. Substantially higher percentages can be detected using better methods for marrow cell collection *(15)*. Chromosomal translocations, which create aberrant expression of a normal gene product or the formation of a hybrid gene, are the best-studied chromosomal abnormality in ALL. Hybrid genes are transcribed into abnormal mRNAs, which are translated into abnormal proteins. Often, these are transcription factors associated with leukemogenesis *(16,17)*.

The Philadelphia chromosome (Ph^{1c}) t(9;22) is the most common translocation in ALL, and is present in more than 30% of adults *(2,18)*. Transcription products may be of different molecular sizes (210 or 190 kDa). Patients may be BCR-ABL-positive by molecular techniques, without demonstration of the Ph^{1c}. Patients with ALL should undergo polymerase chain reaction for BCR-ABL transcripts. The second most common translocation, t(4;11) (q21;q23), is seen in approx 5% of adults with ALL *(19–21)*. This translocation is associated with hyperleukocytosis. The third most common translocation in ALL is t(1;19)(q23:q13), found in pre-B-ALL *(22)*. Specific cytogenetic abnormalities are commonly associated with specific immunophenotypes.

The Ph^{1c} is associated with a dismal prognosis. Adults with a t(9;22) have a complete remission (CR) rate of 60%, with a median duration of remission of 5–10 mo. The survival rate at 3 yr is consistently less than 20% *(23,24)*. Translocations (4;11) and (1;19) are also associated with poor prognoses.

Most studies of the clinical significance of karyotypic abnormality in ALL have been performed in children. These studies have led to risk-adapted therapy, in which treatment is tailored according to subclassification of ALL. Attempts to identify subsets and tailor treatment in adults have been less successful, because of a substantially poorer database and the consistently poor outcome in most studies, regardless of treatment strategy. Some studies in adults have indicated that hyperdyploidy, in the absence of unfavorable structural changes, is a significant indicator of higher potential for cure *(2,12,25)*. Regrettably, routine cytogenetic studies are often not performed, or are inadequate. Many laboratories identify cytogenetic abnormalities in ALL at a much lower frequency than would be expected. Further, cytogenetic analysis underestimates the frequency of BCR-ABL *(12,26,27)*, TCR gene rearrangements involving TAL1 *(28,29)*, t(12;21) *(30,31)*, deletions and mutations of the *p16* gene of chromosome 9 *(32,33)*, and, probably, numerous other genetic rearrangements. In summary, a significant proportion of genetic alterations are unrecognized.

Age has a profound impact on duration of remission and survival *(1,34–36)*. In childhood ALL, CR rate approaches 95%. In adults more than 50 yr old, CRs are approx 40–60% *(37)*, and cure rates are less than 20% *(1)*. Increasing age is a negative prognostic variable, in part, because of disease biology, e.g., an increase in poor prognostic cytogenetics (e.g., Ph⁺). In addition, children tolerate aggressive treatment better than adults, because of a lower incidence of delays caused by marrow toxicity, and because of a lower incidence of extramedullary organ injury.

Numerous other factors influence prognosis. A white blood cell (WBC) count in excess of 30,000/μL is associated with a poor prognosis in B-lineage ALL, but not T-lineage ALL *(3)*. Patients who attain CR in less than 4 wk experience sustained disease free survival at twice the frequency of those who require longer durations to achieve remission *(3)*. Central nervous system (CNS) involvement predicts for a poor prognosis.

3. INDUCTION THERAPY

Induction therapy regimens have been established in children and used in adult ALL. Induction with vincristine, prednisone, asparaginase, and an anthracycline results in CR in more than 70% of adults *(1,3)*. Attempts to further intensify induction treatment in adults have been limited by severe toxicity. CR following induction therapy indicates reduction of the number of leukemic cells to less than that detectable by conventional methods. Molecular techniques commonly detect more than 10^8 residual leukemic cells in the bone marrow of patients in CR. The goal of therapy, once remission is achieved, is to eradicate all malignant cells.

Induction therapy has recently been tailored to biological subsets of ALL. CR rates in T-cell malignancy are higher with higher doses of cyclophosphamide and cytarabine *(38)*. Improved survival has also been demonstrated with the addition of radiation to mediastinal masses associated with T-cell malignancy *(39)*. Mature B-cell neoplasms in both children and adults have responded to high doses of cyclophosphamide, methotrexate, and cytarabine *(40–42)*. In general, prognostic factors exert a much greater effect on remission duration, rather than remission rate.

4. BONE MARROW TRANSPLANTATION FOR ALL

Myeloablative therapy with radiation and CT, or CT alone, followed by allogeneic bone marrow transplantation (allo-BMT) is the most effective method to achieve eradication of leukemic cells. Elimination of malignant cells results from the ablative affect of chemoradiotherapy and the antileukemic activity of the allograft *(43–47)*. The development of graft-vs-host disease (GVHD) is associated with a significant reduction in relapse rate and improved leukemia-free survival *(45,47)*. The International Bone Marrow Transplant Registry (IBMTR) has noted decreased relapse rates in recipients of allografts with acute or chronic GVHD. Patients with both acute and chronic GVHD experienced the most substantial decrease in relapse rate *(47,48)*. The risk of relapse correlated inversely with the severity of GVHD. Compared to individuals with acute myeloid leukemia and chronic myeloid leukemia, acute GVHD had a stronger affect in patients with ALL, and chronic GVHD a lesser affect in ALL *(47)*. Individuals with ALL should have blood drawn for histocompatibility typing prior to initiation of treatment for identification of sibling or unrelated donors, and for procurement of HLA-matched platelet products, if they become refractory to platelet transfusions. Second, marrow specimens should undergo immunophenotypic, cytogenetic, and molecular analysis.

If a CR is achieved, and patients are not treated with allotransplantation while in first CR (CR1), patients who relapse are candidates for allotransplantation. Most patients with ALL can be induced into a second remission, and this should generally be attempted. Patients with an HLA-identical sibling or unrelated donor should be evaluated for transplantation in second remission. Delay of transplantation beyond second remission compromises safety and effectiveness.

In adults with ALL who undergo transplantation in second CR, most studies indicate a LFS rate of approx 30% *(48–51)*. This compares favorably to the dismal results achieved with CT *(1,2)*.

Many patients with ALL undergo transplantation beyond second remission. Transplantation may be the best strategy for patients in more advanced stages of disease. Results are superior to those obtained with CT alone. However, for most individuals, earlier transplantation offers the best chance for cure with the least risk.

Approximately 20% of individuals who fail primary induction therapy achieve sustained LFS following allotransplantation *(52,53)*. The fewer cycles of induction CT patients receive, the more likely a successful outcome. Thus, transplantation should be considered early in patients who fail induction therapy.

Over the past several years, results have improved substantially with allotransplantation *(54)*. Furthermore, in patients who have relapsed, long-term outcome of allotransplantation using matched unrelated donors is similar to those achieved with sibling donors *(55,56)*. The increased incidence of transplant-related mortality (TRM), using unrelated donors, is offset by a lower relapse rate.

5. TRANSPLANTATION IN FIRST REMISSION

Allotransplantation in adults with ALL in first remission is a controversial topic. An easy and frequently asserted answer to the question posed in this chapter's title is that allotransplantation in first remission has not yet been proven to result in a better outcome than CT, and therefore this treatment should not be recommended. The authors do not agree. Variability in results makes a simple conclusion difficult, but critical interpretation of reported studies does permit reasonable conclusions.

It is clear that some adults with ALL benefit from allotransplantation performed early. The best-studied and most widely accepted indication for allo-BMT in first remission is the presence of the Ph^{lc}. It confers a dismal prognosis on patients who undergo treatment with conventional CT *(23,24,57)*. Forman et al. *(58)* reported a LFS of 44% in Ph-positive ALL patients receiving transplant in CR1. The IBMTR reported sustained LFS in nearly 40% of 55 Ph^+ ALL patients who underwent allotransplantation in first remission or after relapse, which is a substantially better result than that reported with CT regimens *(59)*. The Ph^{lc} identifies a group of patients who should routinely undergo transplantation in first remission, if related or unrelated donor sources are available. Translocations such as t(4;11) are known to confer a similarly poor prognosis on patients treated with conventional CT. Patients with this disorder have been cured with allotransplantation (60), and should routinely undergo allotransplants in first CR1, if sibling or matched unrelated donors are available.

Many investigators have used other prognostic factors to identify patients in first CR who are at high risk for relapse, and recommend allotransplantation during first remission in these individuals. However, factors that place patients at high risk for relapse with CT treatment, e.g., high presenting WBC, older age, and slow response to CT, have been reported to adversely affect outcome after transplantation (61–63). For the majority of adults with ALL, transplantation in first remission is not widely accepted as the best treatment. Reports from the IBMTR (61,62), which compared outcome in adults with ALL in first remission who underwent allotransplant, to two German cooperative group trials in which patients received intensive postremission CT, provide the most frequently quoted justification for not performing transplantation in first remission. Similar probabilities for 5-yr LFS were achieved (61,62), but this was not a randomized trial. Compared to other published data, the CT-treated patients chosen experienced an unusually favorable outcome, and the group of patients undergoing transplantation had a strikingly high TRM of nearly 53% (95% CI, 45–61%).

A more recent retrospective analysis compared CT subjects from the Japan Adult Leukemia Study Group to a cohort from the IBMTR, aged 15–55 yr, diagnosed between 1988 and 1990 (64). The stated goal of this study was "to compare treatment-related mortality, relapse, and leukemia-free survival after chemotherapy versus transplantation after adjusting for . . . confounding variables. . . ." The overall difference in LFS was not reported; however, it appears to have been in excess of 15%, despite a higher proportion of patients with high WBCs and the Ph^{lc} in the transplant group. Instead, based on preliminary evaluation of data, further analyses were stratified by age. Relapse probabilities in patients treated with CT were 69% (50–84%) in patients ≤30 yr, and 70% (53–85%) in patients >30 yr. LFS at 5 yr was significantly better in patients ≤30 yr who underwent transplantation (53% [44–63%] vs 30% [15–48%]), but the 26% (13–41%) LFS with CT was not significantly worse than that in transplanted older patients (30% [20–41%]). The absence of a demonstrable significant improvement was clearly related to an high mortality rate (57% [43–69%]) among patients >30 yr who underwent transplantation. The relapse rate in the transplant group was similar, at 22%, to many single and multi-institutional studies (65–71).

The most striking result from this study was the high incidence of TRM, particularly among patients >30 yr. The authors would agree that a TRM rate approaching 60% should steer patients and clinicians away from allotransplant in first CR, in all but the most dire circumstances. However, many investigators have reported substantially lower mortality rates (65–71), especially for allotransplants performed recently. The European Bone Marrow Transplantation Group found a substantial reduction in 3-yr TRM, from 39 to 25% (p = 0.0001), and a corresponding improvement in LFS, from 45 to 54% (p = 0.0001), for patients transplanted after 1986, vs those transplanted before 1986 (54). The lower TRM was attributable to better supportive care, and was not associated with loss of antileukemic activity. The improvement occurred despite the older age of patients transplanted after 1986. Although the mortality rate in older patients was higher, it did not appear to approach that reported by the IBMTR. Several studies (72–75) have reported low mortality rates in older patients undergoing allotransplantation for a variety of disorders. Many institutions and study groups have noted substantially lower mortality rates than that reported from the IBMTR. The role of patient selection, preparative therapy, clinical care, and other factors in these differences merits further study.

A prospective randomized study by the French Group for Therapy of Adult ALL assigned allotransplantation for patients who had histocompatible sibling donors and either autotransplant or CT in those who did not. The group undergoing allo-BMT had a 5-yr disease-free survival of 45%; the others had a 5-yr disease-free survival of 31% *(76)*. All analyses were performed on an intention-to-treat basis. In the BMT group, only 81% were actually transplanted; 14 relapsed prior to BMT, six patients refused transplantation, and four were judged to be in poor physical condition. The intention-to-treat analysis, in this study and in others, dilutes the effectiveness of transplantation, by including patients who do not undergo BMT in the analysis. Patients who refuse transplant, relapse prior to transplant, or are judged to be too sick to transplant, are not relevant to the determination of the relative effectiveness of transplantation. The failure of this study to detect a statistically significant difference in outcome does not merit the conclusion that there is no difference in survival or LFS between the two groups. The absence of a statistically significant difference is a result of the size of the trial and the limitations of the intention-to-treat analysis, as well as the relative effectiveness of the treatment arms. In fact, the study found substantially better 5-yr survival rate in the transplant arm, 48% (38–58%) than the control arm, 35% (27–42%) ($p = 0.08$), even by intention-to-treat. The conclusion that allotransplant does not improve survival is unjustified. The trial was inadequately designed to assess this. By design, the trial could detect only a huge difference in outcome. The data actually suggest that transplantation improved LFS in this group of patients. This study did define a group of high-risk patients with the Ph^{1c}, null or undifferentiated, or c-ALL with age >35 yr or WBC >30 × 10^9 L, or time to achieve CR >4 wk. Among high-risk patients, LFS was significantly better among patients who underwent allotransplants.

Vey et al. *(77)*, in Marseilles, have, since 1981, routinely considered all adult ALL patients for allo- or autotransplant. Seventy-one percent of these patients had ≥1 poor-risk factor, i.e., age >30 yr, non-T-cell ALL with WBC ≥30 × 10^9 L, CNS involvement, or biphenotypic ALL, Ph$^+$, or t(4;11), and/or two more induction courses to CR. The autologous group had a relapse rate of 68%, and a 10-yr probability of LFS of 28%. The allogeneic group had a relapse rate of 12% and a 10-yr probability of LFS of 58%. High-risk factors were reported to adversely effect prognosis after autologous BMT, but not after allo-BMT.

The label "high-risk" is relative. A disease with a cure rate of less than 20% and a relapse rate of 70% places virtually everyone at high-risk for relapse. Allotransplantation clearly and substantially reduces relapse rate in all studies, and should be considered in all adult patients. Studies that have identified older individuals as high-risk have found significant benefit to transplantation. For patients older than 30 yr, individual programs should balance the reduction in relapse rates with institutional TRM. It is difficult to reconcile the low risk of TRM in numerous large single and multi-institutional trials, even in older patients with advanced disease, with the high mortality rates reported by the IBMTR studies. It is overly simplistic to attempt to explain such differences purely on numbers of transplant performed. Investigators should analyze their center's individual results in ALL, particularly with regard to TRM. When data indicate mortality rates in excess of 40%, referral to centers where adequate data exists for assessment of risk, and where mortality rates are low, is appropriate.

Current policy at many centers reserves allotransplantation in CR1 for patients with only the most dismal prognostic profiles, e.g., Ph$^+$. This strategy raises several questions. Why should poor results, e.g., high TRM rates in older patients, at some centers, limit transplantation at large centers with favorable results in older patients? Why should results using unfamiliar preparative regimens or supportive care techniques (e.g., in some multi-institutional trials), in which individual centers may enter only a few patients, be relevant to centers using techniques they have established and studied over many years, and with which they have obtained excellent results? Why should results in patients who undergo transplants, despite characteristics that would make them ineligible at other centers, be relevant at more discriminating centers? These questions do not diminish the importance of data from randomized trials or registry results. They only serve to remind us that all studies, including randomized trials, merit critical review.

Studies of allotransplantation in first remission ALL consistently demonstrate substantially low relapse rates. Using a variety of preparative regimens and supportive care techniques, relapse rates are 40–50% lower with transplantation than with CT. This is balanced, in part, by considerable TRM. However, the mortality rates with allotransplantation for ALL in first remission have improved considerably over the past several years. The substantial improvement in relapse rates justifies the procedure, if it can be performed safely. It is therefore reasonable that the majority of patients with ALL, who have appropriate sibling donors, undergo allotransplantation in first remission. This should be applied to virtually all patients, with the possible exception of those at exceedingly low risk of relapse, e.g., adolescents who have no high-risk prognostic factors, such as extramedullary disease, WBC count greater than 30,000, unfavorable cytogenetics, or delay in achieving CR, and who have undergone adequate evaluation. For patients who have inadequate cytogenetic analysis, transplantation is probably advisable, since a substantial proportion will have abnormal cytogenetics, most of which are unfavorable. Patients who are at increased risk for transplantation, because of functional status, transaminitis, or significant cardiopulmonary or renal disease, should not generally have allotransplant in CR1. Furthermore, with the exception of the aforementioned cytogenetic abnormalities associated with dismal prognosis, matched unrelated transplantation should probably be recommended for second remission.

A study between the Eastern Cooperative Oncology Group and the Medical Research Council in Britain is currently in progress, comparing the rates of HLA-matched sibling allo-BMT vs either conventional CT or autotransplantation in patients with ALL in first remission. In this large prospective randomized study, all patients will receive the identical induction and intensification CT. They will be stratified according to prognostic factors (age, WBC at presentation, time to CR, immunophenotype, karyotype, and CNS involvement). This study may help determine the best therapy for ALL in first remission, stratified according to prognostic variables.

This chapter may convince clinicians of the need for continued clinical research in adult ALL, and of the importance of placing patients on appropriate clinical studies. Proctor has eloquently summarized limitations in our current trials, and suggested "a strategic shift in study approach" (2). For reasons presented in this chapter, and in Proctor's review, the authors concur. At present, however, it appears that most adults with ALL who achieve CR will relapse with conventional therapy. The number of cured patients can be improved by allotransplantation in patients with sibling donors. Present philosophy places the burden of proof on the demonstration of specific high-risk features for consideration of transplantation. Failure to adequately characterize ALL, e.g., by cytogenetic and molecular testing, results in a substantial proportion of patients who are not appropriately identified as destined to relapse. The burden of proof should be on the treating clinician, to reliably demonstrate that a patient is at low risk for relapse, before deciding that allotransplantation in first remission is not indicated.

REFERENCES

1. Copelan EA and McGuire EA. Biology and treatment of ALL in adults, *Blood*, **85** (1995) 1151–68.
2. Proctor SJ. Acute lymphoblastic leukaemia in adults: the case for a strategic shift in study approach, *Br. J. Hematol.*, **88** (1994) 229–233.
3. Forman SJ. Allogeneic transplantation for acute lymphoblastic leukemia in adults. In Thomas ED, Blume KG, and Forman SJ (eds.), *Hematopoietic Cell Transplantation*, 2nd ed. Blackwell, Malden, MA, 1998, pp. 849–858.
4. Loeffler H, Kayser W, Schmitz N, et al. Morphological and cytochemical classification of adult acute leukemias in two multicenter studies in the Federal Republic of Germany, *Haemotol. Blood Transfusion*, **30** (1987) 21.
5. Pui, C-H, Behm FG, and Crist WM. Clinical and biological relevance of immunologic marker studies in childhood acute lymphoblastic leukemia, *Blood*, **82** (1993) 343–362.
6. Crist W, Pullen J, Boyett J, et al. Acute lymphoid leukemia in adolescents: clinical and biologic features predict a poor prognosis: a Pediatric Oncology Group Study, *J. Clin. Oncol.*, **6** (1988) 34–43.
7. Kersey J, Nesbit M, Hallgren H, Sabad A, Yunis E, and Gajl-Peczalska K. Evidence of origin of certain childhood acute lymphoblastic leukemia and lymphoma in thymus-derived lymphocytes, *Cancer*, **36** (1975) 1348–1352.
8. Reinherz EL, Kung PC, Goldstein G, Levey RH, and Schlossman SF. Discrete stages of human intrathymic differentiation. Analysis of normal thymocytes and leukemic lymphoblasts of T-cell lineage, *Proc. Natl. Acad. Sci. USA*, **77** (1980) 1588–1592.
9. Theil E, Kranz BK, Raghavachar A, et al. Prethymic phenotype and genotype of pre-T (CD7$^+$/ER$^-$) cell leukemia and its clinical significance within acute lymphoblastic leukemia, *Blood*, **73** (1989) 1247.
10. Boucheix C, David B, Sebban C, et al. Immunophenotype of adult acute lymphoblastic leukemia, clinical parameters, and outcome: an analysis of a prospective trial including 562 tested patients (LALA87). French Group on Therapy for Adult Acute Lymphoblastic Leukemia, *Blood*, **84** (1994) 1603–1612.
11. Bloomfield CD, Secker-Walker LM, Goldman AI, et al. Six-year follow-up of the clinical significance of karyotype in acute lymphoblastic leukemia, *Cancer Genet. Cytogenet.*, **40** (1989) 171–185.
12. Faderl S, Kantarjian HM, Talpaz M, and Estrov Z. Clinical significance of cytogenetic abnormalities in adult acute lymphoblastic leukemia, *Blood*, **91** (1998) 3995–4019.
13. Bloomfield CD, Lindquist LL, Arthur D, et al. Chromosome abnormalities and their clinical significance in acute lymphoblastic leukemia (for the Third International Workshop on Chromosomes in Leukemia), *Cancer Res.*, **43** (1986) 868.
14. Bloomfield CD, Goldman AI, Alimena G, et al. Chromosome abnormalities identify high-risk and low-risk patients with acute lymphoblastic leukemia, *Blood*, **67** (1986) 415–420.
15. Williams PL, Ramondi SC, Rivera G, et al. Presence of clonal abnormalities in virtually all cases of acute lymphoblastic leukemia, *N. Engl. J. Med.*, **313** (1985) 640.
16. Rabbitts TH. Translocations, mastergenes and difference between origins of acute and chronic leukemias, *Cell*, **67** (1991) 641–644.
17. Nichols J and Nimer SD. Transcription factors, translocations, and leukemia, *Blood*, **80** (1992) 2953–2963.
18. Bloomfield CD, Lindquist LL, Brunning RD, Yunis JJ, and Coccia PF. Philadelphia chromosome in acute leukemia, *Virchows Arch. (B)* **29** (1978) 81–91.
19. Arthur DC, Bloomfield CD, Lindquist LL, and Nesbit ME Jr. Translocation 4; 11 in acute lymphoblastic leukemia: clinical characteristics and prognostic significance, *Blood*, **59** (1982) 96–99.

20. Levin MD, Michael PM, Garson OM, Tiedemann K, and Firkin FC. Clinical pathological characteristics of acute lymphoblastic leukemia with the 4:11 chromosome translocation, *Pathology*, **16** (1984) 63–66.

21. Pui C-H. Acute leukemias with the t(4;11)(q21•3), *Leukemia Lymphoma*, **7** (1992) 173–179.

22. Michael PM, Levin MD, and Garson OM. Translocation 1:19: a new cytogenetic abnormality in acute lymphoblastic leukemia, *Cancer Genet. Cytogenet.*, **12** (1984) 333–341.

23. Secker-Walker LM, Craig JM, Hawkins JM, and Hoffbrand AV. Philadelphia positive acute lympho-blastic leukemia in adults: age distribution, bcr break-point, and prognostic significance, *Leukemia*, **5** (1991) 196–199.

24. Lestingi TM and Hooberman AL. Philadelphia positive acute lymphoblastic leukemia, *Hematol. Oncol. Clin. North Am.*, **7** (1993) 161–175.

25. Bloomfield CD, Secker-Walker LM, Goldman AI, et al. Six-year follow-up of the clinical significance of karyotype in acute lymphoblastic leukemia, *Cancer Gene Cytogenet.*, **40** (1989) 171–185.

26. Westbrook Ca, Hooberman L, Spino C, et al. Clinical significance of the bcr-abl fusion gene in adult acute lymphoblastic leukemia: a Cancer and Leukemia Group B Study (8762), *Blood*, **80** (1992) 2983–2990.

27. Tuszynski A, Dhut S, Young BD, et al. Detection and significance of bcr-abl mRNA transcripts and fusion proteins in Philadelphia-positive adult acute lymphoblastic leukemia, *Leukemia*, **7** (1993) 1504–1508.

28. Janssen JWG, Ludwig W-D, Sterry W, and Bartram CR. SIL-Tal1 deletion in T-cell acute lymphoblastic leukemia, *Leukemia*, **8** (1993) 1204–1210.

29. Bash RO, Hall S, Timmons CF, Crist WM, Amylon M, Graham Smith R, and Baer R. Does activation of the TAL1 gene occur in a majority of patients with T-cell acute lymphoblastic leukemia? A Pediatric Oncology Group Study, *Blood*, **86** (1995) 666–676.

30. Rubnitz JE, Downing JR, Pui C-H, et al. TEL gene rearrangement in acute lymphoblastic leukemia: a new genetic marker with prognostic significance, *J. Clin. Oncol.*, **15** (1997) 1150–1157.

31. Shurtleff SA, Bujis A, Behm FG, et al. TEL/AML1 fusion resulting from a cryptic t(12;21) is the most common genetic lesion in pediatric ALL and defines a subgroup with an excellent prognosis, *Leukemia*, **9** (1995) 1985–1989.

32. Haidar MA, Cao X-B, Manshouri T, et al. p16^{INK4A} and p15^{INK4B} gene deletions in primary leukemias, *Blood*, **86** (1995) 311–315.

33. Quesnel B, Preudhomme C, Philippe N, et al. p16 gene homozygous deletions in acute lymphoblastic leukemia, *Blood*, **85** (1995) 657–663.

34. Hammond D, Sather H, Nesbit M, et al. Analysis of prognostic factors in acute lymphoblastic leukemia, *Med. Pediatr. Oncol.*, **14** (1986) 124–134.

35. Sather HN. Age at diagnosis in childhood acute lymphoblastic leukemia, *Med. Pediatr. Oncol.*, **14** (1986) 166–172.

36. Leumert JT, Burns CP, Wiltse CG, Armitage JO, and Clark WA. Prognostic information of pretreatment characteristics in adult acute lymphoblastic leukemia, *Blood*, **56** (1980) 510.

37. Hoelzer D. Change in treatment strategies for adult acute lymphoblastic leukemia (ALL) according to prognostic factors and minimal residual disease, *Bone Marrow Transplant.*, **6(S1)** (1990) 66–70.

38. Hoelzer D. Therapy of the newly diagnosed adult with acute lymphoblastic leukemia. In Bloomfield CD, Herzig GP (eds.), *Hematology/Oncology Clinics of North America*, W.B. Saunders, Philadelphia, 1993, pp. 139–160.

39. Hoelzer D, Thiel E, Löffler H, et al. Intensified chemotherapy and mediastinal irradiation in adult T-cell acute lymphoblastic leukemia. In Gale RP, Hoelzer D (eds.), *Acute Lymphoblastic Leukemia*, Liss, New York, 1990, pp. 221–229.

40. Schwenn MR, Blattner SR, Lynch E, and Weinstein HJ. HiC-COM: A 2-month intensive chemotherapy regimen for children with stage III and IV Burkitt's lymphoma and B-cell acute lymphoblastic leukemia, *J. Clin. Oncol.*, **9** (1991) 133–138.

41. Reiter A, Schrappe M, Ludwig W-D, et al. Favorable outcome of B-cell acute lymphoblastic leukemia in childhood: a report of three consecutive studies of the BFM group, *Blood*, **80** (1992) 2471–2478.

42. Pees HW, Radtke H, Schwamborn J, and Graf N. The BFM-protocol for HIV-negative Burkitt's lymphomas and L₃ ALL in adult patients: a high chance for cure, *Ann. Hematol.*, **65** (1992) 201–205.

43. Barrett AJ, Horowitz MM, Gale RP, et al. Marrow transplantation for acute lymphoblastic leukemia: factors affecting relapse and survival, *Blood*, **74** (1989) 862–871.

44. Bortin MM, Truitt RL, Rimm AA, and Bach FH. Graft-versus-leukaemia reactivity induced by alloimmunisation without augmentation of graft-versus-host reactivity, *Nature*, **281** (1979) 490–491.

45. Weisdorf DJ, Nesbit ME, Ramsay NCK, et al. Allogeneic bone marrow transplantation for acute lymphoblastic leukemia in remission: prolonged survival associated with acute graft-versus-host disease, *J. Clin. Oncol.*, **5** (1987) 1348–1355.

46. Doney K, Fisher LD, Appelbaum FR, et al. Treatment of adult acute lymphoblastic leukemia with allogeneic bone marrow transplantation. Multivariate analysis of factors affecting acute graft-versus-host disease, relapse, and relapse-free survival, *Bone Marrow Transplant.*, **7** (1991) 453–459.

47. Horowitz MM, Gale RP, Sondel PM, et al. Graft-versus-leukemia reactions after bone marrow transplantation, *Blood*, **75** (1990) 555–562.

48. Blume KG, Forman SJ, Krance RA, Henke M, Findley DO, and Hill LR. Bone marrow transplantation for acuate leukemia, *Hematol. Blood Transfusion*, **29** (1985) 39–41.

49. Gratwhol A, Hermans J, Zwaan F, for the EBMT. Bone marrow transplantation for ALL in Europe. In Gale RP and Hoelzer D (eds.), *Acute Lymphoblastic Leukemia*, Liss, New York, 1990, pp. 271.

50. Herzig RH, Barrett AJ, Gluckman E, et al. Bone marrow transplantation in high-risk acute lymphoblastic leukaemia in first and second remission, *Lancet*, (1987) 786–789.

51. Butturini A and Gale RP. Chemotherapy versus transplantation in acute leukaemia, *Br. J. Hematol.*, **72** (1989) 1–8.

52. Forman S, Schmidt G, Nademanee A, et al. Allogeneic bone marrow transplantation as therapy for primary induction failure for patients with acute leukemia, *J. Clin. Oncol.*, **9** (1991) 1570–1574.

53. Biggs JC, Horowitz MM, Gale RP, et al. Bone marrow transplants may cure patients with acute leukemia never achieving remission with chemotherapy, *Blood*, **80** (1992) 1090–1093.

54. Frassoni F, Lobopin M, Gluckman E, et al. Results of allogeneic bone marrow transplantation for acute leukemia have improved in Europe with time: a report of the acute leukemia working party of the European group for blood and marrow transplantation (EBMT), *Bone Marrow Transplant.*, **17** (1996) 13–18.

55. Kernan MA, Bartsch G, Ash RC, et al. Retrospective analysis of 462 unrelated marrow transplants facilitated by the National Marrow Donor Program for treatment of acquired and congenital disorders of the lymphohematopoietic system and congenital metabolic disorders, *N. Engl. J. Med.*, **328** (1993) 592–.

56. Beatty PG, Hansen JA, Longton GM, et al. Marrow transplantation from HLA-matched unrelated donors for treatment of hematologic malignancies, *Transplantation*, **51** (1991) 443–447.

57. Champlin R and Gale RP. Acute lymphoblastic leukemia: recent advances in biology and therapy, *Blood*, **73** (1989) 2051–2066.

58. Forman SJ, O'Donnell MR, Nademanee AP, et al. Bone marrow transplantation for patients with Philadelphia chromosome-positive acute lymphoblastic leukemia, *Blood*, **70** (1987) 587–588.

59. Barrett AJ, Horowitz MM, Ash RC, et al. Bone marrow transplantation for Philadelphia chromosome-positive acute lymphoblastic leukemia, *Blood*, **79** (1992) 3067–3070.

60. Copelan EA, Kapoor N, Murcek M, Theil K, and Tutschka PJ. Marrow transplantation following busulfan and cyclophosphamide as treatment for translocation (4;11) acute leukemia, *Br. J. Haematol.*, **70** (1988) 127–128.

61. Horowitz MM, Messerer D, Hoelzer D, et al. Chemotherapy compared with bone marrow transplantation for adults with acute lymphoblastic leukemia in first remission, *Ann. Intern. Med.*, **115** (1991) 13–18.

62. Zhang MJ, Hoelzer D, Horowitz MM, et al. Long-term follow-up of adults with acute lymphoblastic leukemia in first remission treated with chemotherapy or bone marrow transplantation. The Acute Lymphoblastic Leukemia Working Committee, *Ann. Intern. Med.*, **123** (1995) 428–431.

63. Slovak ML, Kopecky KJ, Wolman SR, et al. Cytogenetic correlation with disease status and treatment outcome in advanced stage leukemia post bone marrow transplantation: a Southwest Oncology Group Study (SWOG-8612), *Leukemia Res.*, **19** (1995) 381–388.

64. Oh H, Gale RP, Zhang M-J, et al. Chemotherapy vs HLA-identical sibling bone marrow transplants for adults with acute lymphoblastic leukemia in first remission. *Bone Marrow Transplant.*, **22** (1998) 253–257.

65. Blume KG, Forman SJ, Snyder DS, et al. Allogeneic bone marrow transplantation for acute lymphoblastic leukemia during first complete remission, *Transplantation*, **43** (1987) 389–392.

66. Vernant JT, Marit G, Maraninchi D, et al. Allogeneic bone marrow transplantation in adults with acute lymphoblastic leukemia in first complete remission, *J. Clin. Oncol.*, **6** (1988) 227–231.

67. Blaise D, Gespard MH, Stoppa AM, et al. Allogeneic or autologous bone marrow transplantation for acute lymphoblastic leukemia in first complete remission, *Bone Marrow Transplant.*, **5** (1990) 7–12.

68. Forman SJ. Role of allogeneic bone marrow transplantation in the treatment of high-risk acute lymphocytic leukemia in adults, *Leukemia*, **11** (1997) S18–S19.

69. Sebban C, Lepage E, Vernant JP, et al. Allogeneic bone marrow transplantation in adult acute lymphoblastic leukemia in first complete remission: a comparative study, *J. Clin. Oncol.*, **12** (1994) 2580–2587.

70. Vey N, Blaise D, Stoppa AM, et al. Bone marrow transplantation in 63 adult patients with acute lymphoblastic leukemia in first complete remission, *Bone Marrow Transplant.*, **14** (1994) 383–388.

71. Attal M, Blaise D, Marit G, et al. Consolidation treatment of adult acute lymphoblastic leukemia: a prospective, randomized trial comparing allogeneic versus autologous bone marrow transplantation and testing the impact of recombinant interleukin-2 after autologous bone marrow transplantation, *Blood*, **86** (1995) 1619–1628.

72. Klingemann HG, Storb R, Fefer A, et al. Bone marrow transplantation in patients aged 45 years and older, *Blood*, **67** (1986) 770–776.

73. Copelan EA, Kapoor N, Berliner M, and Tutschka PJ. Bone marrow transplantation without total-body irradiation in patients aged 40 and older, *Transplantation*, **48** (1989) 65–68.

74. Appelbaum FR, Clift R, Radich J, Anasetti C, and Buckner CD. Bone marrow transplantation for chronic myelogenous leukemia, *Semin. Oncol.*, **22** (1995) 405–411.

75. Copelan E, Penza S, Theil K, et al. Allogeneic marrow transplantation with $BuCy_2$ in patients with chronic myelogenous leukemia, *Blood*, **92S1** (1998) 285a.

76. Fiere D, Lepage E, Sebban C, et al., for the French Group on Therapy for Adult Acute Lymphoblastic Leukemia. Adult acute lymphoblastic leukemia: a multicentric randomized trial testing bone marrow transplantation as postremission therapy, *J. Clin. Oncol.*, **11** (1993) 1990–2001.

77. Vey N, Stoppa AM, Faucher C, et al. Bone marrow transplantation (BMT) for acute lymphoblastic leukemia (ALL) in first complete remission (CR1): Long-term outcome of 88 patients treated in a single institution. Proceedings of the IBMTR-ABMTR ASBMT Tandem Meetings, Keystone, CO, February 28–March 6, 1999, p. 35. Abstract C-1.

8

What Is the Curative Potential of Refractory Leukemia with Related and Unrelated Allogeneic Transplants?

Matt E. Kalaycio, MD

CONTENTS

1. INTRODUCTION

Acute leukemia was uniformly fatal until the development of effective therapeutic chemotherapy (CT) regimens in the early 1970s. Combination CT for acute leukemia induced complete remission (CR) in the majority of patients, but postremission therapy was inadequate to prevent relapse *(1)*. Relapsed patients, and those who failed to achieve CR, invariably died from their leukemia.

In 1977, the Fred Hutchinson Cancer Research Center reported their results with human leukocyte antigen (HLA)-matched sibling, allogeneic bone marrow transplantation (allo-BMT) in 100 patients with relapsed and refractory acute leukemia *(2)*. Of these 100 patients, 56 were adults, the oldest being 56-yr-old. All were considered end-stage, but 10 (18%) were alive at least 330 d post-BMT. All were treated with total body irradiation (TBI) with or without CT. Of the 12 adults going into BMT in poor clinical condition ("advanced relapse, and/or refractory to random platelets, and/ or febrile on broad-spectrum antibiotics, very poor clinical condition") *(2)*, two (17%) survived. These results were obtained without modern cytomegalovirus (CMV) prophylaxis, without cyclosporine for graft-vs-host disease (GVHD) prophylaxis, and without antifungal prophylaxis. Most of the surviving patients were still alive 5-yr later *(3)*, clearly demonstrating that BMT can cure otherwise incurable patients with acute leukemia.

From: *Current Controversies in Bone Marrow Transplantation*
Edited by: B. Bolwell © Humana Press Inc., Totowa, NJ

Yet, since the publication of those early results, the non-BMT therapy of acute leukemia has also improved *(4,5)*. Some subgroups of untreated acute leukemia can now be cured with modern intensive CT protocols *(4)*. Long-term disease-free survival (DFS) has been achieved, even in relapsed and refractory patients, with high-dose cytarabine *(6–10)*. In fact, for patients whose first remissions' duration exceeds 2 yr, the long-term DFS with salvage CT is approx 20%, similar to the results seen with BMT *(11,12)*.

Despite occasional long-term survivors, the vast majority of patients who fail to respond to initial CT or relapse after an initial remission, are not curable with CT alone *(13–16)*. BMT is usually recommended for these patients, but the curative potential of BMT in this setting is not generally appreciated by either those recommending the procedure or those receiving one. Given the wider availability of matched donors made possible by large international registries of unrelated volunteer marrow donors, clinicians caring for patients with acute leukemia need a clear understanding of the curative potential of BMT in refractory disease.

2. PRIMARY REFRACTORY ACUTE LEUKEMIA

Patients who fail to achieve CR with initial induction CT have a poor prognosis with salvage CT alone. Following induction CT with 1–2 cycles of cytarabine (100–200 mg/m^2/d as a continuous infusion for 7 d) and idarubicin (12 mg/m^2/d for 3 d), approx 30% of patients under the age of 60 yr will fail to achieve remission *(17–19)*. Although some of these patients may achieve remission with salvage high-dose cytarabine (2–3 g/m^2 every 12 h for 3–6 d), cure is rare *(6,7)*. For patients treated initially with high-dose cytarabine, refractory disease portends an even worse prognosis, with a low probability of even achieving a remission to salvage CT *(12)*. Similar statistics exist for patients with acute lymphoblastic leukemia (ALL) receiving standard induction with vincristine-based regimens *(5,13)*.

BMT potentially cures primary refractory acute leukemia. In a study from 1991, Forman et al. *(20)* described a series of 21 patients (children and adults) treated with HLA-matched sibling BMT for primary refractory leukemia. All but three patients were treated with a TBI-containing preparative regimen. Nine patients (seven adults) survived at least 556 d, with an estimated 10-yr DFS of 40%. Approximately one-half of the patients who did not survive died from leukemic relapse, not BMT complications.

In another study of 24 patients with primary refractory acute leukemia treated with BMT, 17/20 evaluable patients (85%) achieved a CR *(21)*. Ten of these patients subsequently died of transplant-related complications, but three (17%) survived at least 2 yr. These three began their preparative regimens with 39–90% blasts in the bone marrow, indicating that truly CT-resistant leukemia is potentially curable with BMT.

The International Bone Marrow Transplant Registry (IBMTR) published their results of HLA-matched sibling BMT in 126 patients with refractory acute leukemia *(22)*. Most patients (83%) were treated with TBI-containing preparative regimens. Various GVHD prophylaxis schedules were employed, but most (56%) included cyclosporine. Although approx 60% of patients relapsed, the estimated 3-yr DFS was 21%, with no significant differences seen between those treated for acute myeloid leukemia (AML) and those treated for ALL.

Results for matched unrelated donor (MUD) BMT are less readily available. The few patients treated for primary refractory leukemia are usually considered in the same group as those with resistant relapse or active leukemia. Although cure is described within this group of patients, the specific results for primary refractory disease are unavailable in published reports. As of September 14, 1998, only 78 patients had been reported to the IBMTR as being treated for primary refractory acute leukemia with MUD BMT. The 3-yr probability of leukemia-free survival in these patients was 11%. The relapse rate of 67% is similar to that noted with sibling BMT.*

The high relapse rates noted following BMT strongly suggest that myeloablative therapy with radiation and/or CT is often inadequate to eradicate leukemia. Thus, minimal residual disease probably persists following the preparative regimen. The persistence of subclinical disease has been clearly demonstrated following BMT for chronic myeloid leukemia, and may predict for subsequent relapse (23,24). Emerging evidence suggests that the minimal residual disease present following BMT may be eliminated by immunologic manipulations, such as adoptive immunotherapy (25), immunomodulation with cytokines (26), and gene therapy (27). Although these therapies are currently experimental, they hold promise for reducing relapse rates, and for improving outcome.

Most authorities recommend BMT for patients with primary refractory acute leukemia (4,12,13). However, physicians must anticipate the possibility of refractory disease at initial diagnosis, for expedient application of BMT. HLA-typing, donor assessment, virological screening, and insurance verification require time to complete. The patient who has failed a second induction cycle of CT has already been neutropenic and transfusion-dependent for weeks. Any extra time used to secure a donor increases the likelihood of an infectious complication and possible death. Securing an unrelated donor is even more problematic. Unfortunately, many patients are not HLA-typed at diagnosis, and consultations with a transplant center often do not begin until the patient is already refractory. Optimal results from BMT will only become manifest when patients with refractory disease are evaluated for BMT early in their treatment course.

3. RELAPSED ACUTE LEUKEMIA

At the onset of relapse, patients for whom a marrow donor is identified and available may either proceed immediately to BMT or receive salvage CT in an attempt to induce a second CR. Which of these two options is the optimal strategy is not clear.

In an early retrospective report by the Fred Hutchinson Cancer Research Center, 62 patients with an initial relapse of AML were treated with TBI-containing preparative regimens and HLA-matched sibling BMT (28). Long-term DFS of patients treated with immediate BMT was 29%, which compared favorably with results achieved in patients treated first with salvage CT, then treated with BMT in persistent relapse (10% DFS) or second remission (20% DFS). This small, retrospective study suggested no advantage for salvage CT with intent to induce a second remission prior to BMT, compared to immediate BMT. A larger, updated retrospective review confirmed the utility of immediate HLA-matched sibling BMT for untreated relapse of AML, compared to those first

*The data presented here were obtained from the Statistical Center of the IBMTR. The analysis has not been reviewed or approved by the Advisory Committee of the IBMTR.

Table 1
Results of HLA-matched Sibling BMT for Relapsed AML

	n	Transplant-related mortality	Relapse	5-yr survival (%)
Untreated	54	36	10	28
Second remission	49	34	9	31
Resistant relapse	29	22	9	24

Adapted with permission from ref. 29.

receiving salvage CT (Table 1; 29). Finally, the Seattle experience, treating active, relapsed AML with BMT, was recently updated (30). A variety of preparative regimens were used to treat 126 patients. The early mortality rate was high, with 20 patients dying before d 30 post-BMT, but 26 patients (21%) survived at least 2 yr post-BMT. The chief cause of death was relapse, which occurred in 48 patients (38%). Two cohorts of patients in this study differed only by their GVHD prophylactic regimen. One group was treated with cyclosporine and methotrexate; the other was treated with methotrexate alone. The risk of GVHD was lower in the cohort treated with cyclosporine, but the risk of relapse increased leading to a similar overall survival between the two groups. The association of GVHD with a decreased risk of relapse supports the findings of other studies, which suggest a graft-versus-leukemia (GVL) effect exists for AML (31).

Often, however, many patients cannot proceed immediately to BMT upon relapse. Reasons vary, but may include lack of foresight in securing a matched donor, active and life-threatening relapse requiring immediate intervention, and lack of guaranteed insurance coverage. For these patients, salvage CT is administered in an attempt to induce a second remission before proceeding to BMT. In fact, most patients are treated with salvage CT before proceeding to BMT. However, salvage CT will not always result in remission. The likelihood of second remission is directly proportional to the duration of first remission (Table 2). Therefore, patients who are treated with salvage CT will come to BMT in remission, or (just as often) with active, CT-resistant disease.

BMT for patients achieving a second remission, results in leukemia-free survival of 25–50%, whether the source of stem cells is a relative (32–36) or unrelated donor (37–39). Given that only rare cases of relapsed adult acute leukemia are curable with CT alone, allo-BMT is recommended for selected (normal cardiorespiratory function, normal hepatic and renal function, and no significant co-morbid illness) patients less

Table 2
Results of Salvage CT for AML

	CR Rate (%)
First Salvage CT	
CR > 2 yr	73
CR > 1 yr, < 2 yr	47
CR < 1 yr	14
Second Salvage CT	
First CR < 1 yr	0

Data from ref. 61.

than 60 yr of age in second remission, who have an HLA-matched donor *(14,40)*. Patients failing to achieve remission have a worse prognosis with BMT. One could reasonably ask this question: Is BMT indicated in the patient with acute leukemia who fails to achieve remission after relapse?

In an early report *(41)*, 33 patients with acute leukemia treated with matched-sibling BMT were analyzed for outcome. Of these patients, eight had active disease at the time of BMT and six had more than 25% blasts in their bone marrow. All were treated with TBI-containing preparative regimens, but only methotrexate was given for GVHD prophylaxis. Only one of the eight patients with active disease survived >276 d; none of the others survived beyond 165 d post-BMT. None of the patients with >25% marrow blasts survived. In contrast, patients treated identically, but in remission, experienced a survival rate greater than 50%.

Similar poor results were reported in another series of 26 patients with active, relapsed AML treated with TBI-containing regimens, and HLA-matched sibling BMT *(34)*. Sixteen of these patients had relapsed from an initial second remission, and 10 failed to respond to salvage CT. Although three patients (10%) were alive and in remission from 17–44 mo post-BMT, no refractory patients survived.

The results of these studies suggest that patients with AML are best treated in remission, in contrast to the conclusions reached by the Seattle studies *(29)*. Data supporting the Seattle group's position comes from a European case series *(32)*. Thirty-eight patients were treated with TBI and high-dose VP-16-213, followed by matched, related-donor BMT. Of four patients with AML and four patients with ALL treated for refractory relapse, five survived without relapse 219–1078 d post-BMT. Two of the survivors were adults (22 and 42 yr of age).

Results similar to those achieved in AML have been reported for ALL. Using TBI-containing preparative regimens, 103 adult patients with active ALL were treated with matched-sibling BMT in another series reported by the Seattle group *(42)*. These patients had either primary refractory ($n = 10$) or relapsed (first relapse $n = 37$; second or greater relapse $n = 50$) disease. Compared to a group of patients treated similarly, but in remission, the patients with active disease experienced a similar incidence of transplant-related complications, but an increased incidence of relapse. The long-term DFS of less than 20% was similar in both groups. Many deaths were attributed to interstitial fibrosis, a complication less commonly encountered with modern treatment protocols. The presence of extramedullary disease (leukemic meningitis) did not predict for worse outcome in multivariate analysis.

Clearly, the results of matched, related-donor BMT for resistant relapse of acute leukemia are poor. Cure, however, is possible with BMT for these otherwise incurable patients. Unfortunately, BMT is not even an option for the majority of patients lacking a related, histocompatible marrow donor. For these patients, MUD BMT holds some potential appeal.

Few patients have been treated for relapsed, refractory acute leukemia with MUD BMT. Only 77 adult patients with adult leukemia treated with MUD BMT were reported as "not in remission" to the IBMTR as of 1991 *(43)*. In case series, these few patients are usually considered together with other groups of high-risk patients, making analysis of their specific outcome difficult *(44,45)*. However, some studies have classified patients treated for acute leukemia with MUD BMT into those in remission and those with active disease at the time of BMT.

In a review of 462 MUD transplants facilitated by the National Marrow Donor Program (NMDP), 153 patients with acute leukemia were described *(37)*. The patients treated in first or second remission had a 2-yr DFS of 45%, compared to 19% survival for patients treated with more advanced disease, including those with active disease at the time of BMT.

In another reported series, 55 patients with acute leukemia were treated with various preparative regimens, followed by MUD BMT *(38)*. The patients were subgrouped into those treated in remission and those treated with active disease. The patients treated in remission had a 3-yr DFS of 33%, compared to a survival of 15% in patients treated with active disease. The risk of relapse was 24%, indicating that mortality in this series was largely attributable to complications arising from BMT, such as GVHD.

The largest series of patients with acute leukemia treated with MUD BMT was recently reported *(46)*: 168 patients were treated with TBI and cyclophosphamide, and six were treated with CT only. All patients were either matched (identical at HLA-A,D, and D/DRD1 loci) or minor mismatched (single disparity at a class I antigen belonging to the same crossreactive group, or a single disparity for D/DRB1 subtype alleles within the same DR specificity). All minor-mismatched patients were less than 36 yr old. Standard GVHD prophylaxis with cyclosporine and methotrexate was given after BMT *(47)*.

Although 16 patients died before engraftment could be fully assessed, 99% of the remaining 158 patients achieved sustained donor engraftment *(46)*. BMT was complicated by severe acute GVHD in 47% of patients. Although faster engraftment was associated with a larger marrow cell dose, severe GVHD occurred less often with larger cell doses.

At the time of BMT, patients were classified as either in remission or with active disease. The relapse rate was greater than 40% for patients receiving BMT with active disease, compared to less than 30% in those patients treated in remission *(46)*. Of those patients with active disease, patients with more than 30% marrow blasts had a relapse risk >60%, compared to a risk of about 40% in those with <30% marrow blasts.

Survival also depended on the status of disease at the time of BMT. Although only 19% of patients enjoyed long-term leukemia-free survival, the survival of those patients treated in remission was 27% for AML and 37% for ALL *(46)*. The survival rate of patients treated with active disease was only 11%. Within this poor prognostic group, however, patients beginning their preparative regimen with less than 30% blasts in their marrow, and no circulating blasts, had a significantly better survival, compared to those who had more than 30% blasts in their marrow or circulating peripheral blasts. There was no significant difference in survival when comparing patients receiving BMT in untreated relapse (12%; *n* = 50) vs those in CT-resistant relapse (5%; *n* = 44).

At the time of relapse, adult patients with acute leukemia and no histocompatible relatives are often entered into the NMDP, in an attempt to locate a MUD. Especially for Caucasians, a donor is usually found. For those patients achieving a second remission, cure is possible in 30–40% of patients who go on to MUD BMT (Table 3). For those who fail to achieve remission or relapse before beginning BMT, however, cure is possible in 10–20% of cases, which is similar to results achieved with BMT for primary refractory acute leukemia utilizing HLA-matched sibling donors. For selected young patients, especially those who relapse within 2 yr of achieving CR, MUD BMT offers

Table 3
Results of MUD BMT for Patients with Relapsed Acute Leukemia

	Status	n	Leukemia-free survival (%)	Ref
NMDP	Remission	55	45	37
	Relapse	98	19	
UCLA	Remission	28	33	38
	Relapse	26	15	
Fred Hutchinson Cancer Research Center	Remission	66	27–37[a]	46
	Relapse	94	10–12[a]	

[a]Results for AML and ALL, respectively.

a chance for cure not otherwise possible. Such a chance should be offered to appropriate patients, along with a frank discussion of potential risks.

4. GRAFT VERSUS ACUTE LEUKEMIA EFFECT

The most common reason for failure of BMT to cure refractory acute leukemia is relapse. To improve the curative potential of BMT, the relapse rate must be reduced. There are two major components to BMT that can impact on the relapse rate. One is the preparative regimen. Standard myeloablative regimens, whether busulfan- or TBI-based, effectively destroy recipient hematopoiesis, yet the leukemic clone often survives. Alterations of the preparative regimen, such as adding new drugs, intensifying the dose, and specific targetting of blast cell antigens, have not yet improved the outcome of BMT to a significant degree. The intrinsic resistance of the leukemic clone to both CT and radiation suggests that new, innovative approaches are needed, if the true potential of BMT is to be ultimately met.

The second component capable of eradicating leukemia is the so-called GVL effect. There is substantial evidence that a donor-lymphocyte-mediated graft-versus-acute-leukemia (GVAL) effect exists, and can potentially be harnessed for exploitation. The first line of evidence supporting a GVAL effect comes from early studies that indicated a lower relapse rate in patients who developed GVHD *(31)*. In their series of patients with AML treated by sibling BMT, the Seattle Group noted a larger reduction in the rate of relapse among patients who developed chronic GVHD, compared to those who developed acute GVHD *(29)*. In contrast, acute GVHD appeared to significantly reduce the relapse rate in patients treated for ALL *(42)*. An IBMTR report noted a protective effect of any GVHD against ALL relapse, but only chronic GVHD against AML relapse *(48)*. Other series *(35)* support the observation that acute GVHD does not appear to reduce the relapse rate in AML.

Studies of T-cell-depleted (TCD) BMT provide contradictory evidence of a GVAL effect. TCD reduces the incidence and severity of GVHD. Therefore, donor T-cells appear to mediate GVHD. If GVHD prevents relapse, one would predict higher relapse rates in patients treated with TCD BMT. This prediction is demonstrably true for chronic myeloid leukemia (CML) *(49)*. An increased relapse rate following TCD was noted by the IBMTR in AML, but not in ALL *(48)*. More recent series *(50–52)*, however, have failed to indicate a higher incidence of relapse for the acute leukemias following TCD BMT. The confusing results obtained from reviewing studies of TCD BMT may result from differences in preparative regimen, additional GVHD prophylaxis, and patient selection. Only prospective studies will ultimately determine whether or not TCD influences relapse rate and survival.

The results of syngeneic BMT represent a third line of evidence supporting the existence of a GVAL effect. The relapse rate of patients receiving syngeneic BMT for high-risk acute leukemia is higher than in patients with GVHD after allo-BMT *(31,53)*.

Finally, the most compelling evidence for a GVAL effect comes from cases of acute leukemia relapsed after allo-BMT. In this situation, a reduction in immunosuppression can lead to remission, without the requirement for cytotoxic CT. When this maneuver fails to elicit either GVHD or remission, an infusion of donor lymphocytes (DLI) may provide the desired effect. DLI may induce remission in as many as 30% of patients with relapsed AML, but the effect on ALL has been less pronounced *(54,55)*. Clearly, however, a GVAL effect exists, and potentially can be exploited to reduce relapse rates in acute leukemia.

Unfortunately, the beneficial effect of GVAL is undermined by its association with GVHD, which can be very debilitating, and is often fatal *(56)*. The separation of GVAL from GVHD promises to improve the curative potential of refractory acute leukemia. Several approaches to achieve this elusive goal are under active investigation *(57)*. One of these approaches attempts to selectively deplete donor marrow of lymphocytes that mediate GVHD, while retaining those that might mediate GVAL. An infusion of CD8[+] TCD DLI results in GVL effects similar to unmanipulated DLI, without incurring a high incidence of GVHD in patients with CML *(58)*. Similar results have been noted in several series utilizing CD8[+] TCD BMT for hematologic malignancies *(52,59,60)*. All demonstrate a reduction in GVHD without an increase in relapse rates. These observations suggest that GVAL can potentially be separated from GVHD.

Another approach to separate GVHD from GVAL utilizes gene transduction technology. Donor lymphocytes are transduced with *Herpes simplex* virus thymidine kinase, rendering the cells sensitive to treatment with ganciclovir. These transduced cells can be infused into a recipient with relapsed leukemia, in an attempt to generate a GVL effect. If unwanted, severe GVHD develops instead, ganciclovir is administered, effectively destroying the transduced donor lymphocytes *(27)*. This and other innovative approaches promise to separate GVAL from GVHD for therapeutic exploitation.

5. CONCLUSIONS

This chapter was written to help clinicians treating critically ill patients with acute leukemia who are refractory to standard CT, to determine the potential role of BMT. For the clinician biased against BMT in this situation, evidence is given to support their position. Clearly, most patients with refractory leukemia will either die as a result of BMT or relapse in spite of it. No prospective study will ever document improved leukemia-free survival with BMT, compared to standard treatments alone. The toxicity of BMT is extreme, and the cost is exorbitant. Some will conclude that these considerations indicate the procedure is not justified, and, therefore, need not be offered.

Transplant physicians, in contrast, will review the same data, note a defined cure rate, and conclude that all patients should not only be offered, but encouraged to receive a BMT. Most patients are either referred to transplant physicians by like-minded community oncologists, or are in search of cure at any cost. Even the most optimistic of transplant physicians, however, must accept the somber reality of a limited benefit of BMT in the setting of refractory acute leukemia.

Neither the view of the therapeutic nihilist nor the opinion of the aggressive transplanter is absolutely correct. The field of BMT is not static. New findings and insights emerge almost daily. Not to offer cure when new therapies and ideas are being tested would be to accept the current state of affairs, and to stifle progress. To continue current treatment protocols without modification seems equally short-sighted. The curative potential of BMT rests in innovative treatment strategies that seek to take advantage of the leads provided by previous clinical studies and new basic research. Patients should be exhorted to follow the example set by the pioneers who volunteered for the initial trials of BMT in Seattle. Some of those patients are alive today, because of their conquering spirit and the timely application of available technology.

The author is often asked, "When will you be able to cure leukemia?" The cure is available now. Although only occasional patients will survive the procedure as administered today, the curative potential of BMT for refractory acute leukemia is 100%. The challenge is for clinicians to achieve that potential by seizing on the advances already made, and to develop innovative methods to capitalize on them.

REFERENCES

1. Rosenthal DS and Moloney WC. Treatment of acute granulocytic leukemia in adults, *N. Engl. J. Med.*, **277** (1992) 1176–1177.
2. Thomas ED, Buckner CD, Banaji M, et al. One hundred patients with acute leukemia treated by chemotherapy, total body irradiation, and allogeneic bone marrow transplantation, *Blood*, **49** (1977) 511–533.
3. Thomas ED. Marrow transplantation for malignant diseases, *J. Clin. Oncol.*, **1** (1983) 517–531.
4. Stone RM and Mayer RJ. Treatment of the newly diagnosed adult with de novo acute myeloid leukemia, *Hematol. Oncol. Clin N. Am.*, **7** (1993) 47–64.
5. Hoelzer D. Treatment of acute lymphoblastic leukemia, *Semin. Hematol.*, **31** (1994) 1–15.
6. Hines JD, Oken MM, Mazza JJ, et al. High-dose cytosine arabinoside and m-AMSA is effective therapy in relapsed acute nonlymphocytic leukemia, *J. Clin. Oncol.*, **2** (1984) 545–549.
7. Herzig RH, Lazarus HM, Wolff SN, et al. High-dose cytosine arabinoside therapy with and without anthracycline antibiotics for remission reinduction of acute nonlymphoblastic leukemia, *J. Clin. Oncol.*, **3** (1985) 992–997.
8. Freund M, Diedrich H, Ganser A, et al. Treatment of relapsed or refractory adult acute lymphocytic leukemia, *Cancer*, **69** (1992) 709–716.
9. Milpied N, Gisselbrecht C, Harousseau JL, et al. Successful treatment of adult acute lymphoblastic leukemia after relapse with prednisone, intermediate-dose cytarabine, mitoxantrone, and etoposide (PAME) chemotherapy, *Cancer*, **66** (1990) 627–631.
10. Giona F, Testi AM, Annino L, et al. Treatment of primary refractory and relapsed acute lymphoblastic leukaemia in children and adults: the GIMEMA/AIEOP experience. Gruppo Italiano Malattie Ematologiche Maligne dell'Adulto. Associazione Italiana Ematologia ed Ocologia Pediatrica, *Br. J. Haematol.*, **86** (1994) 55–61.
11. Archimbaud E, Thomas X, Leblond V, et al. Timed sequential chemotherapy for previously treated patients with acute myeloid leukemia: long-term follow-up of the etoposide, mitoxantrone, and cytarabine-86 trial, *J. Clin. Oncol.*, **13** (1995) 11–18.
12. Estey E. Treatment of refractory AML, *Leukemia*, **10** (1996) 932–936.
13. Copelan EA, McGuire EA. The biology and treatment of acute lymphoblastic leukemia in adults, *Blood*, **85** (1995) 1151–1168.
14. Appelbaum FR. Allogeneic hematopoietic stem cell transplantation for acute leukemia, *Semin. Oncol.*, **24** (1997) 114–123.

15. Champlin R, Gale RP. Acute myelogenous leukemia: recent advances in therapy, *Blood*, **69** (1987) 1551–1562.

16. Schiller GJ. Treatment of resistant disease, *Leukemia*, **12** (1998) S20–S24.

17. Wiernik PH, Banks PL, Case DC Jr, et al. Cytarabine plus idarubicin or daunorubicin as induction and consolidation therapy for previously untreated adult patients with acute myeloid leukemia, *Blood*, **79** (1992) 313–319.

18. Vogler WR, Velez-Garci E, Weiner RS, et al. A phase III trial comparing idarubicin and daunorubicin in combination with cytarabine in acute myelogenous leukemia: a Southeastern Cancer Study Group Study, *J. Clin. Oncol.*, **10** (1992) 1103–1111.

19. Berman E, Heller G, Santorsa J, et al. Results of a randomized trial comparing idarubicin and cytosine arabinoside with daunorubicin and cytosine arabinoside in adult patients with newly diagnosed acute myelogenous leukemia, *Blood*, **77** (1991) 1666–1674.

20. Forman SJ, Schmidt GM, Nademanee AP, et al. Allogeneic bone marrow transplantation for primary induction failure for patients with acute leukemia, *J. Clin. Oncol.*, **9** (1991) 1570–1574.

21. Mehta J, Powles R, Horton C, et al. Bone marrow transplantation for primary refractory acute leukemia, *Bone Marrow Transplant.*, **14** (1994) 415–418.

22. Biggs JC, Horowitz MM, Gale RP, et al. Bone marrow transplants may cure patients with acute leukemia never achieving remission with chemotherapy, *Blood*, **80** (1992) 1090–1093.

23. Drobyski WR, Endean DJ, Klein JP, et al. Detection of BCR/ABL RNA transcripts using the polymerase chain reaction is highly predictive for relapse in patients transplanted with unrelated marrow grafts for chronic myelogenous leukaemia, *Br. J. Haematol.*, **98** (1997) 458–466.

24. Hochhaus A, Reiter A, Skladny H, et al. Molecular monitoring of residual disease in chronic myelogenous leukemia patients after therapy, *Recent Results Cancer Res.*, **144** (1998) 36–45.

25. Porter DL, Roth MS, Lee SJ, et al. Adoptive immunotherapy with donor mononuclear cell infusions to treat relapse of acute leukemia or myelodysplasia after allogeneic bone marrow transplantation, *Bone Marrow Transplant.*, **18** (1996) 975–980.

26. Fefer A, Robinson N, Benyunes MC, et al. Interleukin-2 therapy after bone marrow or stem cell transplantation for hematologic malignancies, *Cancer J. Sci. Am.*, **3** (1997) S48–53.

27. Bonini C, Ferrari G, Verzeletti S, et al. HSV-TK gene transfer into donor lymphocytes for control of allogeneic graft-versus-leukemia, *Science*, **276** (1997) 1719–1724.

28. Appelbaum FR, Clift RA, Buckner CD, et al. Allogeneic marrow transplantation for acute nonlymphoblastic leukemia after first relapse, *Blood*, **61** (1983) 949–953.

29. Clift RA, Buckner CD, Thomas ED, et al. The treatment of acute nonlymphoblastic leukemia by allogeneic bone marrow transplantation, *Bone Marrow Transplant.*, **2** (1987) 243–258.

30. Clift RA, Buckner CD, Appelbaum FR, et al. Allogeneic marrow transplantation during untreated first relapse of acute leukemia, *J. Clin. Oncol.*, **10** (1992) 1723–1729.

31. Weiden PL, Flournoy N, Thomas ED, et al. Antileukemic effect of graft-versus-host disease in human recipients of allogeneic-marrow grafts, *N. Engl. J. Med.*, **300** (1979) 1068–1073.

32. Schmitz N, Gassmann W, Rister M, et al. Fractionated total body irradiation and high-dose VP 16-213 followed by allogeneic bone marrow transplantation in advanced leukemias, *Blood*, **72** (1988) 1567–1573.

33. Herzig RH, Bortin MM, Barrett AJ, et al. Bone-marrow transplantation in high-risk acute lymphoblastic leukaemia in first and second remission, *Lancet*, **1** (1987) 786–789.

34. Dinsmore R, Kirkpatrick D, Flomenberg N, et al. Allogeneic bone marrow transplantation for patients with acute nonlymphocytic leukemia, *Blood*, **63** (1984) 649–656.

35. Dinsmore R, Kirkpatrick D, Flomenberg N, et al. Allogeneic bone marrow transplantation for patients with acute lymphoblastic leukemia, *Blood*, **62** (1983) 381–388.

36. Wingard JR, Piantadosi S, Santos GW, et al. Allogeneic bone marrow transplantation for patients with high-risk acute lymphoblastic leukemia, *J. Clin. Oncol.*, **8** (1990) 820–830.

37. Kernan NA, Bartsch G, Ash RC, et al. Analysis of 462 transplantations from unrelated donors facilitated by the National Marrow Donor Program, *N. Engl. J. Med.*, **328** (1993) 593–602.

38. Schiller G, Feig SA, Territo M, et al. Treatment of advanced acute leukaemia with allogeneic bone marrow from unrelated donors, *Br. J. Haematol.*, **88** (1994) 72–78.

39. Sierra J, Storer B, Hansen JA, et al. Transplantation of marrow cells from unrelated donors for treatment of high-risk acute leukemia: the effect of leukemic burden, donor HLA-matching, and marrow cell dose, *Blood*, **89** (1997) 4226–4235.

40. Laport GF, Larson RA. Treatment of adult acute lymphoblastic leukemia, *Semi. Oncol.*, **24** (1997) 70–82.

41. Blume KG, Beutler E, Bross KJ, et al. Bone-marrow ablation and allogeneic marrow transplantation in acute leukemia, *N. Engl. J. Med.*, **302** (1980) 1041–1046.

42. Doney K, Fisher LD, Appelbaum FR, et al. Treatment of acute lymphoblastic leukemia with allogeneic bone marrow transplantation. Multivariate analysis of factors affecting acute graft-versus-host-disease, relapse, and relapse-free survival, *Bone Marrow Transplant.*, **7** (1991) 453–459.

43. Szydlo R, Goldman JM, Klein JP, et al. Results of allogeneic bone marrow transplants for leukemia using donors other than HLA-identical siblings, *J. Clin. Oncol.*, **15** (1997) 1767–1777.

44. Nademanee A, Schmidt GM, Parker P, et al. The outcome of matched unrelated donor bone marrow transplantation in patients with hematologic malignancies using molecular typing for donor selection and graft-versus-host disease prophylaxis regimen of cyclosporine, methotrexate, and prednisone, *Blood,* **86** (1995) 1228–1234.

45. Geller RB, Devine SM, O'Toole K, et al. Allogeneic bone marrow transplantation with matched unrelated donors for patients with hematologic malignancies using a preparative regimen of high-dose cyclophosphamide and fractionated total body irradiation, *Bone Marrow Transplant.*, **20** (1997) 219–225.

46. Sierra J, Storer B, Hansen JA, et al. Transplantation of marrow cells from unrelated donors for treatment of high-risk acute leukemia: the effect of leukemic burden, donor HLA-matching, and marrow cell dose, *Blood,* **89** (1997) 4226–4235.

47. Storb R, Deeg HJ, Whitehead J, et al. Methotrexate and cyclosporine compared with cyclosporine alone for prophylaxis of acute graft versus host disease after marrow transplantation for leukemia, *N. Engl. J. Med.*, **314** (1986) 729–735.

48. Horowitz MM, Gale RP, Sondel PM, et al. Graft-versus-leukemia reactions after bone marrow transplantation, *Blood,* **75** (1990) 555–562.

49. Marmont AM, Horowitz MM, Gale RP, et al. T-cell depletion of HLA-identical transplants in leukemia, *Blood,* **78** (1991) 2120–2130.

50. Soiffer RJ, Fairclough D, Robertson M, et al. CD6-depleted allogeneic bone marrow transplantation for acute leukemia in first complete remission, *Blood,* **89** (1997) 3039–3047.

51. Papadopoulos EB, Carabasi MH, Castro-Malaspina H, et al. T-cell-depleted allogeneic bone marrow transplantation as postremission therapy for acute myelogenous leukemia: freedom from relapse in the absence of graft-versus-host disease, *Blood,* **91** (1998) 1083–1090.

52. Jansen J, Hanks S, Akard L, et al. Selective T cell depletion with CD8-conjugated magnetic beads in the prevention of graft-versus-host disease after allogeneic bone marrow transplantation, *Bone Marrow Transplant.*, **15** (1995) 271–278.

53. Gale RP, Horowitz MM, Ash RC, et al. Identical-twin bone marrow transplants for leukemia, *Ann. Intern. Med.*, **120** (1994) 646–652.

54. Kolb HJ, Schattenberg A, Goldman JM, et al. Graft-versus-leukemia effect of donor lymphocyte transfusions in marrow grafted patients. European Group for Blood and Marrow Transplantation Working Party Chronic Leukemia, *Blood,* **86** (1995) 2041–2050.

55. Collins RH Jr, Shpilberg O, Drobyski WR, et al. Donor leukocyte infusions in 140 patients with relapsed malignancy after allogeneic bone marrow transplantation, *J. Clin. Oncol.*, **15** (1997) 433–444.

56. Vogelsang GB, Hess AD. Graft-versus-host disease: new directions for a persistent problem, *Blood,* **84** (1994) 2061–2067.

57. Champlin R. Graft-versus-leukemia without graft-versus-host disease: an elusive goal of bone marrow transplantation, *Semin. Hematol.*, **29** (1992) 46–52.

58. Giralt S, Hester J, Huh Y, et al. CD8-depleted donor lymphocyte infusion as treatment for relapsed chronic myelogenous leukemia after allogeneic bone marrow transplantation, *Blood,* **86** (1995) 4337–4343.

59. Champlin R, Ho W, Gajewski J, et al. Selective depletion of CD8$^+$ T lymphocytes for prevention of graft-versus-host disease after allogeneic bone marrow transplantation, *Blood,* **76** (1990) 418–423.

60. Nimer SD, Giorgi J, Gajewski JL, et al. Selective depletion of CD8$^+$ cells for prevention of graft-versus-host disease after bone marrow transplantation: a randomized trial, *Transplantation,* **57** (1994) 82–87.

61. Estey E, Thall P, David C. Design and analysis of trials of salvage therapy in acute myelogenous leukemia, *Cancer Chemother. Pharmacol.*, **40** (1997) S9–12.

9 What Is the Role of Autologous Stem Cell Transplantation for Leukemia?

Selina M. Luger, MD, and
Edward A. Stadtmauer, MD

CONTENTS

From: *Current Controversies in Bone Marrow Transplantation*
Edited by: B. Bolwell © Humana Press Inc., Totowa, NJ

1. INTRODUCTION

At first glance, autologous stem cell transplantation (ASCT) for a bone marrow (BM) disease such as leukemia makes little intuitive sense. Regardless of the eradication of leukemia by high-dose chemotherapy (CT), stem cells previously collected, either in remission or at time of active disease, will almost certainly be contaminated by a population of tumor cells. Viable cells will logically result in relapse. If, however, there are no viable tumor cells present at the time of the transplant, then one would wonder whether high-dose therapy (HDT) is really necessary. Long-term survivors after ASCT are perhaps only those who would have been cured by therapy received prior to the SCT. This chapter investigates the truth or fallacy of the above statements.

If HDT and SCT is to be successful as a curative therapy for leukemia, then one or more of the following must be true:

1. HDT overcomes drug resistance, and therefore converts patients in remission to cure, and thereby improves outcome.
2. The processing and purging of stem cells is capable of eliminating the contaminating leukemia cells from the graft, thereby resulting in cure.
3. There is some not-well-understood difference between high-dose chemotherapy (HDCT) and conventional-dose therapy that stimulates the host immune system to eradicate minimal residual leukemia cells in the form of adoptive immunotherapy.

On the other hand, if SCT does not alter the natural history of leukemia more than does conventional-dose CT, then the numerous promising phase II trials of this modality must be misleading. The most likely reason for this would be the possibility that patients chosen for SCT are different than historical controls, and this selection bias accounts for improved outcome. Phase II and, when available, randomized clinical trials are reviewed, to critically evaluate the role of SCT in leukemia.

2. AUTOLOGOUS SCT FOR ACUTE MYELOID LEUKEMIA

2.1. History

The first report of autologous bone marrow transplantation (AMBT) for acute myeloid leukemia (AML) was published in 1977 by Gorin, et al. *(1)*. This patient with AML in first relapse had marrow collected in first remission, which was stored in liquid nitrogen and infused after a myeloablative regimen at time of relapse. The patient experienced hematopoietic recovery and entered a second remission. Soon thereafter, Fefer et al. *(2)* reported a series of patients with refractory AML who had syngeneic donor transplants, and also demonstrated long-term relapse-free survival (RFS). A number of reports followed, utilizing first remission marrow for hematopoietic rescue after HDT for refractory AML, all demonstrating high response rates, but few cures *(3)*. With these promising reports of activity, the procedure was moved earlier into the course of disease, at first or subsequent remission.

2.2. Rationale

Increased dose and dose intensity of postremission therapy has now been shown to clearly improve outcome in AML. In 1985, Cassileth et al. *(4)* demonstrated that low-dose cytosine arabinoside (Ara-C) maintenance CT was superior to no postremission therapy in first remission AML. Subsequently, a number of trials have demonstrated that higher doses of ara-C, either in a single course or a number of postremission cycles, is superior to lower doses of ara-C postremission therapy *(5,6)*. SCT was the logical progression of this idea: administering myeloablative doses of CT, hopefully so toxic to hematopoietic stem cells (HSC) that replacement was necessary for hematopoietic recovery.

2.3. Prognostic Factors

A number of patient characteristics have now been identified as prognostic factors in the treatment of AML. Interpretation of clinical trials must be made, because of different prognostic subtypes, and a more disease-directed therapeutic approach is evolving. Factors that have consistently been found to predict poor therapeutic outcome with standard CT include: older age, high white blood cell (WBC) count at diagnosis, trilineage morphologic dysplasia, more than one cycle of induction CT to achieve complete remission (CR), poor-risk cytogenetics (including abnormalities of chromosomes 5, 7, 8, 11, and 13), CD34 and MDR-1 expression by flow cytometry, secondary AML arising from a preexisting stem cell disorder or from therapy-related, extramedullary disease, or residual cytogenetic abnormalities present after a course of induction CT. Good prognostic factors include the lack of the above characteristics, but, most particularly, favorable cytogenetic abnormalities, such as the 15:17 translocation in acute promyelocytic leukemia, or the 8;21 translocation and abnormalities of the chromosome 16, thought to involve abnormalities in the core-binding-factor complex.

In general, patients with secondary or therapy-related AML, myelodysplasia, and residual cytogenetic abnormalities are rarely treated with ASCT. All other subgroups have been considered appropriate for clinical trials.

2.4. Methods of SCT

2.4.1. HIGH-DOSE REGIMENS

A number of myeloablative regimens have been used for SCT in AML. The two most common were derived by the pioneering work in AML by the Johns Hopkins *(7)* and Seattle *(8)* groups. To this day, total body irradiation (TBI) and cyclophosphamide (Cy), or the busulfan (Bu) and Cy, are the most common regimens utilized. Bu/Cy consists of 1 mg/kg oral Bu given every 6 h for 16 total doses (16 mg/kg), followed by 2–4 d Cy for a total of 120–200 mg/kg. Most centers utilize the Bu/Cy(2) regimen *(7,8)*. Most recently, Bu dosing has been monitored and adjusted pharmacokinetically by measuring the area-under-the-curve (AUC) *(9)*. Maintenance of AUC levels within a narrow range is being investigated, to determine whether toxicity and survival can be optimized. Additionally, intravenous preparations of Bu may improve the delivery and decrease the toxicity of this agent *(10)*. Radiation is usually given in six fractionated doses of 200 cGy, with the 120 mg/kg Cy dose. No definitive data suggests a clear benefit of a radiation-containing regimen over a CT regimen. VP-16 has been added to both regimens, resulting in increased mucositis and hyperbilirubinema, without clear incremental benefit *(11)*.

2.4.2. STEM CELL SOURCE

Pluripotent HSCs can be derived directly from bone marrow (BM) via numerous percutaneous aspirations or by leukopheresis of cells circulating in the blood. Blood-derived stem cells appear to consistently shorten the time to neutrophil and platelet recovery, compared to BM, but this difference can be substantially reduced by the use of hematopoietic growth factors, and has not clearly been shown to alter outcome. BM-derived stem cells have traditionally been used as the stem cell source of choice for in vitro purging techniques, because of easier logistics.

2.4.3. STEM CELL IN VITRO PURGING

Stem cells derived from BM or blood have a high likelihood of contamination with leukemia. These residual leukemic cells may then contribute to relapse (12). Work by Brenner et al. (13) has demonstrated that leukemic cells in the BM graft are present at the time of relapse. Patients had one-third harvested marrow incubated with LNL-6 retroviral vector, which contains the neomycin-resistant genes. Patients underwent SCT using both marked and unmarked marrows. At the time of relapse, a subset of leukemia cells contained the neomycin-resistant gene, suggesting that at least some component of the relapse was caused by cells from the reinfused product (13)

Ex vivo laboratory studies show that a number of different purging techniques will substantially reduce the contamination of leukemia cells from the harvested product (14,15). However, no study has shown a survival benefit of purged stem cells, compared to unpurged stem cells. In fact, studies of syngeneic BMT for AML show a >50% relapse rate, suggesting that failure of the myeloablative regimen may be a greater reason for failure of transplant than relapse from contaminating tumor cells (16). A number of approaches for stem cell purging have been utilized for AML. Most studies have utilized pharmacological purging with Cy-derived compounds of 4-hydroperoxy-cyclophosphamide (4-HC) or mafosfamide (17,18). Cy requires the liver for metabolism into the volatile metabolite, hydroxycyclophosphamide. The purging agents, however, are metabolized intracellularly to phosphoramide mustard, the active agent. VP-16 has also been added to these agents for increased effect (19).

Monoclonal antibodies (mAbs) have also been used to purge contaminating early hematopoietic cells. Anti-CD33, anti-CD15, and anti-CD14 mAbs have been utilized, along with complement fixation (20–23). Other methods that have been utilized include density separation, elutriation, and cytokines, such as interleukin-2. Although no randomized study has yet been performed, comparison of multiple phase II studies suggests that these purging techniques have resulted in a delayed engraftment and resultant increased morbidity from infection and bleeding without clear benefit, compared to unpurged stem cell products. The use of granulocyte colony-stimulating factor and granulocyte-macrophage colony-stimulating factor after purged SCTs has not been studied extensively, and may ameliorate some of these toxicities (24). Alternatively, amifostine has been used as a cytoprotective agent, to allow for sparing of normal HSCs in the graft (25).

Retrospective studies have compared purged marrow to unpurged stem cells for AML patients in first remission. The Autologous Blood and Marrow Registry reviewed 294 patients with AML who underwent ASCT in first and second remission. In a multivariate analysis, patients who received 4-HC-purged stem cells had a significantly lower rate of treatment failure (3 yr leukemia-free survival 56 vs 33% CR1, 39 vs 10% CR2), but without clear benefit in terms of overall survival (OS) (Miller, unpublished data).

Despite a sound rationale and laboratory evidence for efficacy of purging techniques,

Table 1
ABMT for AML in Early Relapse or Second and Subsequent Remission

RF	# Patients	Regimen	Purge	DFS (%)	Relapse (%)
Meloni et al. (26)	60 CR2	BAVC	No	42	58
Chopra et al. (27)	9 ER	Bu/Cy	No	33	70
	25 CR2				
Yeager (28)	82 CR2	Bu/Cy	4 HC	34 CR2	58 CR2
	16 CR3			26 CR3	55 CR3
Korbling et al. (29)	30 CR2	Cu/TBI	Mafosfamide	34	65
Rosenfeld et al. (30)	8 ER	Bu/Cy or	4 HC	19	73
	7 CR2	Cy/TBI			
	9 ≥ CR3				
Ball et al. (31)	23 ER	Cy/TBI or	mAb	30	48
	84 ≥ CR2	Bu/Cy or			
		Bu/VP-16			
Linker et al. (32)	19 CR2	Bu/VP-16	4-HC	56	25
	2 CR3				

BAVC, BCNU, amaserine (AMSA), VP-16, Ara-C; ER, Early relapse.

there remains no definitive evidence of a benefit from any of the purging techniques, compared to unpurged stem cells.

2.5. Clinical Results

2.5.1. PHASE II TRIALS

Numerous phase II trials have demonstrated the efficacy of ASCT as a consolidation therapy for AML in remission. Trials in second and subsequent remission generally demonstrate a 20–30% long-term RFS; studies in first remission show a 34–70% long-term RFS, with mortalities ranging from <5 to 15%. Table 1 reviews phase II studies in patients in early relapse or second and subsequent remissions. In general, in these patients, first relapses occurred after periods of <1 yr. Actuarial disease-free survival (DFS) and relapse rates are based on median follow-ups of 20–40 mo. Although no randomized study has been performed, these results are clearly better than those with standard CT in this patient population.

Numerous phase II studies have subsequently been done in patients in first remission (33–35). Although DFS of up to 70% has been reported, the interpretation of these results is limited by a number of factors. In particular, patients on innovative phase II trials are generally healthier, younger, and in remission longer than historical controls. In addition, studies have different induction CTs, various types and numbers of consolidation therapies prior to transplantation, variable durations of remission prior to transplantation, short follow-up times at time of publication, different stem cell manipulations, and different high-dose myeloablative regimens. Prospective randomized trials are needed to compare these results to the results of standard-dose CT and allo-SCT.

2.5.2. PHASE III RANDOMIZED TRIALS

Table 2 lists the results of prospective randomized trials that have been completed in first-remission AML. All trials have compared assignment to allo-BMT for patients

Table 2
Randomized Trials of ASCT for AML in First Remission

Ref.	Treatment	No. Tx/Intended	EFS %	OS (%)
Zittoun et al. (36)	ABMT	95/128	48	56
	DA	104/126	30	46
	Allo BMT	144/168	55	59
Harousseau et al. (37)	ABMT	75/86	44	50
	IA/RA	71/78	40	54.5
	Allo-BMT	73/78	44	52.5
Burnett et al. (38)	MidAC/ABMT	126/190	53	57
	MidAC	186/191	40	45
Cassileth et al. (39)	ABMT (4 HC-purged)	63/116	37	47
	HDAC	99/118	35	54
	Allo-BMT	105/120	43	46

Tx/Intended, number treated/intended to treat; IA, Idarubicin/ara-C; RA, rubidazone/ara-C; DA, dauon-rubicin/ara-C; HDAC, high-dose ara-C; MidAC, Mitoxantrone, Mid-dose ara-C

with human leukocyte antigen (HLA)-matched sibling donors to a randomization for the rest of the group to ASCT vs conventional-dose CT. All trials except the Eastern Cooperative Oncology Group (ECOG) study used unpurged marrow. Results are all given by intent-to-treat analysis.

The AML-8 European Organization for the Research and Treatment of Cancer-GIMEMA trial included 941 eligible and evaluable patients with newly diagnosed AML: Median age was 33 yr (range 11–59 yr) (36). Patients all received daunorubicin and ara-C induction therapy (3/7) for 1–2 cycles, and, if they achieved CR, received one cycle of high-dose ara-C and amsacrine consolidation. Patients with HLA-matched sibling donors then went on to allo-BMT utilizing Cy/TBI or Bu/Cy(2), and the others were randomized to either ASCT, with the same myeloablative regimens receiving at least 1×10^8 nucleated cells/kg without in vitro purging, or to a final course of high-dose ara-C and daunorubicin consolidation. Sixty-six percent (623) entered CR, with 168 assigned allogeneic transplant (allotransplant), 128 randomized to autologous transplant (autotransplant), and 126 CT. A number of these patients did not complete assigned therapy because of such reasons as early relapse, toxic death, nonlethal toxicities, or refusal of assigned therapy. Ultimately, 144 completed allo transplant, 95 auto transplant, and 104 CT. The time to initiation of assigned therapy was significantly longer for allo-BMT and ABMT vs CT ($p < 0.001$). There was an even distribution of prognostic factors and patient characteristics, except that all patients assigned allotransplant were <45 yr of age; nine patients randomized to autotransplant and 10 patients randomized to CT were between the ages of 46 and 59 yr. The 4-yr RFS estimates were 55, 48, and 30% for allotransplant, autotransplant, and CT, respectively, with no difference between allo- and autotransplant, but both transplants were significantly better than CT ($p = 0.05$). Likelihood of relapse was highest for CT-treated patients; death in first remission was highest for allo-BMT patients. Ultimately, the 4-yr OS was not signifi-cantly different, at 59, 56, and 46%, respectively, suggesting the salvagability of the CT failures with transplantation in second remission. Time to hematopoietic recovery, both for neutrophils and platelets, and length of hospitalization were greatest for ASCT, probably because of the low stem cell numbers infused.

In the Groupe Ouest Est Leucemies Aigues Myeloblastiques (GOELAM) Trial, patients with newly diagnosed AML received induction CT with either idarubicin or rubidazone, with ara-C for 1–2 cycles *(37)*. After achieving remission, patients with HLA-identical sibling donors could receive a single course of amsacrine and ara-C prior to allo-BMT utilizing Bu/Cy(4) or Cy/TBI preparative regimens. Patients without HLA-matched donors went on to a single course of idarubicin or rubidazone and high-dose ara-C consolidation, then were randomized to ABMT with Bu/Cy$_4$ preparative regimen and infusion of a minimum of 1×10^8 nucleated cells/kg nonpurged stem cells or to a single course of amsacrine and VP-16 consolidation. Five hundred and four patients were eligible and evaluable, and 73% (367) achieved CR. Median age was 36 yr (range 15–50 yr), with 88 patients assigned to allo-BMT and 86 patients randomized to ABMT vs 78 randomized to CT. Only 164/267 patients in CR following induction, without sibling donors, were randomized. A subset of patients did not receive assigned therapy, because of early relapse, nonlethal toxicities, or refusal of assigned therapy. Time to initiation of assigned therapy was least for allo-BMT, and all patients receiving allo transplant were <40-yr old. Four-yr RFS and OS were 44 and 52.5% for allo-BMT, 44 and 50% for ABMT, and 40 and 54.5% for CT. These were not significantly different. Time to hematopoietic recovery was similar for autotransplant and CT, except for time-to-platelet recovery, which was significantly longer in autotransplant, once again perhaps related to the low numbers of stem cells infused.

In the Medical Research Council AML 10 Trial *(38)*, newly diagnosed patients with AML were randomly assigned Daunorubicin, Ara-C, 6-Thioguanine (DAT) or Ara-c, Daunorubicin, Etoposide (DAE) for 1–2 cycles. Patients entering CR then received amsacrine, ARA-C, and VP-16, followed by collection of at least 1×10^8 nucleated cells/kg stem cells. Patients then went on to another consolidation consisting of mitoxantrone and high-dose ara-C. Patients with HLA-matched sibling donors went on to allo-BMT utilizing the Cy/TBI regimen. All others were randomized to autotransplantation using the same preparative regimen, or to no further therapy. One thousand five hundred and nine patients (81%) entered CR. Three hundred and seventy-eight were assigned allo-transplant, but, of the 1131 eligible for randomization, 670 were not randomized, with 481 going on to no further therapy, and 79 going on to autotransplantation. One hundred and ninety were randomized to autotransplant, and 191 to no further therapy, and these groups were well-matched for prognostic factors. Ultimately, 126 went on to autotransplant, and 186 remained on the observation arm. With the median follow-up of 4.8 yr, 7-yr RFS and probability of relapse were significantly different in the two randomized groups, at 53 and 37% for autotransplant, and 40 and 58% for the observation group, respectively. Although there was no significant difference in OS at 2 yr, a significant benefit for autotransplant emerged beyond 2 yr. Seven-year OS was 57% for autotransplant and 45% for the observation arm ($p = 0.2$). Again, there was a significant delay in recovery for the autologous arm, and a median number of 2.18 $\times 10^8$ nucleated cells/kg were infused.

The ECOG-led North American Intergroup trial *(39)* enrolled newly diagnosed patients with AML receiving 1–2 cycles of idarubicin and ara-C (3/7), followed by intensification with idarubicin and ara-C (2/5). Patients with HLA-compatible siblings were assigned to allo-BMT; all others in CR were randomized to either high-dose Ara-C (HDAC) consolidation or ABMT using 4-HC-purged marrow and the Bu/Cy$_4$ preparative regimen. 518/740 patients achieved a CR. 120 patients were assigned to allo-BMT; 116 and 120 patients were randomized to ABMT and HDAC consolidation, respectively. Ultimately, 105, 63, and 99 patients went on to receive their assigned allotransplant, autotransplant, or HDAC consolidation, respectively. With a median follow-up of 4 yr, DFS was not significantly different at 43, 37, and 35%, respectively. OS was slightly better in the HDCT arm, at 54%, than in either the allo- or autotransplant arms, at 46 and 47%, respectively ($p = 0.05$).

2.5.3. CONCLUSIONS

The adult patient with AML currently has three effective postremission therapies, including HDAC consolidation, allo-BMT, and ABMT. Four large randomized trials of these postremission therapies demonstrate no clear survival advantage for any of the postremission therapies. Current techniques of blood SCT and hematopoietic growth-factor-stimulated recovery should improve hematopoietic recovery times and decrease morbidity, but are unlikely to have a major impact on OS. In summary, the benefit of ABMT over conventional-dose therapy in first remission AML remains unproven by available randomized studies. The best results, however, have been seen in patients who undergo autotransplant following intensive consolidation. The lack of clear benefit of ASCT for first remission AML suggests that phase II trials suffered from a patient selection bias, or that the incremental benefit was too small to be detected in the randomized trials. The success of CT consolidation, at least in part, is attributable to the salvagability of relapsed patients with either allo- or auto-BMT. Randomized studies are difficult to interpret, because so few patients actually receive their intended treatment. Investigation into improved pretransplant regimens, posttransplant therapies, and stem-cell-purging techniques may improve the outcome. The benefits of ABMT, compared to CT, for patients in second and subsequent remission, appear stronger, and BMT in this setting should be considered a standard of care. There remains a strong need for new phase I and II trials investigating novel therapies in this disease.

3. ASCT FOR CHRONIC MYELOID LEUKEMIA

3.1. History

One of the major advances in leukemia therapy has been the use of allo-BMT as a curative therapy of chronic myeloid leukemia (CML). CML is now the number one indication for allo-BMT in the world, with greater than 50% of patients long-term disease-free survivors. By virtue of the increasing utilization of alternative donors, the majority of patients will find a suitable donor for allotransplantation. In no other disease is there such clear evidence of the beneficial effect of adoptive immunotherapy or the graft-versus-leukemia effect. Therefore, patients with suitable donors should be directed toward allo transplantation. For patients without suitable donors, or who are older than age 55 yr, interferon α (IFN-α) can induce prolonged remissions in 10–20% of patients, although the long-term outcome of these patients remains to be determined. For IFN-α nonresponders, ASCT has been considered.

The first ASCT for CML was conducted in the early 1980s, and was also the first use of blood-derived stem cells for transplantation. Patients had chronic-phase stem cells cryopreserved, and then, at time of blast crisis, received HDCT and reinfusion of chronic-phase stem cells. Most patients achieved chronic phase, but these remissions were of brief duration, limited to 6 mo to 1 yr *(40,41)*.

Table 3
ASCT for CML

Ref.	Purge	No. Patients	CR/PR	Graft failure
Carlo-Stella et al(47)	Mafosfamide	10	6/1	
McGlave et al. (48)	IFN-γ	44	10/12	
Barnett et al. (49)	Long-term culture	22	13/3	5
Coutinho et al. (50)	Long-term culture	9	4/3	2
DeFabritiis et al. (51)	bcr-abl antisense	8	2/0	0
Gewirtz et al. (52)	c-myb antisense	8	1/3	1
Reiffers et al. (53)	None	49	10/5	
Simonsson et al. (54)	In vivo	30	13/10	
Carella et al. (55)	In vivo	30	16/10	0
Verfaillie et al. (56)	In vivo	47	4/9	1

3.2. Rationale

SCT for CML is based on the assumption that, co-existing with Philadelphia chromosome (Ph^1)-positive stem cells are residual normal Ph^1-negative stem cells, and myeloablative therapy with infusion of Ph^1-negative cells may ameliorate disease. Laboratory evidence for this includes: Long-term culture techniques can result in Ph^1-negative colonies identified (42); in vitro colony-forming unit assays show the growth of Ph^1-negative colonies intermixed with Ph^1-positive colonies (43); and at presentation, both Ph^1-positive and -negative cells can be identified (44). Clinical evidence for benign precursors in CML include the observation that IFN-α can induce complete cytogenetic remission in 10–20% of patients (45), and patients in chronic phase or blast crisis, treated with intensive CT regimens, can induce transient Ph^1-negative status (46).

Even if eradication of Ph^1-positive cells is not possible, reduction of such cells may improve survival by a number of mechanisms, including: The BCR-ABL protein may be responsible in part for the evolution of chronic phase to blast crisis, so decreased Ph^1-positive cells, and therefore the production of p210, may be useful for delaying blast crisis; Ph^1-negative cells may also have a growth advantage over the Ph^1-positive cells, and SCT may set the clock back in the natural history of an individual's disease. Based on these assumptions, clinical trials have been initiated utilizing SCT for CML.

3.3. Phase I and Phase II Trials

The field of ASCT for CML is far less advanced than for AML. Most clinical information is derived from small phase I and phase II trials, usually enrolling <50 patients. Most trials included patients in chronic phase or in early accelerated phase, because of the poor results of early studies with blast crisis. Table 3 shows the results of ASCT in chronic-phase CML, using either unpurged or purged stem cell techniques. Partial cytogenetic responses can be achieved after transplant with unselected stem cells, with generally rapid hematopoietic engraftment and low toxicity, but no clear survival advantage, compared to historical controls. Numerous techniques have been utilized in an attempt to decrease the contamination of Ph^1-positive cells in the stem cell product. Mafosfamide and 4-HC have been utilized in a number of studies with early Ph^1-negative engraftment, but virtually all ultimately have progressed (47,57). Interferon-γ (IFN-γ) has been used as a purging agent, but has demonstrated a significant stem cell toxicity, to the extent that many patients have required nonpurged backup marrow to reestablish hematopoietic engraftment, and, again, virtually all patients have progressed *(48)*. Barnett et al. *(49)* treated a series of patients with ex vivo cultured marrow. This study illustrates the potential selection bias of these trials. Eighty-seven patients were enrolled, but only 36 patients collected enough Ph[l]-negative cells after ex vivo culturing techniques, to consider transplantation. Of these patients, 22 underwent SCT, and 13/16 evaluable patients were Ph[l]-negative when first assayed. The majority of these patients had a rapid relapse.

CML stem cells have been one of the first targets for antisense oligodeoxynucleotides (AS-ODN) in the treatment of cancer. These short sequences of DNA, which are the reverse complement of the mRNA encoded by the gene to be disrupted, may lead to specific inhibition of growth of the targeted cells. In CML, bcr-abl-RNA has been targeted because of laboratory studies that showed inhibition of cell proliferation and restored susceptibility to apoptosis of cells when exposed to bcr abl AS ODN in vitro *(50,59)*. Initial clinical trials, however, incubating accelerated-phase BM with anti-bcr-abl AS-ODN, showed little suggestion of therapeutic effects *(51)*.

Gewirtz et al. *(52,60)* has been investigating AS-ODNs to the c-*myb* proto-oncogene which is essential for hematopoiesis, and there appears to be a differential effect in vitro on susceptibility to c-*myb* AS-ODN of malignant and normal HSC. Using a 24-h incubation with c-*myb* antisense, 7/8 patients in chronic-phase CML demonstrated rapid engraftment, with 4/6 evaluable patients demonstrating major cytogenetic response, but most patients experienced rapid progression of disease. With a 72-h purge, 5/5 patients experienced poor engraftment, and required backup unpurged marrow. Studies with a 48-h purge are currently underway.

Perhaps a more promising approach than in vitro purging is the utilization of standard dose CT and/or IFN-α to in-vivo-purge patients to Ph[l]-negativity, and then conduct transplant utilizing in-vivo-purged stem cells. Korbling et al. *(61)* first reported this approach when a patient with chronic-phase CML, who had been induced into cytogenetic remission, was transplanted and recovered with Ph[l]-negative hematopoiesis. A number of trials utilizing this philosophy have ensued. The Swedish–Danish group has reported its results in over 200 patients with CML treated between September 1989 and October 1997 *(54)*. 118 patients were found to have HLA-compatible siblings or unrelated donors, and went on to allo transplant; the remaining 135 patients were treated with IFN-α. If they became Ph[l]-negative, BM and/or stem cell harvest was done. If they remained Ph[l]-positive following a 6-mo trial of IFN, they received up to three different cycles of induction CT. Patients were tested for response after each cycle, and underwent harvest and transplant, if they achieved Ph[l]-negativity. Forty-six patients ultimately underwent autotransplant, three following IFN alone, 21 requiring one cycle of induction CT, 15 requiring two inductions, and seven requiring all three inductions.

Carella et al. *(55)* has reported their experience with the idarubicin, ara-C, VP-16 (ICE) induction regimen, which induced up to 60% of early chronic-phase patients to Ph[l]-negativity, followed by consolidation with SCT. Of nearly 200 patients who received induction, 30 patients were autografted. All engrafted, of which 53% engrafted with Ph[l]-negative BM. This and similar trials have demonstrated that a substantial number of patients do mobilize Ph[l]-negative cells, and that these cells tend to readily engraft, with low treatment-related mortality. However, follow-up is short, and patients in remission >2-yr are few.

3.4. Long-term Results of ASCT for CML

McGlave (62) registered 200 consecutive CML patients undergoing ASCT in North America. The median follow-up was 42 mo, with a range of 9–91 mo, and patients who are transplanted in chronic phase had not reached their median survival. Median survival of patients with accelerated phase was 35.9 mo, and, in blast crisis, 4.1 mo. Currently, an international randomized trial comparing ASCT with unpurged stem cells to prolonged IFN-α therapy is ongoing: Trials similar to this will be necessary to determine the ultimate efficacy of this approach.

3.5. Conclusions

Clinical and laboratory studies in CML suggest Ph[1]-negative stem cells are collectable in CML, and HDCT and SCT can be achieved with reliable engraftment and low mortality. The clinical benefit of this procedure, however, remains unknown, and will require randomized clinical trials; however, pilot studies are encouraging. Currently, the optimal preparative regimen and stem cell manipulation and postremission therapies remain to be determined. Patients with HLA-matched donors should proceed to allo-transplant, and the majority of patients without donors should receive a trial of IFN-α, with the consideration of autologous stem cell harvesting early in the treatment course, should they become Ph[1]-negative.

4. SCT FOR ACUTE LYMPHOBLASTIC LEUKEMIA

4.1. Rationale

Acute lymphoblastic leukemia (ALL) is an uncommon disease of adults. It is very responsive to CT, and the vast majority will enter remission, but relapse is common, and long-term survival is limited to approx 20–30% of patients. Poor prognostic factors include very young or older age, high WBC count at time of diagnosis, and the presence of the Ph[1]. Unlike allo-BMT for myeloid malignancies, there is limited evidence of a beneficial graft-vs-leukemia effect in ALL. The chance for long-term RFS after relapse without transplant, is very limited. ASCT, therefore, has been investigated for the treatment of ALL, because of the responsiveness of ALL to CT, and the possibility of eradicating autologous stem cells of residual disease.

4.2. In Vitro Purging of Stem Cells

mAb purging of HSCs cells has been most extensively studied in ALL, particularly because of the well-known antigens that characterize the disease, and the ability to raise mAbs against these antigens. mAbs against CD9, CD10, CD19, and CD20 have been most commonly used in B-cell ALL, and anti-CD5, and anti-CD7 for T-cell ALL. Similar antibodies have been combined with immunotoxins or magnetic beads, in an attempt to purge marrow. 4-HC has also been used as a purging agent. In vitro laboratory studies demonstrate significant reduction in contaminating tumor cells, but, as with other purging techniques, there has not been clinical evidence to demonstrate the efficacy of this procedure. Most recently, CD34 selection columns have been used to positively select pluripotent HSCs and to passively purge contaminating leukemia cells. The limited degree of selection of these devices, and the possibility of CD34 expression on leukemic blasts, make this approach less promising. In vivo purging with mobilization CT prior to blood stem cell collection is also under investigation in ALL.

4.3. High-dose Regimens

Common regimens for ALL include TBI and cytoxan, with or without the addition of VP-16. Traditionally, the TBI is fractionated, sometimes with an increased dose of 1200–1400 cGy, particularly in the pediatric population. No one regimen has been demonstrated to be superior to another, and, generally, patients have experienced rapid engraftment.

4.4. Phase II Trials

Numerous small phase II trials have been conducted of ABMT for ALL in first CR or in second remission, or with refractory disease. OS has generally ranged between 5 and 20%, for relapsed leukemia, and 2-yr DFS was 30–60%, when transplant is conducted in first CR. Interpretation of these trials suffers from the likely selection bias inherent in phase II trials and the varying pretransplant regimens and prognostic factors of the patients.

4.5. Phase III Trials

Few well-controlled trials compare ASCT to either conventional-dose CT or allo-transplantation in ALL. One prospective trial of high-risk or refractory ALL at the University of Minnesota included 91 patients: 46 underwent transplantation with a matched unrelated donor (MUD), and 45 underwent ASCT using the Cy/TB1 regimen (63). Ultimately, there was no difference in 4-yr OS, with 31% alive after MUD transplant, and 23% alive after autotransplant. Relapse was substantially higher after autotransplant, at 79, vs 9% after MUD transplant.

For first remission patients, one prospective randomized trial (64) randomly assigned patients to ABMT vs CT, with no difference in outcome between the two therapies. In a nonrandomized prospective trial of ALL in the first remission, patients were assigned HLA-matched sibling donor allotransplant vs autotransplant. Forty-three patients underwent allotransplant and 77 autotransplant. Three-yr-DFS was 68% for allotransplant, and 26% for autotransplant, but there was no difference in OS. The two groups were well-matched for prognostic factors. Currently, a national trial of adult ALL is underway. Patients all receive Daunorubicin, Vincristine, Prednisone (DVP)-L-asparaginase induction CT, followed by consolidation therapy. Patients with HLA-identical donors are assigned allotransplant, and the others are randomly assigned long-term maintenance CT vs an ASCT utilizing the TBI/VP-16 regimen, with unmanipulated SCT. This trial is already the largest one of its kind, with a large group of Ph[1]-positive patients, and should add substantially to our understanding of treatment options for ALL.

4.6. Conclusions

A small number of patients with relapsed ALL appeared to be salvaged with ASCT. The benefit of either allo- or auto-SCT, compared to conventional-dose CT in first remission, remains to be determined. Patients should be enrolled on randomized clinical

Table 4
ASCT for CLL

	# Patients	Purge	CR/nCR/PR	SFS	OS (from diagnosis)
Khouri et al. (66)	11	Anti-CD19	6/4/1	4–29 mo	54.4 mo
Rabinowe et al. (67)	12	Anti-CD5	10/0/0	2–31 mo	36 mo

nCR, nodular CR.

trials. Off-study transplantation should be reserved for patients with poor prognostic factors in first remission, or patients in second or subsequent remission.

5. SCT FOR CHRONIC LYMPHOCYTIC LEUKEMIA

5.1. Rationale

The use of BMT for chronic lymphocytic leukemia (CLL) is the least well studied, and the most recent leukemia to have SCT applied. The long natural history of CLL, the older age at diagnosis, and the unclear efficacy of this procedure, and other leukemias, led to this delay. The first allo-BMT, for CLL were conducted in the late 1980s. The largest report of allo-BMT for CLL is from the European Bone Marrow Transplant Registry (65). Fifty-four patients, with a median age of 42 yr, underwent HLA-identical sibling transplants. With a median of 27-mo follow-up, 44% of patients remain alive, with a median time from diagnosis of 40 mo.

5.2. Phase I and Phase II Trials

With more effective combinations of therapy for CLL, including fludarabine in combination with Cy, the likelihood of inducing excellent partial remissions and CRs has improved the likelihood of a less-contaminated stem cell source. Less than 50 patients undergoing ABMT for CLL have been reported in the literature. Two small series are shown in Table 4. Twenty-three patients at MD Anderson and Dana-Farber Cancer Institute have undergone SCT utilizing anti-CD5 and anti-CD19 mAb-purged stem cells. The majority of patients were transplanted with residual disease, and received TBI and cytoxan-preparative regimen. Most patients experienced progressive disease, or had residual disease soon after transplantation.

5.3. Conclusion

The use of either allo-SCT or ASCT for CLL remains in a early investigative stage. Extrapolation from results in low-grade lymphoma and myeloma suggests that a progressive-free survival advantage might be obtained by dose-intensive therapy, though this remains to be determined. Transplantation must be applied very carefully to patients with CLL, who have a chronic disease with a prolonged and natural history that may be cut short by the toxicities of transplantation. Further innovative clinical trials are obviously required to define the role of this modality in this disease.

6. SUMMARY

High-dose CT/radiotherapy and ASCT has been utilized for thousand of patients with leukemia, and many patients are long-term, relapse-free. Patients with relapsed

AML and ALL appear to have the greatest documented benefit, though, even in this setting, the vast majority of those patients will relapse and ultimately succumb to their disease. A number of randomized trials in AML have failed to demonstrate a clear benefit to autotransplant in first remission, and trials remain ongoing for first remission ALL and chronic-phase CML. Pending the results of these trials, the predominant use of ASCT should be within the context of well-designed clinical trials. The same is even more true for CLL, in which the utilization of this technique remains to be justified.

The review of the data suggests that the presumed barriers to the effectiveness of ASCT in primary BM disease may still hold. The inherent resistance of residual leukemia cells present after conventional-dose CT, the likely contamination of stem cell grafts for tumor cells, and the lack of documented additional, meaningful, augmentation of antitumor immune mechanisms remain to be overcome. Though much progress has been made, there is much to learn before mastering human leukemia. Nonetheless, as procedure-related toxicities are decreased, and techniques improve for reducing relapse and stem cell contamination, ASCT is likely to remain an important modality in leukemia therapy.

REFERENCES

1. Gorin NC, Najman A, and Duhamel G. Autologous bone marrow transplantation in acute myelocytic leukemia, *Lancet,* **1** (1977) 1050–.
2. Fefer A, Cheever MA, Thomas ED, et al. Bone marrow transplantation for refractory acute leukemia in 34 patients with identical twins, *Blood,* **57** (1981) 421–430.
3. Dicke KA, Spitzer G, Peters L, et al. Autologous bone-marrow transplantation in relapsed adult acute leukemia, *Lancet,* **1** (1979) 514–517.
4. Cassileth PA, Begg CB, Bennett JM, et al. Randomized study of the efficacy of consolidation therapy in adult acute nonlymphocytic leukemia, *Blood,* **63** (1984) 843–847.
5. Mayer RJ, Davis RB, Schiffer CA, et al. Intensive post-remission chemotherapy in adults with acute myeloid leukemia, *N. Engl. J. Med.,* **331** (1994) 896–903.
6. Cassileth PA, Begg CB, Silber R, et al. Prolonged unmaintained remission after intensive consolidation therapy in adult acute nonlymphocytic leukemia, *Cancer Treat. Rep.,* **71** (1987) 137–140.
7. Santos GW, Tutschka PJ, Brookmeyer R, et al. Marrow transplantation for acute non lymphocytic leukemia after treatment with busulfan and cyclophosphamide, *N. Engl. J. Med.,* **309** (1983) 1347.
8. Tutschka PJ, Copelan EA, Klein JP. Bone marrow transplantation for leukemia following a new busulfan and cyclophosphamide regimen, *Blood,* **70** (1987) 1382.
9. Slattery JT, Clift RA, Buckner CD, et al. Marrow transplantation for chronic myeloid leukemia: the influence of plasma bisulfan levels on the outcome of transplantation, *Blood,* **89** (1997) 3055–3060.
10. Vaughan WP, Cagnoni P, Fernandez H, et al. Decreased incidence of and risk factors for hepatic veno-occlusive disease with an intravenous busulfan (BU) containing preparative regimen for hematopoietic stem cell transplantation (HSCT), *Blood,* **92** (1998) (Suppl): 516a (Abstract).
11. Chao NJ, Stein AS, Long GD, et al. Busulfan/etoposide: initial experience with a new preparatory regimen for autologous bone marrow transplantation in patients with acute non-lymphoblastic leukemia, *Blood,* **81** (1993) 319–323.
12. Miller CB, Zehnbauer BA, Piantadosi S, et al. Correlation of occult clonogenic leukemia drug sensitivity with relapse after autologous bone marrow transplantation, *Blood,* **78** (1991) 1125–1131.
13. Brenner MK, Rill DR, Moen RC, et al. Gene-marking to trace origin of relapse after autologous bone marrow transplantation, *Lancet,* **341** (1993) 85.
14. Sharkis SJ, Santos GW, Colvin M. Elimination of acute myelogenous leukemic cells from marrow and tumor suspensions in the rat with 4-hydroperoxycyclophosphamide, *Blood,* **55** (1980) 521–523.
15. Kushner BH, Kwon JH, Culati SC, et al. Preclinical assessment of purging with VP-16-213: key role for long-term marrow cultures, *Blood,* **69** (1987) 65–71.
16. Gale RP, Horowitz MM, Ash RC, et al. Identical-twin bone marrow transplants for leukemia, *Ann. Intern. Med.,* **120** (1994) 646–652.

17. Kaizer H, Stuart RK, Brookmeyer R, et al. Autologous bone marrow transplantaton in acute leukemia: a phase I study of in vitro treatment of marrow with 4-hydroperoxycyclophosphamide to purge tumor cells, *Blood*, **65** (1985) 1504–1510.

18. Yeager AM, Kaizer H, Santos GW, et al. Autologous bone marrow transplantation in patients with acute nonlymphocytic leukemia, using ex vivo marrow treatment with 4-hydroperoxycyclophosphamide, *N. Engl. J. Med.*, **315** (1986) 141–147.

19. Gulati S, Acaba L, Yahalom J, et al. Autologous bone marrow transplantation for acute myelogenous leukemia using 4-hyroperoxycyclophosphamide and VP-16 purged bone marrow, *Bone Marrow Transplant.*, **10** (1992) 129–134.

20. Lavoie J, Belanger R, Robertson MJ, et al. Autologous bone marrow transplant (BMT) purged with anti-CD33 immunotoxin for patients with acute myeloid leukemia (AML), *Blood*, **92 (suppl)** (1998) 323a (Abstract).

21. Robertson MJ, Soiffer RJ, Freedman AS, et al. Human bone marrow depleted of CD33-positive cells mediates delayed but durable reconstitution of hematopoieseis: clinical trial of MY9 monoclonal antibody-purged autografts for the treatment of acute myeloid leukemia, *Blood*, **79** (1992) 2229–2236.

22. Ball ED, Mills LE, Cornwell GG, et al. Autologous bone marrow transplantation for acute myeloid leukemia using monoclonal antibody-purged bone marrow, *Blood*, **75** (1990) 1199–1206.

23. Selvaggi KJ, Wilson JW, Mills JE, et al. Improved outcome for high-risk acute myeloid leukemia patients using autologous bone marrow transplantation and monoclonal antibody-purged bone marrow, *Blood*, **83** (1994) 1698–1705.

24. Carlo-Stella C, Mangoni L. Use of recombinant human granulocyte-macrophage colony-stimulating factor in patients with lymphoid malignancies transplanted with unpurged or adjusted dose mafosfamide-purged autologous marrow, *Blood*, **80** (1992) 2412–2418.

25. Shpall EJ, Stemmer SM, Hami L, et al. Amifostine (WR-2721) shortens the engraftment period of 4-hydroperoxycyclophosphamide purged bone marrow in breast cancer patients receiving high-dose chemotherapy with autologous bone marrow support, *Blood*, **83** (1994) 3132–3137.

26. Meloni G, Fabritis PD, Petti M, et al. BAVC regimen and autologous bone marrow transplantation in patients with acute myelogenous leukemia in second remission, *Blood*, **75** (1990) 2282–2285.

27. Chopra R, Goldstone GH, McMillan AK, et al. Successful treatment of acute myeloid leukemia beyond first remission with autologous bone marrow transplantation using busulfan/cyclophosphamide and unpurged marrow: the British autograft group experience, *J. Clin. Oncol.*, **9** (1991) 1840–1847.

28. Yeager AM. Autologous bone marrow transplantation for acute myeloid leukemia. In Forman SJ, Blume KG, and Thomas ED (eds.) *Bone Marrow Transplantation*, Blackwell Oxford; (1994) pp. 709–730.

29. Korbling M, Hunstein W, Fliedner TM, et al. Disease-free survival after autologous bone marrow transplantation in patients with acute myelogenous leukemia, *Blood*, **74** (1989) 1898–1904.

30. Rosenfeld C, Shadduck RK, Przepoirka D, et al. Autologous bone marrow transplantation with 4-hydroperoxycyclophosphamide purged marrow for acute nonlymphocytic leukemia in late remission or early relapse, *Blood*, **74** (1989) 1159–1164.

31. Ball ED, Phelps V, Wilson J. Autologous bone marrow transplantation for acute myeloid leukemia in remission on first relapse using monoclonal antibody-purged marrow, *Blood*, **88 (Suppl)**: (1996) 485a (Abstract).

32. Linker CA, Ries CA, Damon LE, et al. Autologous bone marrow transplantation for acute myeloid leukemia using 4-hydroperoxycyclophosphamide purged bone marrow and the busulfan/etoposide preparative regimen: a follow-up report, *Bone Marrow Transplant.*, **22** (1998) 865–872.

33. Sanz MA, de la Rubia J, Sanz GF, et al. Busulfan plus cyclophosphamide followed by autologous blood stem cell transplantation for patients with acute myeloblastic leukemia in first complete remission: a report from a single institution, *J. Clin. Oncol.*, **11** (1993) 1661–1667.

34. Gorin NC, Aegerter P, Auvert B, et al. Autologous bone marrow transplantation for acute myelocytic leukemia in first remission: a European survey of the role of marrow purging, *Blood*, **75** (1990) 1606–1614.

35. Burnett AK, Tansey P, Watkins R, et al. Transplantation of unpurged autologous bone marrow in acute myeloid leukaemia in first remission, *Lancet*, **2** (1984) 1068–1070.

36. Zittoun RA, Mandelli F, Willemze R, et al. Autologous or allogeneic bone marrow transplantation compared with intensive chemotherapy in acute myelogenous leukemia, *N. Engl. J. Med.*, **331** (1995) 217–223.

37. Harousseau JL, Cahan JY, Pignon B, et al. Comparison of autologous bone marrow transplantation

and intensive chemotherapy as postremission therapy in adult acute myeloid leukemia, *Blood*, **90** (1997) 2978–2986.

38. Burnett AK, Goldstone AH, Stevens RM, et al. Randomised comparison of addition of autologous bone-marrow transplantation to intensive chemotherapy for acute myeloid leukaemia in first remission: result of MRC AML 10 trial, *Lancet*, **351** (1998) 700–708.

39. Cassileth PA, Harrington DP, Appelbaum FR, et al. Chemotherapy compared with autologous or allogeneic bone marrow transplantation in the management of acute myeloid leukemia in first remission, *N. Engl. J. Med.*, **339** (1998) 1649–1656.

40. Haines ME, Goldman JM, Worsely AM, et al. Chemotherapy and autografting for chronic granulocytic leukaemia in transformation: probable prolongation of survival for some patients, *Br. J. Haematol.*, **58** (1984) 711–721.

41. Reiffers J, Troutee R, Marit G, et al. Autologous blood stem cell transplantation for chronic granulocytic leukaemia in transformation: a report of 47 cases, *Br. J. Haematol.*, **77** (1991) 339–345.

42. Coulombel L, Kalousek DK, Eaves CJ, et al. Long-term marrow culture reveals chromosomally normal hematopoietic progenitor cells in patients with Philadelphia chromosome-positive chronic myelogenous leukemia, *N. Engl. J. Med.*, **306** (1983) 1493–1498.

43. Chervenick PA, Ellis LD, Pan SF, et al. Human leukemic cells: in vitro growth of colonies containing the Philadelpha (Ph) chromosome, *Science*, **174** (1971) 1134–1136.

44. Verfaillie CM, Bhatia R, Miller W, et al. Benign primitive progenitors can be selected on the basis of the CD34+/IILA-DR-phenotype in early chronic phase but not advanced phase CML, *Blood*, **87** (1996) 4770–4779.

45. Talpaz M, Kantarjian HM, Kurzrock R, et al. Interferon-alpha produces sustained cytogenetic responses in chronic myelogenous leukemia Philadelphia chromosome-positive patients, *Ann. Intern. Med.*, **114** (1991) 532–538.

46. Cunningham I, Gee T, Dowling M, et al. Results of treatment of Ph1-positive chronic myeloid leukemia with an intensive regimen (L-5 protocol), *Blood*, **53** (1979) 375–395.

47. Carlo-Stella C, Mangoni L, Almici C, et al. Autologous transplant for chronic myelogenous leukemia using marrow treated ex vivo with mafosfamide, *Bone Marrow Transplant.*, **14** (1994) 425–432.

48. McGlave PB, Arthur D, Miller WJ, et al. Autologous transplantation for CML using marrow treated ex vivo with recombinant human interferon gamma, *Bone Marrow Transplant.*, **6** (1990) 115–120.

49. Barnett M, Eaves C, Phillipps G, et al. Autografting with cultured marrow in chronic myeloid leukemia: result of a pilot study, *Blood*, **84** (1994) 724–732.

50. Continho LH, Chang J, Brereton ML, et al. Autografting in Philadelphia (Ph)+ chronic myeloid leukemia using cultured marrow: an update of a pilot study, *Bone Marrow Transplant.*, **19** (1997) 969–976.

51. DeFabritiis P, Amadori S, Calabretta B, et al. Elimination of clonogenic Philadelphia-positive cells using BCR-ABL antisense oligodeoxynucleotides, *Bone Marrow Transplant.*, **12** (1993) 261–265.

52. Gewirtz AM, Luger S, Sokol D, et al. Oligodeoxynucleotide therapeutics for human myelogenous leukemia: Interim results, *Blood*, **88 (Suppl 1)** (1996) 270a (Abstract).

53. Reiffers J, Goldman J, Meloni G, et al. Autologous stem cell transplantation in chronic myelogeneous leukemia: a retrospective analysis of the European Group for Bone Marrow Transplantation. Chronic Leukemia Working Party of the EBMT, *Bone Marrow Transplant.*, **14** (1994) 407–410.

54. Simonsson B, Oberg G, Killander A, et al. Intensive treatment in order to minimize the Ph negative/positive clone in chronic myelogenous leukemia, *Stem Cells*, **111 (Suppl 3)** (1993) 73–76.

55. Carella AM, Lerma E, Corsetti MT, et al. Autografting with Philadelphia chromosome-negative mobilized hematopoietic progenitor cells in chronic myelogenous leukemia, *Blood*, **93** (1999) 1534–1539.

56. Verfaillie CM, Bhatia R, Steinbuch M, et al. Comparative analysis of autografting in chronic myelogenous leukemia: effects of priming regimen and marrow or blood origin of stem cells, *Blood*, **92** (1998) 1820–1831.

57. Degliantoni G, Mangoni N, Rizzoli V. In vitro restoration of polyclonal hematopoiesis in a chronic myelogenous leukemia after in vitro treatment with 4-hydroperoxycyclophosphamide, *Blood*, **65** (1985) 753––781.

58. Szczylik C, Skorski T, Nicolaides NC, et al. Selective inhibition of leukemia cell proliferation by BCR-ABL antisense oligodeoxynucleotides, *Science*, **253** (1991) 562–565.

59. deFabritiis P, Skorski T, DePropris MS, et al. Effect of bcr-abl oligodeoxynucleotides on the clonogenic growth of chronic myelogenous leukaemia cells, *Leukemia*, **11** (1997) 811–819.

60. Ratajczak MZ, Hijiya N, Catani L, et al. Acute- and chronic-phase chronic myelogenous leukemia

colony-forming units are highly sensitive to the growth inhibitory effects of c-myb antisense oligodeox-ynucleotides, *Blood,* **79** (1992) 1956–1961.

61. Korbling M, Burke P, Braine H, et al. Successful engraftment of blood derived stem cells in chronic myelogenous leukemia, *Exp. Hematol.,* **9** (1981) 684–690.

62. McGlave PB, DeFabritiis P, Deisseroth et al. Autologous transplants for chronic myelogenous leukemia: results from eight transplant groups, *Lancet,* **343** (1994) 1486–1488.

63. Weisdorf DJ, Billet AL, Hannon P, et al. Autologous versus unrelated donor allogeneic marrow transplantation for acute lymphoblastic leukemia, *Blood,* **90** (1997) 2962–2968.

64. Fiere D, Lepage E, Sebban C, et al. Adult acute lymphoblastic leukemia: a multicentric randomized trial testing bone marrow transplantation as post-remission therapy. The French Group on Therapy for Adult Acute Lymphoblastic Leukemia, *J. Clin. Oncol.,* **11** (1993) 1990–2001.

65. Michallet M, Archimbaud E, Bandini G, et al. HLA-identical sibling bone marrow transplantation in younger patients with chronic lymphocytic leukemia. European Group for Blood and Marrow Transplantation and the International Bone Marrow Transplant Registry, *Ann. Intern. Med.,* **96** (1996) 311–315.

66. Khouri IF, Kantarjian HM, Talpaz M, et al. Results with high-dose chemotherapy and unpurged autologous stem cell transplantation in 73 patients with chronic myelogenous leukemia: the MD Anderson experience, *Bone Marrow Transplant.,* **17** (1996) 775–779.

67. Rabinowe SN, Soiffer RJ, Gribben JG, et al. Autologous and allogeneic bone marrow transplantation for poor prognosis patients with B-cell chronic lymphocytic leukemia, *Blood,* **82** (1993) 1366–1376.

10 Autologous Transplantation for Hodgkin's Disease

Who Benefits?

Craig H. Moskowitz, MD,
and Stephen D. Nimer, MD

CONTENTS

1. INTRODUCTION

The majority of patients with Hodgkin's disease (HD) can be cured with radiation therapy (RT) and/or combination chemotherapy (CT). However, patients who relapse after attaining a complete remission (CR) from CT, and those who fail to achieve a complete response with CT (primary refractory disease), have a poor outcome using conventional-dose second-line or salvage regimens *(1–3)*. Over the past 15 yr, numerous clinical trials using high-dose chemotherapy (HDCT), or chemoradiotherapy, with autologous stem cell transplantation (ASCT) have been reported, and 30–50% of patients appear to be cured using this approach. These results compare favorably with historical data using conventional second-line chemoradiotherapy, and, currently, ASCT is the salvage treatment of choice for many patients with relapsed and primary refractory HD *(4–7)*.

From: *Current Controversies in Bone Marrow Transplantation*
Edited by: B. Bolwell © Humana Press Inc., Totowa, NJ

Two prospective randomized studies have examined the efficacy of high-dose therapy (HDT) in patients with CT refractory and relapsed HD. These studies were performed by the British National Lymphoma Investigation *(8)* and the German HD Study Group (HD-R1 study) *(9)*, and compared mini-BCNU/etoposide/cytosine arabinoside/melphalan (BEAM), or Dexa-BEAM, respectively, in the standard-dose second-line CT arm, to that of 1–2 cycles of mini-BEAM or dexa-BEAM followed by the high-dose BEAM CT regimen, given with autologous bone marrow (BM) or peripheral blood progenitor cell (PBPC) support. Both studies showed statistically significant improvement in event-free survival (EPS) and progression-free survival differences for the patients treated on the HDT arms, but neither study showed an overall survival (OS) advantage for patients treated on the high-dose arm.

Historical data presented in April 1998 at the Fourth International Symposium on HD in Cologne, Germany, from both the European (EBMT) and the American bone marrow transplant (ABMT) registries, demonstrated a 10–15% improvement in survival for HD patients undergoing HDT and ASCT, compared to prior transplant data, which reflected a decrease in transplant-related morbidity, rather than a decreased rate of relapse.

Although HDT and ASCT for patients with HD is safe and efficacious, it is important to determine whether all patients with relapsed HD should be transplanted, RT can be given safely as part of an ASCT conditioning regimen, all patients eligible for HDT and ASCT have a similar prognosis, HDT should be offered to poor-prognosis HD patients as part of their initial therapy, and double transplants should be given to relapsed/refractory patients with poor prognostic features.

2. SHOULD ALL PATIENTS WITH RELAPSED AND REFRACTORY HD RECEIVE HDT AND ASCT?

Although standard-dose second-line-CT for patients with relapsed or refractory HD can achieve a high response rate, the long-term results of this approach are not encouraging. Long-term disease-free survival (DFS) for patients with relapsed disease that was originally treated with mustard, vincristine, procarbazine, prednisone (MOPP) is poor with standard-dose second-line CT, especially for patients whose initial remission lasted less than 1 yr. However, even in the better prognosis group, the results were suboptimal, with a 10-yr DFS of only 24%. The EBMT analyzed data from 139 patients with HD transplanted in first relapse, to determine OS and progression-free survival. In this study, patients who had an initial remission duration of >1 yr ($n = 57$) had a 5-yr survival rate equivalent to that of patients whose initial remission was <1 yr ($n = 63$), 49 vs 44% *(10)*. The authors' institution previously reported data on 146 patients who received high-dose chemoradiotherapy and ABMT from 1985 to 1993, and, using multivariate analysis, found that only a poor response to the standard-dose second CT, and mixed cellularity histology, adversely affected EFS and OS *(11)*. The duration of initial remission was not a prognostic factor; therefore, it is unclear that the length of the first CR should be used to decide who should undergo ASCT *(11)*.

A comparison of conventional-dose second-line CT to HDT with ASCT was recently reported by Yuen et al. *(12)*. Sixty patients with relapsed or refractory disease, treated with nonstandardized cytoreductive CT, followed by ASCT using either cyclophosphamide (Cy), carmustine, and etoposide (CBV) or total body irradiation (TBI), Cy, and etoposide, were compared to 103 patients treated, before the advent of ASCT, with conventional-dose second-line CT. Four-yr EFS and freedom from progression was superior for the patients who received HDT (53 vs 27% and 62 vs 32%, respectively); however, OS was similar (54 vs 47%). In this historical comparison, the application of peripheral blood progenitor cell transplantation (PBPCT) was not uniform, and many patients were not in a state of minimal disease at the time of ASCT. This could account for a lack of an OS difference.

The outcome of PBPCT vs ABMT has been compared in patients with relapsed HD, and, although there is no difference in OS, PBPCT is overwhelmingly the approach of choice today, because of the improved toxicity profile seen when PBPCs are used as the stem cell source *(13)*. In HD patients who are transplanted in second or greater relapse, PBPC collections are commonly suboptimal, because patients either have been heavily pretreated or have received nitrogen mustard and/or procarbazine. We have shown that poorer mobilization of progenitor cells occurs in patients who have received stem-cell-toxic CT, including nitrogen mustard, procarbazine, melphalan, BCNU, or >7.5 g cytarabine CT premobilization, or ≥11 cycles of any previous CT *(14)*. BM harvests can also be inadequate in heavily pretreated patients, making the ASCT impossible.

With modern supportive care, which includes hematopoietic growth factor support, appropriate blood and platelet transfusions, and newer antibiotics and antifungal agents, nearly 95% of patients will survive an ASCT. Therefore, the authors recommend that all patients who relapse, after receiving a standard CT regimen for HD, have primary refractory HD, or who have multiple-relapsed HD, be offered a program that includes a short course of non-stem-cell-toxic cytoreductive therapy, to determine chemosensitivity and mobilize PBPCs, followed by high-dose chemoradiotherapy and ASCT. Transplantation of HD patients with chemorefractory disease is, and should be, the subject of ongoing clinical trials.

3. CAN RT BE GIVEN SAFELY AS PART OF AN ASCT CONDITIONING REGIMEN?

No prospective trials have compared the efficacy of the different transplant-conditioning regimens commonly used in patients with HD (or non-Hodgkin's lymphoma, for that matter). The most commonly used transplant-conditioning regimen in the United States is CBV *(4)*; the BEAM regimen is most commonly used in Europe, yielding results similar to those obtained with CBV *(5)*. The CR rates seen with these regimens range from 46 to 59%, with projected 3–4-yr survivals of 26–45% *(15–17)*. Transplant-related mortality in these studies has ranged between 4 and 11%. Dose escalation of either CBV or BEAM regimens leads to severe nonhematological toxicity *(18,19)*, leading investigators to add thiotepa, mitoxantrone, or cisplatin to the CBV regimen. Generally, these attempts have led to an increase in morbidity, without a demonstrable increase in long-term survival *(20)*.

Ionizing RT is the most effective single agent for the treatment for HD, yet approx one-half of HD patients undergoing ASCT have never been treated with RT *(21–23)*, because of the increasing use of CT in early-stage HD, and the trend toward eliminating consolidative RT in advanced-stage disease. Also, patients who fail to attain a CR to CT usually proceed directly to second-line therapy, even if RT was originally planned as part of an initial combined modality program. Relapse of HD after HDCT tends to occur at sites of initial disease involvement *(24–27),* and this predictability suggests that preemptive RT may decrease the relapse rate post-ASCT.

A number of retrospective series have addressed the pre- or posttransplant use of involved-field RT (IFRT) to areas of significant disease. Chopra et al. *(28)* used IFRT in 45 of 155 patients undergoing HDCT and ASCT. Forty-one patients received RT, because they had not achieved a CR; four patients received RT, because of bulky disease. Local control was attained in 90% of patients. Other programs have used IFRT for similar indications *(29,30),* but, as a result of selection bias, no attempt was made to separately analyze the outcome of patients receiving RT. For example, Mundt et al. *(31)* selected patients who had adverse prognostic features, such as bulky or symptomatic disease, to receive IFRT prior to bone marrow transplantation (BMT); patients who did not attain a CR were irradiated posttransplant. Patients who received IFRT for persistent disease posttransplant had greater progression-free survival (40 vs 12%; $p =$ 0.04) than those who did not. Moreover, patients who converted from a partial response (PR) to a CR by the addition of IFRT had a progression-free survival similar to those patients who achieved a CR with HDCT alone.

Early attempts to integrate larger-field RT into the transplant-conditioning regimen used low-dose TBI, but for small numbers of patients *(31–33).* Concerns about additive toxicities, especially in previously irradiated patients, tended to discourage evaluation of this combined modality approach; however, investigators at the City of Hope *(34,35)* treated 70 patients, who had never received RT, with HDCT and fractionated TBI ± boost RT to bulky sites of disease. The majority of patients had stage IV disease or B symptoms at diagnosis, and 49% of patients had extranodal disease at relapse. The DFS for this poor-prognosis group of patients was 76%, with the last relapse occurring 10 mo post-ASCT *(36).* These results compare favorably to trials using HDCT alone for similar patients.

We have utilized total lymphoid irradiation (TLI), instead of TBI, as part of the transplant-conditioning regimen *(11,37,38)* for patients who have not been previously irradiated. Because relapses after either standard-dose initial CT *(25,26),* or HDCT and ASCT occur in nodal sites initially involved with disease *(32,39,40),* the authors have also given boost-RT pretransplant to sites of bulky disease, or disease that remains postsalvage CT. The use of an accelerated RT schedule has permitted the delivery of TLI and boost-radiation to all commonly involved nodal sites, within a short period of time, prior to ASCT, thus decreasing the risk of tumor-spread during RT, and minimizing the period of marrow aplasia prior to engraftment *(41).* In earlier experience, we administered TLI, 1800 cGy, within 5 d, and added boost-radiation to bulky sites, prior to TLI, so that the dose of RT to these high-risk sites was 3600 cGy. The RT was then followed by HDCT and BM infusion. Eight of 47 patients treated in this manner died of toxicity during the peritransplant period, although 29/39 evaluable patients (74%) attained a CR, and 25 patients (53%) are currently free of disease, with a median follow-up of 9 yr *(42).* Our current program, using mobilized PBPCs as the source of progenitor cells, rather than BM, uniform second-line CT for cytoreduction, and a slight modification in the transplant conditioning regimen, has decreased the toxic mortality from 17 to 3% *(43).* Randomized studies need to be conducted, to determine whether integrating RT, as TLI and/or boost-RT, into a transplant-conditioning regimen can improve long-term event-free survival (EFS) for patients with relapsed and refractory HD.

4. DO ALL PATIENTS HAVE THE SAME PROGNOSIS
WITH HDT AND ASCT?

Data from multiple studies have shown that HDT, followed by ASCT, can cure patients with chemosensitive, relapsed and refractory HD, with EFS ranging from 30–60%. The 10–15% improvement in survival, which has occurred over the past 5 yr appears to be related primarily to better supportive care, the use of mobilized PBPCs as the stem cell source, and possibly changes in patient selection. Response to salvage or second-line CT (i.e., the presence of chemosensitive disease) *(28–30)* has been used as the major selection criteria for proceeding to ASCT, but other prognostic factors may also predict for long-term EFS in these patients. Several reports have described prognostic factors, identifiable prior to the transplant or the presalvage therapy, which predict for a poor outcome with this approach.

In a series of 128 patients treated with CBV, and reported by Bierman et al. *(44)*, a poor performance status, having failed ≥2 CT regimens, and presence of mediastinal disease, were associated with a poor failure-free survival (FFS). The 4-yr FFS for patients who failed >2 regimens was only 10 vs 31% in patients that failed ≤2 prior regimens. Only a poor performance status was predictive of survival in patients treated with ≤2 regimens. A study from the City of Hope, similarly identified >2 prior CT regimens (relative risk 2.5), prior radiation (relative risk 2.1), and extranodal disease at the time of ASCT (relative risk 1.8) to be associated with a poor survival following autotransplantation using CBV or TBI, Cy, and etoposide *(36)*. A study from Stanford, of 119 patients with relapsed and refractory HD, who received TBI, Cy, and etoposide, or CBV, identified B symptoms at relapse, BM or pulmonary involvement with HD, and >2 cm involvement of HD, at the time of ASCT, as poor prognostic factors. Patients with none of these factors had a 4-yr EFS of 85%, compared to 41% in patients with any one factor *(45)*.

The authors analyzed data from 144 patients with HD at Memorial Sloan-Kettering Cancer Center, treated from 1985 to 1993 with TLI, etoposide and Cy, or CBV and ABMT: A poor response to standard-dose second-line CT and mixed cellularity histology predicted for an unfavorable outcome *(42)*. However, analysis of our more recent intent-to-treat study, in which all patients received two cycles of ifosfamide, carboplatin, and etoposide (ICE), for cytoreduction prior to PBPC mobilization (and only patients with chemosensitivity subsequently received HDT), identified two pre-ICE CT factors that predicted for EFS: B symptoms, and extranodal disease. Patients with neither adverse factor had an EFS of 83%; patients with a single risk factor had an EFS of 59%, and patients with both factors had an EFS of only 12% *(43)*. Thus, prognostic factors, other than chemosensitivity, shown to predict for a poor outcome posttransplant in multiple studies, include heavy pretreatment, presence of B symptoms, poor performance status, and presence of extranodal disease.

5. SHOULD UPFRONT HDT BE OFFERED TO POOR PROGNOSIS
PATIENTS AS PART OF THEIR INITIAL THERAPY?

The international prognostic index for intermediate grade non-Hodgkin's lymphoma can be used to separate patients into four distinct prognostic groups. Four-yr EFS rates are 80, 55, 42, and 23%, depending on the number of prognostic factors a given patient has *(46)*. Whether upfront HDT and ASCT for patients with NHL and three or more poor prognostic factors will improve survival is an area of active clinical investigation. A randomized trial of methotrexate, adriamycin, cyclophosphoramide, vincristine, prednisone, bliomycin (MACOP)-B CT vs sequential HDCT with stem cell support, showed a trend toward a survival advantage for the transplanted poor-prognosis patients (47).

A prognostic score for advanced-stage HD was recently published, based on 5141 patients treated with combination CT with or without RT. Using freedom from progression (FFP) as the end point, a prognostic score was calculated, based on the number of adverse prognostic factors present at diagnosis. Seven factors had an independent effect: serum albumin <4 g/dL, hemoglobin <10.5 g/dL, male sex, age >45 yr, stage IV disease, WBC >15,000/μL, and lymphopenia <600 μL. FFP ranged from 80% for patients with 0–2 factors, to 55% for patients with three factors, to 40–50% for patients with >3 factors (48). Whether upfront HDT and ASCT, for patients with three or more poor prognostic factors, will improve FFP is the subject of numerous clinical trials.

An alternative to upfront ASCT in HD is the use of more intensive initial therapy, and, since 1992, two new combined modality treatment programs for advanced-stage HD have been reported. The Stanford V regimen (49), a 12-wk regimen that maintains the dose intensity of the most active agents, yet shortens the duration of therapy, has generated promising results, and may reduce the cumulative toxicity of the alkylating agents that are given. Stanford V CT was followed by RT to all initial sites of disease >5 cm. The actuarial 3-yr FFS for patients was 87%. The authors have treated 50 patients with this treatment program, and 47 patients are failure-free at a median follow-up of 21 mo (50). A second new treatment program is (BEACOPP), and its variant, escalated BEACOPP, which are dose-escalated versions of COPP/ABVD (cyclophosphamide, vincristine, procarbazine, prednisone/adriamycin, bleomycin, vinblastine, dacrabazine). A three-arm randomized trial comparing COPP/ABVD, vs BEACOPP, vs escalated BEACOPP was conducted by the German Hodgkin's disease study group (51). The BEACOPP regimen is a shorter and more intense regimen than COPP/ABVD, and the escalated version of BEACOPP is more intense than BEACOPP, and is given with granulocyte colony-stimulating factor support. At a median follow-up of 23 mo, the freedom from treatment failure, for patients receiving either of the BEACOPP treatment arms, is 84%, which is similar to the results obtained with the Stanford V regimen. These newer regimens need to be compared prospectively to ABVD, which is the standard CT treatment for HD in much of the world (52). Nonetheless, the apparent success of these regimens makes it unlikely that upfront HDT for advanced-stage HD will benefit more than a rare patient with HD.

6. IS THERE RATIONALE FOR PERFORMING DOUBLE TRANSPLANTS IN PATIENTS WITH HD?

Several prognostic factors predict for a poor outcome following HDT and ASCT, but it is currently unclear whether such poor prognosis patients can be cured using the autotransplant approach. One published report addresses the use of double autotransplants in patients with HD. Ahmed et al. (53) evaluated the efficacy of performing a second transplant, with a different conditioning regimen, for patients with refractory HD who had neither disease progression nor excessive toxicity associated with the first. Of 83 patients with refractory disease, 14 died during the first peritransplant period; 23 had progressive disease after the first ASCT. Thirty-eight patients achieved a CR or PR with the first ASCT, but only 11 of the 19 patients who achieved a PR to the first ASCT agreed to undergo a second transplant. Thus, the question of whether double ASCT is effective in patients with HD cannot be answered by this data. We have identified patients with B symptoms and extranodal disease prior to second-line therapy as having a very poor outcome with a single ASCT (12% EFS), and thus have decided to investigate the role of double ASCT only in these poor-prognostic patients.

7. CONCLUSIONS

Despite advances in the management of HD, up to 40% of patients with advanced-stage disease, and 20% of patients with early-stage disease, will relapse or have primary refractory disease. The data suggests that, independent of the initial remission duration, HDT and ASCT provides a longer EFS, compared to standard-dose CT or RT approaches, and should be recommended. The use of RT as part of the transplant-conditioning regimen, either as boost-radiation to bulky sites of disease or as TLI or TBI, may provide real benefit, compared to CT-only regimens. All patients with chemosensitive disease do not have the same prognosis when treated with HDT, and treatments for poor-prognosis patients should be evaluated as part of a clinical trial. More effective first-line standard-dose chemoradiotherapy regimens are being evaluated, which may make the role of upfront HDT for HD patients of little importance. The results of randomized, autotransplant trials may provide firmer evidence to support current practice guidelines.

REFERENCES

1. Bonfante V, Santoro A, Viviani S, et al. Outcome of patients with Hodgkin's disease failing after primary MOPP-ABVD, *J. Clin. Oncol.,* **15** (1997) 528–534.
2. Longo D, Duffey P, Young R, et al. Conventional-dose salvage combination chemotherapy in patients relapsing with Hodgkin's disease after combination chemotherapy: the low probability for cure, *J. Clin. Oncol.,* **10** (1992) 210–218.
3. Yahalom J. Management of relapsed and refractory Hodgkin's disease, *Semin. Radiat. Oncol.,* **6** (1996) 210–224.
4. Bierman PJ and Armitage JO. Role of autotransplantation in Hodgkin's disease, *Hematol. Oncol. Clin. North Am.,* **7** (1993) 591–611.
5. Goldstone AH, McMillan AK: Place of high-dose therapy with haemopoietic stem cell transplantation in relapsed and refractory Hodgkin's disease, *Ann. Oncol.,* **4** (1993) 21–27.
6. Armitage JO, Bierman PJ, Vose JM, et al. Autologous bone marrow transplantation for patients with relapsed Hodgkin's disease, *Am. J. Med.,* **91** (1991) 605–611.
7. Carella AM, Congiu AM, Gaozza E, et al. High-dose chemotherapy with autologous bone marrow transplantation in 50 advanced resistant Hodgkin's disease patients: an Italian study group report, *J. Clin. Oncol.,* **6** (1988) 1411–1416.
8. Linch DC, Winfield D, Goldstone AH, et al. Dose intensification with autologous bone-marrow transplantation in relapsed and resistant Hodgkin's disease: results of a BNLI randomised trial, *Lancet,* **341** (1993) 1051–1054.
9. Schmitz N, Sextro M, Hasenclever D, et al. HD-R1: First results of a randomized trial comparing aggressive chemotherapy with high-dose therapy (HDT) and hematopoietic and stem cell transplantation (HSCT) in patients with chemosensitive relapse of Hodgkin's disease, *Blood,* **90 (Suppl 1)** (1997) 115a(Abstract).
10. Sweetenham JW, Taghipour G, Milligan D, et al. High-dose therapy and ASCT for patients with HD in first relapse after chemotherapy: results from the EBMT, *Bone Marrow Transplant.,* **20** (1997) 745–752.
11. Yahalom J, Gulati SC, Toia M, et al. Accelerated hyperfractionated total lymphoid irradiation, high-dose chemotherapy, and autologous bone marrow transplantation for refractory and relapsing patients with Hodgkin's disease, *J. Clin. Oncol.,* **11** (1993) 1062–1070.

12. Yuen AR, Rosenberg SA, Hoppe RT, et al. Comparison between conventional salvage therapy and high-dose therapy with autografting for recurrent or refractory Hodgkin's disease, *Blood,* **89** (1997) 814–822.

13. Schmitz N, Linch DC, Dreger P, et al. Randomized trial of filgrastim-mobilized PBPCT vs. ABMT in lymphoma patients, *Lancet,* **347** (1996) 353–357.

14. Moskowitz CH, Glassman JR, Wuest D, et al. Factors affecting mobilization of PBPCs in patients with lymphoma, *Clin. Cancer Res.,* **4** (19   ) 311–316.

15. Jagannath S, Armitage JO, Dicke KA, et al. Prognostic factors for response and survival after high-dose cyclophosphamide, carmustine, and etoposide with autologous bone marrow transplantation for relapsed Hodgkin's disease, *J. Clin. Oncol.,* **7** (1989) 179–185.

16. Moormeier JA, Williams SF, Kaminer LS, et al. Autologous bone marrow transplantation followed by involved field radiotherapy in patients with relapsed or refractory Hodgkin's disease, *Leukemia Lymphoma,* **5** (1991) 243–246.

17. Carella A, Carlier P, Congiu A, et al. Nine years' experience with ABMT in 128 patients with Hodgkin's disease: an Italian study group report, *Leukemia,* **5** (1991) 68–71.

18. Wheeler C, Antin JH, Churchill WH, et al. Cyclophosphamide, carmustine, and etoposide with autologous bone marrow transplantation in refractory Hodgkin's disease and non-Hodgkin's lymphoma. A dose-finding study, *J. Clin. Oncol.,* **8** (1990) 648–856.

19. Zulian GB, Selby P, Mllan S, et al. High-dose melphalan, BCNU and etoposide with autologous bone marrow transplantation for Hodgkin's disease, *Br. J. Cancer,* **59** (1989) 631–635.

20. Reece DE, Connors JM, Spinelli JJ, et al. Intensive therapy with cyclophosphamide, carmustine, etoposide +/− cisplatin, and autologous bone marrow transplantation for Hodgkin's disease in first relapse after combination chemotherapy, *Blood,* **83** (1994) 1193–1199.

21. Poen JC, Hoppe RT, and Horning SJ. High-dose therapy and autologous bone marrow transplantation for relapsed/refractory Hodgkin's disease: the impact of involved field radiotherapy on patterns of failure and survival, *Int. J. Radiat. Oncol. Biol. Phys.,* **36** (1996) 3–12.

22. Wirth A, Corry J, Laidlaw C, et al. Salvage radiotherapy for Hodgkin's disease following chemotherapy failure, *Int. J. Radiat. Oncol. Biol. Phys.,* **39** (1997) 599–607.

23. Pezner RD, Lipsett JA, Vora N, et al. Radical radiotherapy as salvage treatment for relapse of Hodgkin's disease initially treated by chemotherapy alone: prognostic significance of the disease-free interval, *Int. J. Radiat. Oncol. Biol. Phys.,* **30** (1994) 965–970.

24. Biti G, Cimino G, Cartoni C, et al. Extended-field radiotherapy is superior to MOPP chemotherapy for the treatment of pathologic stage I–IIA Hodgkin's disease: eight-year update of an Italian prospective randomized study, *J. Clin. Oncol.,* **10** (1992) 378–382.

25. Young R, Canellos G, Chabner B, et al. Patterns of relapse in advanced Hodgkin's disease treated with combination chemotherapy, *Cancer,* **42** (1978) 1001–1007.

26. Yahalom J, Ryu J, Straus D, et al. Impact of adjuvant radiation on the patterns and rate of relapse in advanced-stage Hodgkin's disease treated with alternating chemotherapy combinations, *J. Clin. Oncol.,* **9** (1991) 2193–2201.

27. Brizel D, Winer E, Prosnitz L, et al. Improved survival in advanced Hodgkin's disease with the use of combined modality therapy, *Int. J. Radiat. Oncol. Biol. Phys.,* **19** (1991) 535–542.

28. Chopra R, McMillan AK, Linch DC, et al. The place of high-dose BEAM therapy and autologous bone marrow transplantation in poor-risk Hodgkin's disease. A single-center eight-year study of 155 patients, *Blood,* **81** (1993) 1137–1145.

29. Anderson JE, Litzow MR, Appelbaum FR, et al. Allogeneic, syngeneic, and autologous marrow transplantation for Hodgkin's disease: the 21-year Seattle experience, *J. Clin. Oncol.,* **11** (1993) 2342–2350.

30. Crump M, Smith AM, Brandwein J, et al. High-dose etoposide and melphalan, and autologous bone marrow transplantation for patients with advanced Hodgkin's disease: importance of disease status at transplant, *J. Clin. Oncol.,* **11** (1993) 704–711.

31. Mundt AJ, Sibley G, Williamks S, et al. Patterns of failure following high-dose chemotherapy and autologous bone marrow transplantation with involved field radiotherapy for relapsed/refractory Hodgkin's disease, *Int. J. Radiat. Oncol. Biol. Phys.,* **33** (1995) 261–270.

32. Phillips GL, Wolff SN, Herzig RH, et al. Treatment of progressive Hodgkin's disease with intensive chemoradiotherapy and autologous bone marrow transplantation, *Blood,* **73** (1989) 2086–2092.

33. Gianni AM, Siena S, Bregni M, et al. Prolonged disease-free survival after high-dose sequential chemo-radiotherapy and haemopoietic autologous transplantation in poor prognosis Hodgkin's disease, *Ann. Oncol.,* **2** (1991) 645–653.

34. McMillan A, and Goldstone A. What is the value of autologous bone marrow transplantation in the treatment of relapsed or resistant Hodgkin's disease? *Leukemia Res.,* **15** (1991) 237–243.

35. Petersen FB, Appelbaum FR, Hill R, et al. Autologous marrow transplantation for malignant lymphoma: a report of 101 cases from Seattle, *J. Clin. Oncol.,* **8** (1990) 638–647.

36. Nadermanee A, O'Donnell MR, Snyder DS et al. High-dose chemotherapy with or without TBI followed by ASCT for patients with relapsed and refractory HD: results of 85 patients and analysis of prognostic factors, *Blood,* **85** (1995) 1381–1390.

37. Roach M, Kapp D, Rosenberg S, et al. Radiotherapy with curative intent: an option in selected patients relapsing after chemotherapy for advanced Hodgkin's Disease, *J. Clin. Oncol.,* **5** (1987) 550–555.

38. Mauch P, Tarbell N, Skarin A, et al. Wide-field radiation therapy alone or with chemotherapy for Hodgkin's disease in relapse from combination chemotherapy, *J. Clin. Oncol.,* **5** (1987) 544–549.

39. Gribben JG, Linch DC, Singer CR, et al. Successful treatment of refractory Hodgkin's disease by high-dose combination chemotherapy and autologous bone marrow transplantation, *Blood,* **73** (1989) 340–344.

40. Reece DE, Barnett MJ, Connors JM, et al. Intensive chemotherapy with cyclophosphamide, carmustine, and etoposide followed by autologous bone marrow transplantation for relapsed Hodgkin's disease [published erratum appears in *J. Clin. Oncol.* **10** (1992) 170], *J. Clin. Oncol.,* **9** (1991) 1871–1879.

41. Yahalom J. Integrating radiotherapy into bone marrow transplantation programs for HD, *Int. J. Radiat. Oncol. Biol. Phys.,* **33** (1995) 525–528.

42. Yahalom J, Moni J, Gulati SC, et al. Salvage therapy of Hodgkin's disease with intensive total lymphoid irradiation, cyclophosphamide and etoposide followed by autologous bone marrow transplantation: 10-year results, *Proc. ASCO,* **16** (1997) 24.

43. Moskowitz CH, Nimer SD, Portlock CS, et al. Ifosfamide, carboplatin, and etoposide (ICE) cytoreduction followed by high-dose chemoradiotherapy and ASCT for refractory and relapsed Hodgkin's disease: an intent to treat study, *Blood,* **90 (Suppl 1)** (1997) 233a.

44. Bierman PJ, Bagin RG, Jagannath S, et al. High-dose chemotherapy followed by ASCT in HD: long-term follow-up in 128 patients, *Ann. Oncol.,* **4** (1993) 767–773.

45. Horning SJ, Chao NJ, and Negrin RS. High-dose therapy and ASCT for recurrent or refractory HD: analysis of the Stanford University results and prognostic indices, *Blood,* **89** (1997) 801–813.

46. Shipp MA, Harrington DP, Anderson JR, et al. Predictive model for aggressive NHL, *N. Engl. J. Med.,* **329** (1993) 987–992.

47. Gianni AM Bregni M, Sienna S, Brambilla C, et al. High-dose chemotherapy and ABMT compared with MACOP-B in aggressive B cell lymphoma, *N. Engl. J. Med.,* **1290** (1997) 336–341.

48. Hansenclever D and Diehl V. Prognostic score for advanced HD, *N. Engl. J. Med.,* **339** (1998) 1506–1514.

49. Barlett NL, Rosenberg SA, Hoppe RT, et al. Brief chemotherapy, Stanford V, and adjuvant radiotherapy for bulky or advanced stage Hodgkin's disease, *J. Clin. Oncology.,* **13** (1995) 1080–1088.

50. Moskowitz CH, Yahalom J, Straus D, et al. The use of Stanford V overcomes poor prognostic features in patients with advance stage HD, *Blood,* **92** (1998) 2579.

51. Tesch H, Diehl V, Lathan B, et al. Moderate dose escalation for advanced-stage Hodgkin's disease using bleomycin, etoposide, adriamycin, cyclophosphamide, vincristine, procarbazine and prednisone scheme and adjuvant radiotherapy. A study of the German Hodgkin's Lymphoma Study Group, *Blood,* **92** (1998) 4560–4567.

52. Canellos GP, Anderson JR, Propert KJ, et al. Chemotherapy of advanced stage Hodgkin's disease with MOPP, ABVD or MOPP alternating with ABVD, *N. Engl. J. Med.,* **327** (1992) 1478–1484.

53. Ahmed T, Lake DE, Beer M, et al. Single and double autotransplants for relapsing/refractory HD: results of two consecutive trials, *Bone Marrow Transplant.,* **19** (1997) 449–454.

11 Hematopoietic Stem Cell Transplantation for Mantle Cell Lymphoma

Brad Pohlman, MD

CONTENTS

1. INTRODUCTION

Mantle cell lymphoma (MCL) is a unique subtype of non-Hodgkin's lymphoma (NHL). In the past, this lymphoma was classified (or misclassified) as diffuse small-cleaved-cell lymphoma or follicular small-cleaved-cell lymphoma, in the International Working Formulation *(1–3);* as centrocytic lymphoma, in the Kiel classification *(4);* as lymphocytic lymphoma of intermediate differentiation *(5);* as intermediate cell lymphoma *(5);* or as mantle zone lymphoma *(6).* The term "mantle cell lymphoma" was proposed in 1992 *(7)* and was defined by the Revised European-American Lymphoma Classification in 1994 *(8).* MCL has a distinct morphology, histology, and immunophenotype (CD5[+], CD19[+], CD20[+], CD10[−], CD23[−]), which are now widely accepted, and increasingly recognized. This lymphoma and subset of patients is more specifically defined by a distinct translocation, t(11;14)(q13;32), which results in the rearrangement of the *bcl-1* locus, and overexpression of cyclin D1 protein.

From: *Current Controversies in Bone Marrow Transplantation*
Edited by: B. Bolwell © Humana Press Inc., Totowa, NJ

Table 1
Failure-free Survival (FFS) and Overall Survival (OS) Among 83 Patients
with MCL According to the International Prognostic Index (IPI) *(9)*

IPI	Median FFS (yr)	Median OS (yr)
Total (*n* = 83)	~1.1	~2.8
0 or 1 (*n* = 19)	~2	~5
2 or 3 (*n* = 45)	~1	~3
4 or 5 (*n* = 19)	~0.5	~1.5

MCL accounts for approx 6–11% of patients with NHL *(1–3,9)*. In a review of 13 small studies *(10)* involving 575 patients with MCL, the median age at diagnosis was 58 yr. Bone marrow (BM) involvement was reported in 53–93% of patients, and lymphocytosis was reported in 10–69% of patients. In a more recent analysis of another 83 MCL patients *(9)*, 80% had advanced-stage disease and 79% had a Karnofsky score ≥80%.

In 12 trials with conventional chemotherapy (CT), the overall response rate was 84%, but only 46% achieved a complete remission (CR) *(10)*. The median progression-free survival (PFS) was 20 mo, and the median overall survival (OS) was 36 mo. A comparison of two European Organization for the Research and Treatment of Cancer trials suggested that doxorubicin (Dox)-based CT regimens offer no significant survival advantage, compared to non-Dox-based CT regimens *(2)*. Only one prospective, randomized study compared a Dox-based to a non-Dox-based CT regimen *(11)*. In this trial, 63 patients with centrocytic lymphoma (in the Kiel classification) were randomized to receive either cyclophosphamide (Cy), vincristine, and prednisone (COP) or Cy, Dox, vincristine, and prednisone (CHOP) CT. The COP vs CHOP overall response rate (84 vs 88%), CR rate (41 vs 58%), median relapse-free survival (10 vs 7 mo), and the median OS (32 vs 37 mo) were not significantly different. These studies provide no evidence that patients with MCL are cured with conventional CT. In fact, very few patients remain alive 10 yr after diagnosis *(1)*.

Investigators have evaluated many potential prognostic characteristics. Among MCL patients treated with conventional CT, older age, male sex, poor performance status, B symptoms, splenomegaly, anemia, elevated lactate dehydrogenase (LDH), bulky disease, advanced stage, extranodal sites, marrow and/or blood involvement, elevated β_2-microglobulin, failure to achieve CR, blastoid variant, high mitotic index, and p53 mutations have all been reported to predict a worse outcome in patients treated with conventional CT *(10)*. In one large retrospective series, the International Prognostic Index (IPI) predicted both failure-free survival (FFS) and OS (Table 1; *9*).

Because of their relatively young age (most are less than 60 yr) and good performance status, yet dismal prognosis with conventional CT, these MCL patients are potentially excellent candidates for high-dose therapy (HDT) with hematopoietic stem cell transplantation (HSCT). Undoubtedly, patients with MCL have been included in early transplant series, but were simply not recognized, or not reported as a distinct group. With the evolution of specific diagnostic criteria and the recognition of these patients, the results from several transplant series are now available.

2. AN OVERVIEW OF TRANSPLANTATION
FOR MANTLE CELL LYMPHOMA

A review of the literature identified 16 series with five or more MCL patients who received HDT with HSCT. In addition, this report includes another 11 patients transplanted at the Cleveland Clinic Foundation, for a total of nearly 300 patients (Table 2). Approximately 40% of patients were transplanted in first CR or partial remission (PR); 60% of patients were transplanted after they failed to respond to, or progressed, following initial therapy. The majority received a myeloablative regimen that contained total body irradiation (TBI). Almost 90% of patients received autologous HSCT. Among this group, approx 20% received autologous bone marrow transplantation (ABMT), and the rest received autologous blood stem cell transplantation (ABSCT). The transplant-related mortality was generally very low; eight series reported no transplant-related fatalities. The disease-free survival (DFS) (event-free [EFS], failure-free, or progression-free) and OSs ranged from 12 to 100% and 23 to 100%, respectively.

3. AUTOLOGOUS TRANSPLANTATION

In 1995, Stewart et al. *(12)* from the University of Nebraska published the first series of MCL patients to receive HDT with autologous HSCT. Nine patients with relapsed MCL received one of four different high-dose regimens. Two patients received ABMT, and seven patients (with unsuitable BM) received ABSCT. Only three of 12 patients remained in remission at 7, 12, and 25 mo posttransplant. The 2-yr FFS and OS were both 34%.

The following year, Haas et al. *(13)*, from Germany, reported 13 patients with advanced-stage MCL, who received HDT with ABSCT. One patient was in first CR, and eight patients were in first PR. Seven patients had BM involvement at the time of stem cell mobilization with CT and granulocyte colony-stimulating factor (G-CSF). Twelve patients received TBI and Cy. One patient died of interstitial pneumonitis 17 d posttransplant. Two patients, who were transplanted in second remission, relapsed 10 and 11 mo posttransplant, respectively. Ten patients (including all nine patients transplanted in first remission) were alive and in remission, with a median follow-up of 18 (range 10–47) mo. The Kaplan-Meier estimate of DFS and OS was 76 and 92%, respectively.

3.1. Prognostic Factors

Several studies have attempted to identify prognostic factors in patients receiving HDT with ABSCT *(14,19,21,24)*. Ketterer et al. *(16)*, from France, reported 16 patients with MCL, who received an ABMT and/or ABSCT. Most patients were in second or third remission, and had BM involvement at the time of BM and/or blood stem cell (BSC) harvest. Three patients died from hemorrhage prior to platelet recovery. With a median follow-up of 22 (range 12–90) mo, only five patients were alive without progression, and only three patients remained in CR. The expected EFS and OS at 3 yr were both 24%. A longer, but, statistically, not significantly different, OS was observed in patients intensified in first CR or PR, and in those intensified during the

Table 2
Series of Five or More Patients with MCL who Received High-dose Therapy with Autologous or Allogeneic Follow-up Hematopoietic Stem Cell Transplantation

Ref.	No. Pts	Median age (range) (yr)	Disease status (n)	TBI no.	Type of Transplant (n)	TRM (%)	CR, %	(range) (mo)	Posttransplant DFS/EFS/FFS/PFS (%)	OS (%)
Stewart et al., 1995 (12)	9	54 (35–64)	RC (4), RU (4), u (1)	2	ABMT (2), ABSCT (7)	u	u	12 (2–33)	FFS 34 @ 2 yr	34 @ 2 yr
Haas et al., 1996 (13)	13	49 (30–60)	R1 (9), R2+ (4)	12	ABSCT (13)	8	u	18 (10–47)	DFS 76	92
Dreger et al., 1997 (14)	9	47 (38–60)	R1 (6), R2+ (3)	7	ABSCT[a] (6)	0	100	12 (3–33)	100	100
Gressin et al., 1997 (15)	5	53 (51–66)	CR2+ (4), ref (1)	5	ABSCT (5)	0	80	<13 (7–22)	80	80
Ketterer et al., 1997 (16)	16	u	R1 (6), R2+ (10)	12	ABMT (2), ABSCT[b] (14)	19	54	22 (12–90)	EFS 24 @ 3 yr	24 @ 3 yr
Khouri et al., 1997 (17)*	18	u	R1 (18)	18	ABSCT (u), allo-BMT (u)	u	94	12 (5–33)	FFS 100 @ 2 yr	100 @ 2 yr
Romaguera et al., 1997 (18)*	13	u	R2+ (13)	13	ABSCT (8)	25	u	u	FFS 50	50
					AlloBSCT (5)	40	u	u	FFS 60	60
Blay et al., 1998 (19)	18[c]	50 (25–64)	R1 (8), R2+ (10)	11	ABMT (7), ABSCT (11)	0	89	32 (10–139)	PFS 75 @ 2 yr	91 @ 2 yr
Conde et al., 1998 (20)*	55	49 (21–64)	CR1/2 (15/9), RC (28), ref (3)	12	ABMT (10), ABSCT (45)	5	80	u	DFS 26 @ 9 yr	58 @ 9 yr
Freedman et al., 1998 (21)	28	u	R1 (8), R2+ (20)	28	ABMT[d] (28)	0	u	24 (10–135)	DFS 31 @ 4 yr	62 @ 4 yr
Khouri et al., 1998 (22)*	13[e]	53 (38–58)	CR (3), PR (7), ref (3)	10	Allo-SBCT (13)	23	92	21 (4–44)	FFS 67 @ 3 yr	67 @ 3 yr
Kröger et al., 1998 (23)	9[f]	47 (28–61)	R1 (7), R2+ (2)	6	ABSCT[g] (8), allo-BMT (1)	0	100	22 (9–64)	100	100
Milpied et al., 1998 (24)	18	47 (40–60)	R1 (10), R2 (5), ref (3)	13	ABMT (4), ABSCT (13), allo-BMT (1)	0	72	36 (13–80)	DFS 49 @ 3 yr	81 @ 4 yr
Molina et al., 1998 (25)*	24	52 (32–61)	R1 (13), R2+ (4), ref (7)	17	ABSCT (18), allo-BMT (6)	4	u	18 (2–43)	DFS 78 @ 2 yr	77 @ 2 yr
Sohn et al., 1998 (26)*	28	47 (38–67)	R1 (3), R2+ (18), ref (7)	u	ABSCT (16)	13	86	36 (12–132)	EFS 54 @ 3 yr	63 @ 3 yr
					Allo-BMT (12)	58	75	u	EFS 12 @ 3 yr	23 @ 3 yr
Suzan et al., 1998 (27)*	9	53 (46–61)	R1 (8) u (1)	1	ABSCT (9)	0	78	u	FFS 78	89
Pohlman et al., 1999	11	56 (34–69)	R1 (4), R2+ (8)	0	ABSCT (9), allo-BMT (2)	0	60	13 (1–30)	PFS 82	91

[a]ASC were CD34 selected in 5 patients.
[b]ABMT and ABSCT in 1 patient.
[c]Includes 9 patients with diffuse small cleaved cell lymphoma.
[d]Purged autologous bone marrow.
[e]May include some patients from references 17 and 18.
[f]Includes 2 patients from reference 14.
[g]ASC were CD 34 selected in 2 patients.
*Abstract only.

ABMT, autologous bone marrow transplantation; ABSCT, autologous blood stem cell transplantation; allo-BMT, allogeneic bone marrow transplantation; allo-BSCT, allogeneic blood stem cell transplantation; ASC, autologous stem cells; CR, complete remission; CR1/2, first/second complete remission; DFS, disease-free survival; EFS, event-free survival; FFS, failure-free survival; PFS, progressive-free survival; PR, partial remission; Pts, patients; R1, first complete or partial remission; R2+, second or greater complete or partial remission; RC, relapsed and chemosensitive; ref, refractory; RU, relapsed and untreated; TBI, number of patients who received TBI-based preparative regimen; TRM, transplant-related mortality; u, unknown or not provided.

first year after diagnosis, compared to patients intensified after progression, or after more than 1 yr of follow-up.

Blay et al. *(19),* from France, described nine patients with diffuse centrocytic, and nine patients with immunophenotypically confirmed, MCL, who received an ABMT or ABSCT. The results between those patients with diffuse centrocytic and with confirmed MCL did not differ. With a median follow-up of 32 (range 10–139) mo posttransplant, the 2-yr PFS and OS were 75 and 91%, respectively. In contrast to the previous study, the PFS was 53% among patients in first CR or PR, and 82% among patients in second CR or PR. The OS was 66% among patients in first CR or PR, and 89% among patients in second CR or PR. Neither of these differences was statistically significant. Furthermore, the PFS and OS were not associated with age, performance status, stage, LDH, IPI, BM involvement, preparative regimen, or stem cell source.

Milpied et al. *(24),* from France, described 18 patients with MCL. Seventeen patients received an ABMT or ABSCT, and one patient with refractory disease received an allogeneic bone marrow transplantation (allo-BMT) from an HLA-identical sibling. No pathologic or clinical characteristic predicted response to transplant. With a median follow-up 36 (range 13–80) mo posttransplant, 15 patients were alive, and 11 had not progressed. The projected DFS and OS after transplant were 49 and 81%, respectively. The allo-BMT patient relapsed, and did not respond to donor leukocyte infusion. He received involved-field radiation therapy, and subsequently remained in CR. Another patient relapsed 11 mo after BCNU, etoposide, cytosine, valovisine, melphalan (BEAM) and ABMT, achieved a second PR, and then received a TBI-based allo-BMT from an HLA-identical sibling. This patient was alive and well 38 mo after the second transplant. The investigators evaluated a variety of potential prognostic characteristics. Patients with blastic variant had a worse DFS, compared to other patients (33 vs 64% at 3 yr; $p = 0.06$). Patients who received a TBI-based conditioning regimen had an improved DFS (71 vs 0% at 3 yr, $p < 0.0001$), and OS (89 vs 60% at 4 yr, $p = 0.07$). Patients in first PR appeared to have a better 3-yr DFS (80 vs 18%) and 4-yr OS (90 vs 66%), although these differences were not statistically significant. The authors noted that the only two patients in first PR who relapsed after transplant, received a CT-based preparative regimen.

3.2. Transplantation Product Contamination

Despite aggressive CT, patients with MCL frequently have morphologic, flow cytometric, or molecular evidence of residual disease in the blood and/or BM at the time of BM harvest or peripheral blood stem cell (PBSC) collection *(14,28,29).* This residual lymphoma may contaminate peripheral blood or BM autografts, and, potentially, may contribute to subsequent disease relapse. Dreger et al. *(14),* from Germany, reported nine patients with stage III and IV MCL who received HDT with ABSCT: Two patients were newly diagnosed, four were in first remission, and three were in first relapse. For cytoreduction and stem cell mobilization, patients received 1–2 courses of Dexa-BEAM with G-CSF: Five patients achieved a CR and four patients achieved a PR. Flow cytometry detected $CD5^+CD19^+$ B-cells in 2/9 BSC harvests, and polymerase chain reaction (PCR) detected clonal rearrangements of the immunoglobulin heavy chain gene in at least one leukapheresis product from 6/9 patients.

Corradini et al. *(28),* from Italy, evaluated the leukapheresis products and harvested BM of eight MCL patients. They received sequential high-dose CT ([APO] × 2, dexamethasone, cytarabine, and cisplatin [DHAP] × 1–2, VP-16 × 1, methotrexate × 1, dexamethasone × 3), and then stem cells were mobilized with high-dose Cy and G-CSF. At the start of treatment, lymphoma cells were detectable in the BM by histology in seven patients, and by PCR in all eight patients. The one patient without overt marrow involvement at the start of treatment had no PCR-detectable lymphoma in the two leukapheresis products or harvested marrow. The other seven patients had PCR-detectable lymphoma in every leukapheresis product and harvested marrow. In contrast, 13/19 patients with follicular lymphoma who were treated on the same protocol, had at least one PCR-negative leukapheresis product.

Jacquy et al. *(29)*, from Belgium, described 14 patients with stage III or IV, t(11;14)-positive MCL, who were initially treated with polychemotherapy and G-CSF. Autologous BSCs were then mobilized, using either Cy and etoposide or Dexa-BEAM with G-CSF. Using a semiquantitative method, peripheral blood cells were tested at the time of regeneration from the first polychemotherapy or the mobilizing regimen, for the presence of PCR-detectable patient-specific lymphoma DNA. In most cases, blood cells collected at regeneration, from the combination CT and mobilizing CT, contained more lymphoma cells than steady-state blood or BM. Furthermore, the peripheral blood contamination in patients with MCL was greater than in patients with diffuse large B-cell lymphoma. Although the CT used to mobilize stem cells prior to autologous transplantation (autotransplantation) reduced the patient's tumor load, the authors *(29)* suggested that this benefit was lost by massively mobilizing malignant cells into the stem cell collections, and actually reinfusing more lymphoma with CT-mobilized stem cells than with unmanipulated autologous BM.

3.3. Purging or Selection of Transplantation Products

Because most patients are only in PR and have residual BM involvement at the time of BM harvest or BSC collection, several groups have attempted to purge the BM or positively select CD34⁺ cells from either blood or BM *(14,21,23,30–32)*. Freedman et al. at the Dana-Farber Cancer Institute in Boston described 28 patients with newly diagnosed or relapsed MCL in CR or a minimal disease state (lymph nodes <2 cm and BM <20% involvement) following induction or salvage CT *(21)*. These patients received Cy and TBI followed by purged ABMT. At the time of BM harvest, only 18% of patients were in CR, and most had residual marrow involvement with lymphoma. With a median follow-up of 24 mo, only nine of the 28 patients remained in continuous CR. The DFS and OS were estimated to be 31 and 62%, respectively, at 4 yr posttransplant. The eight patients transplanted in first remission experienced better DFS than the 20 patients transplanted after relapse; the median DFS for the eight patients in first remission and the 20 patients beyond first remission was 49 and 21 mo, respectively (*p* = 0.03). However, Cox proportional hazards regression model, identified no variable (age, sex, stage, histologic subtype, mass >10 cm, BM involvement, extranodal disease, presence of B symptoms, splenic involvement, interval from diagnosis to AMBT, splenectomy, ABMT in first or subsequent remission, and remission status at harvest) that was associated with an improved DFS or OS. They appreciated no plateau in DFS and observed a significant number of relapses beyond 2 yr.

In a separate paper, the investigators at DFCI reported the difficulty in purging the BM of tumor cells in patients with MCL *(30)*. They identified a molecular marker (either *bcl*-1/immunoglobulin H translocation or clonal rearranged immunoglobulin

IMPORTANT DOSAGE CORRECTION

In Current Controversies in Bone Marrow Transplantation, edited by Brian Bolwell, Chapter 11, "Hematopoietic Stem Cell Transplantation for Mantle Cell Lymphoma"

ON PAGE 153, UNDER SUBHEADING 3.4, "PRETRANSPLANTATION CHEMOTHERAPY," IN PARA-GRAPH TWO, REPLACE SENTENCE TWO WITH THE FOLLOWING:

Investigators from MD Anderson Cancer Center (MDACC) in Houston have recently reported (33) the use of an aggressive sequential CT regimen: HyperCVAD alternating with methotrexate and cytarabine (HCVAD/MA). This regimen consists of 300 mg/m^2 Cy over 3 h bid on d 1–3; 50 mg/m^2 Dox over 48 h starting on d 4; 1.4 mg/m^2 vincristine (max. 2 mg) on d 4 and 11; 40 mg/d dexamethasone on d 1–4 and 11–14 alternating with 1 gram/m^2 methotrexate (with leucovorin rescue) infused over 24 h on d 1 and 3 grams/m^2 cytarabine over 2 h bid on d 2 and 3.

heavy-chain gene), which was detectable by PCR in 19 pretransplant MCL patients. Their harvested BM was purged with anti-B-cell monoclonal antibodies and complement-mediated lysis. Five of 19 patients had no morphologic evidence of lymphoma in BM at the time of harvest, but all 19 patients had PCR-detectable disease in the BM. After immunologic purging, no B-cells were detected by flow cytometry; however, all but two patients still had PCR-detectable disease in the BM. These results were in contrast to their patients with follicle center lymphoma and chronic lymphocytic leukemia, in which approx 50% were successfully purged using the same immunologic method.

Only a few investigators have analyzed the ability of CD34-positive selection to reduce or eliminate detectable mantle cells from the autograft. In one patient, who received nine cycles of biweekly CHOP and still had circulating lymphoma cells detectable by flow cytometry, CD34$^+$ selection of G-CSF-mobilized peripheral blood progenitor cells resulted in a three-log reduction of PCR-detectable lymphoma cells *(31)*. In another study, CD34$^+$ cells were positively selected from the leukapheresis products of five MCL patients *(14)*. Prior to CD34$^+$ selection, MCL was detectable by flow cytometry in the products of two patients, and by PCR in six patients. Although no analysis of the leukapheresis products was performed after CD34$^+$ selection, none of the nine patients had PCR-detectable disease in blood and/or BM following transplant.

3.4. Pretransplantation Chemotherapy

Other investigators have attempted to purge in vivo by developing pretransplant CT programs that might successfully minimize or eradicate residual disease from the blood and/or BM prior to stem cell collection or BM harvest *(17,18,27,28)*. Suzan et al. *(27)*, from Paris, described nine evaluable patients with MCL, who were treated on a prospective protocol. Patients received four cycles of CHOP CT. Those patients who achieved at least a PR had PBSCs mobilized with 4.5 g/m^2 Cy and 450 mg/m^2 etoposide with 5 μg/kg/d G-CSF. If a CR was still not achieved, patients received four cycles of DHAP, and PBSCs were harvested after the first two cycles. Patients subsequently received a TBI-based conditioning regimen with ABSCT. None of the patients achieved a CR after CHOP or Cy/etoposide. Eight patients subsequently received four cycles of DHAP, with stem cells collected during recovery from the second cycle. Five of these patients had a CR, and three patients had a good PR (>75%). After transplant, the patient who did not receive DHAP remained in PR; the other eight patients were in CR. Eight patients were still alive, and seven patients remained in CR at the time of the report.

Investigators from MD Anderson Cancer Center (MDAC) in Houston have recently reported *(33)* the use of an aggressive sequential CT regimen: Hyper CVAD alternating with methotrexate and cytarabine (HCVAD/MA). This regimen consists of 300 mg/ m^2 Cy over 3 h bid on d 1–3; 50 mg/m^2 Dox over 48 h, starting on d 4; alternating with 1.4 mg/m^2 vincristine (max 2 mg) on d 4 and 11; 40 mg/d dexamethasone on d 1–4 and 11–14; 1 g/m^2 methotrexate (with leucovorin rescue), infused over 24 h on d 1; and 3 g/m^2 cytarabine over 2 h bid on d 2 and 3. They presented 33 evaluable patients with previously untreated MCL *(17)*. Patients less than 65 yr old received four cycles of HCVAD/MA, followed by consolidation with Cy/TBI and ASCT or allo-SCT. Patients over age 65 yr, and any others not eligible for transplant, completed eight cycles of HCVAD/MA. The median age of the entire group was 57 yr. Thirty (91%) patients were stage IV, and 27 (82%) had BM involvement. Of the 33 patients, 23 patients were eligible for consolidation with transplant, but only 18 patients received it. The median follow-up was 12 (range 5–33) mo. The outcome of this entire group of previously untreated patients was compared to a similar group of previously untreated patients with MCL (median age 54 yr, stage IV = 86%, BM involved = 86%), treated at MDACC from 1986 to 1992 with CHOP or a CHOP-like regimen. The current group of patients had a higher CR rate (HCVAD/MA 87% vs CHOP 21%, $p < 0.0001$), 2-yr FFS (82 vs 32%, $p = 0.002$), and 2-yr OS (81 vs 68%, $p = 0.34$). The 18 patients who were transplanted had a CR rate, 2-yr FFS and OS of 94, 100, and 100%, respectively; the 15 patients who were not transplanted (10 because of age greater than 65 yr) had a CR rate, 2-yr FFS, and OS of 67, 56, and 62%, respectively.

In a separate report, this same group described 19 patients with previously treated MCL who failed frontline therapy, mostly with CHOP (18). The treatment plan was exactly as described above for previously untreated patients. Sixteen (84%) patients achieved a CR, three (15%) achieved only a PR, and one failed to respond. Thirteen patients subsequently received allo-SCT ($n = 5$) or ASCT ($n = 8$). The median follow-up was 13 (range 6–38) mo. Among the entire group, the 2-year FFS was 45%, and the OS was 52%. Of five allograft recipients, two died from complications, and none relapsed. Of the eight autograft recipients, two relapsed and two died from complications of the transplant.

3.5. Posttransplantation Residual Disease

A few groups have evaluated residual disease, using PCR following autotransplantation (14,28,30). For example, the nine patients reported by Dreger et al. (14), who were in clinical remission following transplant, also had no PCR-detectable monoclonal immunoglobulin heavy chain gene in the blood or marrow. Of the eight patients reported by Corradini et al. (28), four actually received the planned HDT with ABSCT. One patient had no PCR-detectable lymphoma in the BM at 12, 29, and 35 mo posttransplant, and remained in clinical remission. One patient, who was only evaluated at 9 mo posttransplant, had no PCR-detectable lymphoma in the BM, and was also in clinical remission. The other two patients were evaluated 10–34 and 44–58 mo posttransplant, and had persistently PCR-positive BM. One of these patients clinically relapsed.

Anderson et al. (30) evaluated BM and/or blood samples from 17 patients posttransplant. Eight of 11 patients, who had PCR-detectable MCL in the first BM and/or blood sample obtained soon after ABMT, relapsed by 2 yr posttransplant; one other patient relapsed nearly 6 yr posttransplant. Seven of 9 patients, with PCR-detectable MCL in every post-ABMT BM and/or blood sample, relapsed. Two patients had persistently PCR-positive BM and/or blood, but had not clinically relapsed at 2 yr post-ABMT. Two patients initially had PCR-negative BM and/or blood post-ABMT, subsequently became PCR-positive, and then clinically relapsed within 16 mo of converting. Four patients remained persistently PCR-negative post-ABMT, and only one has relapsed 4 yr post-ABMT.

4. ALLOGENEIC TRANSPLANTATION

Several investigators have reported the results of allotransplantation, and some have documented an apparent graft-vs-lymphoma effect (17,18,22–26,34–36). For example, Adkins et al. (35) described a 55-yr-old man with the blastic variant of MCL, who had failed four prior CT regimens. This patient then received high-dose etoposide, Cy, and TBI, followed by a BMT from an HLA-matched sibling. Following the transplant, blastic cells persisted in the patient's peripheral blood. On d 20 posttransplant, however, a dramatic decrease in circulating leukemia cells occurred, and by d 27 posttransplant, no circulating tumor cells were identifiable. Evaluation (including variable number of tandem repeats) on d 69 posttransplant confirmed a CR, with complete donor engraftment. Corradini et al. *(36)* described a 32-yr-old man with MCL (including diffuse lymphadenopathy, splenomegaly, leukocytosis, and 70% marrow involvement), who received aggressive induction CT (APO × 2, DHAP × 2, and cytarabine/mitoxantrone), yet 40% marrow infiltration persisted. He subsequently received high-dose thiotepa and Cy and G-CSF-mobilized, HLA-identical sibling BSCs. He had no acute graft-vs-host disease (GVHD) but did develop mild chronic GVHD. Tumor-specific immunoglobulin gene DNA was undetectable by PCR at 12 mo post-BMT and the patient remained in remission 16 mo post-BMT.

Sohn et al. *(26),* from Fred Hutchinson Cancer Center in Seattle, presented 12 MCL patients (median age 45 yr), who received HDT and allo-BMT. Prior to transplant, 92% had BM involvement, and 42% had blood involvement. Only 17% achieved a CR with initial treatment, and 33% were refractory to salvage therapy at the time of transplant. Nine of 12 evaluable patients achieved a CR with transplant. With a median follow-up of 3 (range 1–11) yr, eight patients died (one of relapse, three of infection, one of chronic GVHD, two of pulmonary complications, and one of hepatitis). OS and EFS at 3 yr were 23 and 12%, respectively.

Khouri et al. *(22)* recently reported the results of allotransplantation at MDACC in Houston. Thirteen patients ≤60 yr of age received HCVAD/MA cytoreduction (as described above), followed by matched-sibling donor PBSCT. The median age was 53 yr (range 38–58 yr). All had stage IV disease with marrow involvement. Nine were previously treated: Five failed induction therapy, and one failed a prior autotransplant. At the time of transplant, three had refractory disease, seven were in PR, and three were in CR. Ten patients received Cy and TBI; three other patients received BEAM. Twelve achieved a CR, and one achieved a good PR. With a median follow-up of 21 (range 4–44) mo, none of the patients relapsed. One died at 3 mo post-BMT, because of acute GVHD/sepsis, and two others died, also, in CR from chronic GVHD. OS and FFS at 3 yr were both 67%.

Two additional patients received a nonmyeloablative preparative regimen (25 mg/m^2/d × 4 cisplatin; 30 mg/m^2/d × 2 fludarabine; and 1000 mg/m^2/d × 2 cytarabine) *(22)*. One patient, transplanted in first remission, had graft failure, and subsequently relapsed and died 4 mo later. The other patient was 57 yr old, was refractory to three prior conventional CT regimens, and had no response in the marrow to pretransplant induction therapy. At the time of transplant and 1 mo posttransplant, the patient had lymphadenopathy and 50–85% marrow involvement, with lymphoma. Three mo posttransplant, the patient developed GVHD, and, by 8 mo posttransplant, the lymphadenopathy resolved and the BM involvement decreased to 5%.

5. THE CLEVELAND CLINIC FOUNDATION EXPERIENCE

Eleven patients with MCL were identified in the database of the Cleveland Clinic Foundation BMT Program (Table 3). Eight patients were diagnosed prospectively, according to standard criteria. Three patients initially had a diagnosis of diffuse small-cleaved-cell lymphoma, and were retrospectively diagnosed with MCL. The median age was 55 yr (range 34–68 yr). All had stage IV disease, with BM involvement. The IPI was 1 in three patients and 2–3 in the rest. Eight patients had received 2–3 prior CT regimens. Only three patients had received one prior CT regimen, and were transplanted as part of the initial planned therapy. At the time of transplant, the median age was 56 yr (range 34–69 yr), and a median of 12 mo (range 4–62) had elapsed since diagnosis. All patients were in PR at the time of transplant, and at least eight had persistent BM involvement. The preparative regimen consisted of 14 mg/kg busulfan, 50–60 mg/kg etoposide, and 120 mg/kg Cy (37). Two patients received HLA-identical sibling BM, and nine patients received hematopoietic, growth-factor-mobilized, autologous BSCs. Seven patients achieved a CR. One patient relapsed 12 mo after transplant, and one patient died from pulmonary fibrosis 4 mo after transplant (and 66 mo after diagnosis). Nine patients remain alive, without evidence of disease progression, 3–34 (median 11) mo after transplant.

6. LONG-TERM FOLLOWUP

The PFS and OS in these series varied widely. These differences may reflect the heterogeneous biologic behavior of MCL, the variable status of disease at the time of transplant, and the specific selection criteria used by different transplant centers. The follow-up, in the majority of these studies, was short. Only four studies had a median follow-up of 2 yr or more (19,21,24,26). Among the 134 autograft patients in these four studies, the number of patients that remained in remission varied inversely to the duration of follow-up. The estimated DFS (or EFS or PFS), from the time of transplant, was 75% at 2 yr (19), 54 and 49% at 3 yr (24,26), and 31% at 4 yr (21). The estimated OS in these same four studies was 91% at 2 yr (19), 63% at 3 yr (26), and 81 and 62% at 4 yr (21,24). Although the data are limited, the long-term results in these four studies suggest that the extraordinary results reported in some of the other studies may show that follow-up was too short, and that the majority of patients will eventually relapse. Nevertheless, the survival duration following autotransplant appears substantially longer than expected or reported with conventional CT. Whether this observation is the result of a selection bias, or an alteration of the natural history of the disease, is uncertain.

7. SUMMARY AND CONCLUSIONS

Data from these and other studies suggest that MCL has an intrinsically low sensitivity to conventional CT, and that remissions occur slowly. Adequate pretransplant remissions may not be achieved with standard alkylator- and/or anthracycline-based CT (e.g., CHOP). High-dose cytarabine-based regimens may be more effective. The presence of MCL in the blood, BM, and leukapheresis products, following conventional CT and prior to autotransplantation, is an obvious concern. Although the clonogenic potential is not proven, these residual malignant cells probably contribute to posttransplant disease relapse. The optimal method to rid the blood, BM, and/or leukapheresis products of potentially contaminating malignant cells is unknown. Purging BM appears ineffective, and CD34 selection is inadequately studied.

Table 3
Patients with MCL who Received High-dose CT with Autologous or Allogeneic Hematopoietic Cell Transplantation at the Cleveland Clinic Foundation

	Diagnosis									Transplant							Posttransplant		
Patient	Sex	Age	Stage	PS>1	>1ES	LDH	BM	IPI	Treatment	Dx→Tx (mo)	Age	Status	BM	LDH	Transplant	Response	Follow-up (mo)	Progression?	Alive?
1	F	43	IV	–	+	↑	+	3	Splenectomy CVP × 6 CHOP × 3	20	45	PR 2	+	nl	MSD BMT	CR	34	No	Yes
2	M	65	IV	–	–	nl	+	2	CHOP × 6 MINE × 3	12	66	PR 2	u	nl	ABSCT	CR	31	No	Yes
3	M	52	IV	–	+	u	+	2 or 3	CHOP × 2 P-C × 4 ESHAP × 2	12	53	PR 1	+	nl	ABSCT	PR	37	No	Yes
4	M	58	IV	–	+	u	+	2 or 3	CHOP × 9 DHAP × 2	11	59	PR 1	+	nl	ABSCT	PR	17	No	Yes
5	M	59	IV	–	+	↑	+	3	Fl-M × 6 CHOP × 2	22	61	PR 2	–	↑	ABSCT	CR	17	Yes @ 12 mo	Yes
6	F	34	IV	–	–	nl	+	1	CHOP × 4	4	34	PR 1	+	nl	ABSCT	CR	11	No	Yes
7	F	55	IV	–	+	u	+	2 or 3	CHOP × 6 DHAP × 3	12	56	PR 1	+	↑	ABSCT	CR	11	No	Yes
8	M	43	IV	–	–	↑	+	2	CHOP × 8	7	44	PR 1	+	↑	ABSCT	CR	3	No	Yes
9	M	51	III	–	–	nl	–	1	CVP × 6 Fl-M × 2, CHOP × 6	15	52	PR 2	+	nl	MSD BMT	CR	9	No	Yes
10	M	57	II	–	–	nl	–	1	Excision/RT Excision Fl × 3, CHOP × 8, DHAP × 3	62	62	PR 3	+	↑	ABSCT	PR	4	No	No/PF
11	M	68	IV	–	+	nl	+	3	CHOP × 6	6	69	PR 1	–	↑	ABSCT	PR	3	No	Yes

ABSCT, autologous blood stem cell transplantation; BM, bone marrow; CR, complete remission; Dx↑Tx (mo), time from diagnosis to transplant (months); ES, extranodal sites; Fl, fludarabine; IPI, International Prognostic Index; LD, lactate dehydrogenase; M, mitoxantrone; mo, months; nl, normal; PF, pulmonary fibrosis; MSD BMT, HLA-matched sibling donor BMT; PR, partial remission; Pt, patient, u, unknown; ↑, elevated.

Allotransplantation is particularly promising. Anecdotal reports have demonstrated and proven the importance of a graft-versus-lymphoma effect in achieving CRs and potential cures. Several series include one or more patients that failed autotransplantation, but subsequently experienced continuous DFS following allotransplantation. Although the morbidity and mortality are high, only 15% of the allotransplant patients reported in the literature have relapsed.

HDT and HSCT should be discussed with all MCL patients, preferably at the time of diagnosis. Patients in first, especially complete, remission are the best candidates for autologous hematopoietic transplantation. On the other hand, young patients and patients with relapsed or refractory disease, who have an HLA-matched donor, might benefit more from an allotransplantation.

REFERENCES

1. Fisher RI, Dahlberg S, Nathwani BN, Danko PM, Miller TP, and Grogan TM. A clinical analysis of two indolent lymphoma entities: mantle cell lymphoma and marginal zone lymphoma (including the mucosa-associated lymphoid tissue and monocytoid B-cell subcategories): a Southwest Oncology Group study, *Blood*, **85** (1995) 1075–1082.

2. Teodorovic I, Pittaluga S, Kluin-Nelemans JC, et al. Efficacy of four different regimens in 64 mantle-cell lymphoma cases: clinicopathologic comparison with 498 other non-Hodgkin's lymphoma subtypes, *J. Clin. Oncol.*, **13** (1995) 2819–2826.

3. Pittaluga S, Bignens L, Teodorovic I, et al. Clinical analysis of 670 cases in two trials of the European Organization for the Research and Treatment of Cancer Lymphoma Cooperative Group subtyped according to the Revised European-American Classification of Lymphoid Neoplasms: a comparison with the Working Formulation, *Blood*, **87** (1996) 4385–4367.

4. Lennert K, Mohri N, Stein H, et al. The histopathology of maligiant lymphoma, *Br. J. Haematol.*, **31 (Suppl)** (1975) 193–203.

5. Beard CW and Dorfman RF. Histopathology of malignant lymphoma. In Rosenberg SA (ed), *Clinics in Hematology*, WB Saunders, London, **3** (1974) 39.

6. Weisenburger DD, Nathwani BN, Diamond LW, Winberg CD, and Rappaport H. Malignant lymphoma, intermediate lymphocytic type: a clinicopathologic study of 42 cases, *Cancer*, **48** (1981) 1415–1425.

7. Banks PM, Chan J, Clear ML, et al. Mantle cell lymphoma: a proposal for unification of morphologic, immunologic, and molecular data, *Am. J. Surg. Pathol.*, **16** (1992) 637–640.

8. Harris NL, Jaffe ES, Stein H, et al. A revised European-American classification of lymphoid neoplasms: a proposal from the International Lymphoma Study Group, *Blood*, **84** (1994) 1361–1392.

9. Armitage JO, Weisenburger DD, for the Non-Hodgkin's Lymphoma Classification Project. New approach to classifying non-Hodgkin's lymphomas: clinical features for the major histologic subtypes, *J. Clin. Oncol.*, **16** (1998) 2780–2740.

10. Press OW, Grogan TM, and Fisher RI. Evaluation and management of mantle cell lymphoma, *Adv. Leukemia Lymphoma.*, **6** (1996) 3–11.

11. Meusers P, Engelhard M, Bartels H, et al. Multicentre randomized therapeutic trial for advanced centrocytic lymphoma: anthracycline does not improve the prognosis, *Hematol. Oncol.*, **7** (1989) 365–380.

12. Stewart DA, Vose JM, Weisenburger DD, et al. Role of high-dose therapy and autologous hematopoietic stem cell transplantation for mantle cell lymphoma, *Ann. Oncol.*, **6** (1995) 263–266.

13. Haas R, Brittinger G, Neusers P, et al. Myeloablative therapy with blood stem cell transplantation is effective in mantle cell lymphoma, *Leukemia*, **10** (1996) 975–979.

14. Dreger P, von Neuhoff N, Kuse R, et al. Sequential high-dose therapy and autologous stem cell transplantation for treatment of mantle cell lymphoma, *Ann. Oncol.*, **8** (1997) 401–403.

15. Gressin R, Legouffe E, Leroux D, et al. Treatment of mantle-cell lymphomas with the VAD +/– chlorambucil regimen with or without subsequent high-dose therapy and peripheral blood stem-cell transplantation, *Ann. Oncol.*, **8 (Suppl. 1)** (1997) 103–106.

16. Ketterer N, Salles G, Espinouse D, et al. Intensive therapy with peripheral stem cell transplantation in 16 patients with mantle cell lymphoma, *Ann. Oncol.*, **8** (1997) 701–704.

17. Khouri I, Romaguera J, Kantarjian H, et al. Preliminary report of an active regimen for mantle cell lymphoma, *Blood,* **90 (Suppl. 1)** (1997) 1092(Abstract).
18. Romaguera J, Khouri J, Hagemeister FB, et al. HCVAD/Ara-C-MTX with or without high-dose chemotherapy and stem cell transfusion as salvage for relapsed or refractory diffuse/nodular mantle cell lymphoma, *Blood,* **90 (Suppl. 1)** (1997) 834(Abstract).
19. Blay JY, Sebban C, Surbiguet C, et al. High-dose chemotherapy with hematopoietic stem cell transplantation in patients with mantle cell or diffuse centrocytic non-Hodgkin's lymphomas: a single center experience on 18 patients, *Bone Marrow Transplant.,* **21** (1998) 51–54.
20. Conde E, Bosch F, Arranz R, et al. Autologous stem cell transplantation for mantle cell lymphoma. The experience of the GEL/TAMO Spanish Cooperative Group, *Blood,* **92 (Suppl. 1)** (1998) 1915(Abstract).
21. Freedman AS, Neuberg D, Gribben JG, et al. High-Dose chemoradiotherapy and anti-B-cell monoclonal antibody-purged autologous bone marrow transplantation in mantle-cell lymphoma: no evidence for long-term remission, *J. Clin. Oncol.,* **16** (1998) 13–18.
22. Khouri I, Korbling M, Albitar M, et al. Allogeneic stem cell transplantation for mantle cell lymphoma (MCL): evidence of graft-versus-lymphoma effect (GVL), *Blood,* **90 (Suppl. 1)** (1998) 2708(Abstract).
23. Kröger N, Hoffknecht M, Dreger P, et al. Long-term disease-free survival of patients with advanced mantle-cell lymphoma following high-dose chemotherapy, *Bone Marrow Transplant.,* **21** (1998) 55–57.
24. Milpied N, Gaillard F, Moreau P, et al. High-dose therapy with stem cell transplantation for mantle cell lymphoma: results and prognostic factors, a single center experience, *Bone Marrow Transplant.,* **22** (1998) 645–650.
25. Molina A, Nademanee A, O'Donnell MR, et al. Autologous (auto) and allogeneic (allo) stem cell transplantation (SCT) for poor-risk mantle cell lymphoma (MCL): the City of Hope (COH) experience, *Blood,* **92 (suppl 1)** (1998) 1894(Abstract).
26. Sohn SK, Bensinger W, Holmberg L, et al. High-dose therapy with allogeneic or autologous stem cell transplantation for relapsed mantle cell lymphoma: the Seattle experience, *Proc. ASCO.,* **17** (1998) 64(Abstract).
27. Suzan F, Belanger C, Ribrag V, et al. Preliminary report of a strategy assessing a CHOP-regimen and high dose ara-C (DHAP) followed by high-dose chemotherapy with autologous peripheral blood stem cell transplantation (APBSCT) for mantle cell lymphoma (MCL), *Blood,* **92 (Suppl. 1)** (1998) 1916(Abstract).
28. Corradini P, Astolfi M, Cherasco C, et al. Molecular monitoring of minimal residual disease in follicular and mantle cell non-Hodgkin's lymphomas treated with high-dose chemotherapy and peripheral blood progenitor cell autografting, *Blood,* **89** (1997) 724–731.
29. Jacquy C, Soree A, Bosly A, Ferrant A, Bron D, and Martiat P. Peripheral blood stem cells contamination in diffuse large cell (DLCL) and mantle cell (MCL) lymphomas: a quantitative comparison, *Blood,* **92 (Suppl. 1)** (1998) 976(Abstract).
30. Andersen NS, Donovan JW, Borus JS, et al. Failure of immunologic purging in mantle cell lymphoma assessed by polymerase chain reaction detection of minimal residual disease, *Blood,* **90** (1997) 4212–4221.
31. Uehira K, Kagami Y, Ogura M, et al. A high dose chemoradiotherapy and peripheral blood stem cell support combined with the CD34(+)-selection method in cyclin D1(+)-mantle cell lymphoma, *Int. J. Hematol.,* **67** (1998) 187–190.
32. Di Nicola M, Magni M, Milanesi M, et al. Successful elimination of follicular or mantle non-Hodgkin lymphoma cells from hematopoietic progenitor cell transplants by high-dose chemotherapy and ex-vivo purging of CD19+ cells, *Blood,* **92 (Suppl. 1)** (1998) 2677(Abstract).
33. Romaguera J, Khouri I, Champlin R, et al. HCVAD/MTX-ARAC: A new effective regimen for diffuse and nodular mantle cell lymphoma (MCL), *Blood,* **88 (Suppl. 1)** (1996) 2261(Abstract).
34. Tongol JM, Carrum G, Udden MM, Lynch G, Williams G, McCarthy PL. Successful allogeneic transplantation in a patient with mantle cell lymphoma, *Proc. ASCO.,* **14** (1995) 11(Abstract).
35. Adkins D, Brown R, Goodnough LT, Khoury H, Popovic W, and DiPersio J. Treatment of resistant mantle cell lymphoma with allogeneic. Bone marrow transplantation, *Bone Marrow Transplant.,* **21** (1998) 97–99.
36. Corradini P, Ladetto M, Astolfi M, et al. Clinical and molecular remission after allogeneic blood cell transplantation in a patient with mantle-cell lymphoma, *Br. J. Haematol.,* **94** (1996) 376–378.
37. Copelan E, Penza S, Pohlman B, et al. A novel Bu/Cy/VP-16 regimen in non-Hodgkin's lymphoma, *Blood,* **92 (Suppl. 1)** (1998) 2737(Abstract).

12 Is Autologous Transplantation for Non-Hodgkin's Lymphoma Underutilized?

Brian J. Bolwell, MD

CONTENTS

1. INTRODUCTION

Thousands of patients with a variety of malignancies have received high-dose chemotherapy (HDCT) with autologous bone marrow transplantation (ABMT)/peripheral blood progenitor cell transplantation (PBPCT) over the past two decades. The use of ABMT in non-Hodgkin's lymphoma (NHL) is an unequivocal success. AMBT now represents state-of-the-art care for many lymphoma patients, and has changed the standard of care for such patients worldwide. In the 1980s, clinical trials showed that ABMT potentially salvaged patients with relapsed/refractory NHL, who were otherwise destined to die of their disease. The superiority of transplantation over conventional therapy for relapsed intermediate and high-grade NHL has been confirmed in a landmark prospective randomized trial (Subheading 2.1). This data has confirmed the proof of

From: *Current Controversies in Bone Marrow Transplantation*
Edited by: B. Bolwell © Humana Press Inc., Totowa, NJ

principle that HDCT may, in fact, overcome tumor cells resistant to conventional-dose CT, and cure some patients who are otherwise incurable. With current techniques utilizing hematopoietic growth factors and PBPCs, mortality risks have decreased to 1–3%. The well-documented efficacy, coupled with decreased morbidity and mortality, have led to clinical research studies utilizing autologous stem cell transplantation (ASCT) for additional groups of patients with NHL, including those with intermediate- and high-grade NHL with poor prognostic factors in first remission, as well as those with poor-prognosis follicular NHL. This chapter briefly reviews autologous transplantation (autotransplantation) in NHL from a historical prospective, then discusses current indications for patients with relapsed/refractory intermediate- and high-grade NHL, and examines the potential utility of autotransplantation in follicular NHL, as well as for those patients with intermediate- and high-grade NHL with poor prognostic features at presentation.

2. ABMT FOR RELAPSED/REFRACTORY NHL

Patients with aggressive histologies of NHL relapsing after primary chemotherapy (CT) are essentially incurable, and generally have a life expectancy measured in months. Those who respond poorly to initial CT have an even grimmer prognosis. Thus, despite the morbidity of ABMT in the 1980s, patients with relapsed or refractory NHL were felt to be candidates for clinical trials of ABMT, because of their otherwise poor prognosis. Table 1 shows the results of some of the early phase II trials of ABMT for such relapsed/refractory patients. These, and other studies, led to several important observations. First, durable remissions were clearly possible in this group of patients, who had no hope for durable remissions with any conventional therapy: 20–40% of patients with refractory disease achieved continuous complete remissions (CR). Second, prognostic variables of transplant outcome could be identified for patients pretransplant. Patients had a worse outcome with transplantation if they entered the transplant with an elevated lactic dehydrogenase (LDH), if they had undergone histologic transformation to a more aggressive histology, or if they had refractory disease. Philip et al. *(1)* introduced the concept of "sensitive relapse," and found that transplant outcome correlated with a patient's response to re-treatment with CT at the time of relapse. Those continuing to respond to CT had a 36% chance of a continued CR after ABMT; those patients having an initial response to CT, but who were no longer responding at the time of transplant, had a 14% chance of continued CR; and those patients never responding to CT had a 0% chance of a continued CR. Subsequent studies have shown that even refractory patients do have a low, but finite, chance of durable remission with autotransplantation *(5–8)*.

Most subsequent series showed that 25–45% of patients with relapsed/refractory NHL achieved extended remissions, and were probably cured with ABMT *(5–11)*. The Cleveland Clinic found that the evaluation of patients 2 yr posttransplant was of great interest. The author et al. *(12)* examined a group of relapsed/refractory NHL patients in CR 2 yr after ABMT *(12)*. These CR patients were then followed for an additional 2–6 yr, and it was found that all patients with high-grade histologies in CR 2 yr posttransplant remained in CR with extended follow-up, i.e., none of these patients subsequently relapsed. Eighty percent of those with intermediate grade NHL in CR 2 yr posttransplant remained so with additional follow-up. The study, therefore, represents

Table 1
ABMT in NHL: Early Trials

Source	No. patients	Preparative regimen	Induction mortality (%)	Outcome
Philip et al. 1987 (1)	100 recurrent/ refractory intermediate or high-grade	39 TBI and CT 61 CT alone	21	0% CCR refractory 14% CCR-resistant relapse 36% CCR-sensitive relapse
Appelbaum et al. (1987) (2)	100 recurrent NHL 36 high-grade 46 intermediate grade (18 HD)	24 autologous Cy/TBI 13 syngeneic 60 allogeneic	36 (Including complications of allo-BMT)	24% CCR (no difference in allo-BMT or ABMT) Best if done in CR2 (sensitive relapse)
Takvorian et al. 1987 (3)	49 responsive to chemotherapy 29 high-grade 14 intermediate 6 low-grade	Cy/TBI mAb purge	4	65% CCR at 1 yr
Vose et al. 1989 (4)	25 recurrent/ refractory intermediate or high-grade	18 TBI and CT 7 CT	24	5-yr DFS 40% Poor prognosis factors: Mass > 10 cm; ↑ LDH; histologic transformation

Abbreviation: TBI, total body irradiation; CCR, continuous complete remission; NHL, non-Hodgkin's lymphoma; HD, Hodgkin's disease; CY/TBI, cyclophosphamide plus total body irradiation; BMT, bone marrow transplantation; CR2, second complete remissions; mAb, monoclonal antibody; DFS, disease-free survival; LDH, lactate dehydrogenase.

further evidence that, not only are CRs possible after ABMT for relapsed/refractory NHL patients, but they are durable, because the vast majority of patients remain in CR with extended follow-up.

Thus, from 1985 through 1994, multiple clinical research studies showed that 25–45% of the patients with relapsed/refractory intermediate- and high-grade NHL were probably cured with ABMT/ASCT in phase II studies. This led to the design of phase III, prospective randomized trials.

2.1. The Parma Trial

The landmark prospective randomized trial showing the clear superiority of autotransplantation over conventional CT for relapsed/refractory NHL is the Parma Trial (13). 215 patients, with relapsed intermediate- or high-grade disease, were enrolled in this trial from July 1987 through June 1994. All patients had been treated with a doxorubicin-containing CT regimen, and all patients had an initial CR to CT. At the time of relapse, all patients received one course of dexamethasone, cisplatin, and cytarabine (DHAP). The patients then underwent a bone marrow harvest. After a second course of DHAP, patients achieving a response were randomized to continue four courses of DHAP or ABMT (peripheral stem cells were not used in this study). The transplant-preparative regimen was carmustine, etoposide, cytarabine, and cyclophosphamide (Cy). With a median follow-up of 63 mo, the overall response rate was 84% after BMT, and 44% after standard-dose CT without transplantation. With follow-up of 5 yr, the rate of event-free survival was 46% in the transplantation group and 12% in the group receiving CT without transplantation ($p = 0.001$). The overall survival (OS) rates were 53 and 32%, respectively ($p = 0.04$).

One of the important aspects of the study was the outcome of patients treated in the conventional treatment group: 45/54 patients relapsed. Only 18/45 relapsed patients subsequently received ABMT; 14/18 died; two survived with relapses; and only two were alive and free of disease 1–3 yr after bone marrow transplantation (BMT).

In May 1998, the Parma Trial was updated at the annual meeting of the American Society of Clinical Oncology *(14)*. With a median follow-up of 100 mo, the 8-yr event-free survival rate was 36%, and the ABMT arm and 11% in the DHAP arm ($p < 0.002$) and the rates of OS were 47 and 27%, respectively ($p = 0.04$),

This study represents concrete evidence that ABMT is the treatment of choice for patients with relapsed intermediate- and high-grade histology NHL. It also underscored the importance of the timeliness of ABMT, and the fact that repeated cycles of conventional-dose CT are potentially deleterious in the overall outcome of this patient population.

2.2. Commentary: Is ABMT Underutilized for Intermediate/High-grade Patients with Relapsed/Refractory Disease?

Approximately 57,000 patients will be diagnosed with NHL in the United States in 1999. Of these, approx 35% will be low-grade lymphomas, 38% intermediate-grade, and 17% high-grade *(26)*. Approximately 65% of those with intermediate-grade will be ≤65 yr of age, and 80% of those with high-grade will be <65 yr old. This means that approx 22,000 patients will be diagnosed with intermediate- or high-grade lymphoma who are less than 65 yr. Approximately 85% (19,000) of these patients will be stage II, III, or IV. No CT for these patients has ever been shown to be superior to Cy, doxorubicin, vincristine, and prednisone (CHOP) in conventional doses *(15)*. With long-term follow-up, CHOP cures 30% of patients with diffuse large-cell NHL *(16)*. This means that approx 5600 of the original 19,000 patients will be cured with CHOP; 13,000 are destined to relapse. The treatment of choice for such patients is ASCT. A distinct minority of these patients even come to transplantation. ABMT can potentially cure approx 40% of these patients. The fact that a minority of these patients ever come to transplant means that thousands of patients with relapsed/refractory intermediate/high-grade NHL die because they never will receive an ABMT/ASCT. Clearly, ABMT is underutilized in relapsed/refractory aggressive/intermediate-grade NHL.

3. BMT/SCT FOR FOLLICULAR LYMPHOMA

3.1. Introduction

One of the chief reasons why ABMT was utilized in patients with intermediate and aggressive subtypes of NHL in the 1980s was the uniformly poor prognosis of patients with relapsed or refractory disease. The fact that low-grade lymphoma patients have a more indolent course made the risks of BMT in the 1980s prohibitive. With the advent of hematopoietic growth factor therapy, and the use of primed PBPC, the mortality risk of auto-PBPC transplantation is now approx 2% *(17–20)*, and there has been a recent re-examination of ABMT/ASCT in the treatment of follicular NHL. Newer data allows an examination of patients with follicular lymphoma (FL) who may have a poor prognosis, and who, therefore, may be candidates for more aggressive therapy; additionally, more mature data is available concerning long-term outcomes of both autologous and allogeneic BMT/SCT.

3.2. Can We Identify Patients with FL with a Poor Prognosis?

Survival for follicle-center NHL is often reported to be 5–10 yr from diagnosis. Recent data indicates, however, that it is possible to identify subtypes of patients with a worse prognosis. The International Prognostic Index (IPI) for aggressive lymphomas has been a useful device to segregate patients into low-risk, low-intermediate risk, high-intermediate risk, or high-risk *(21)*. This index is based on the following variables: age (≤60 yr vs >60 yr), performance status (Eastern Cooperative Oncology Group [ECOG], 0 or 1 vs 2–4), Ann Arbor Stage (1–2 vs 3–4), extranodal involvement (<2 vs ≥2 sites), and serum LDH level (normal vs high). Patients with 0–1 unfavorable risk factors are considered to be of low-risk, those with two are low-intermediate risk, those with three are high-intermediate risk, and those with 4–5 adverse factors are considered to be high-risk. This index has been shown to be useful as a prognostic tool for patients with low-grade lymphoma as well. One study found 10-yr OS rates correlated strongly with the IPI for patients with follicular lymphomas, ranging from 74% for those with a low IPI score to 0% for those with a high IPI *(22)*. Additionally, the Non-Hodgkin's Lymphoma Classification Project recently completed a clinical evaluation of the International Study Group Classification of non-Hodgkin's lymphoma *(23)* and found that survival correlated strongly with the IPI for patients with FLs: 5-yr OS and failure-free survival (FFS) for those with a low IPI score was 84 and 55%, compared with 17 and 6% for those with a high IPI. These authors made a point of stating that patients with FL with a high IPI had a far worse overall FFS than did patients with diffuse large-cell B-cell lymphoma and a low IPI. Therefore, patients with FL with a high IPI score have a very poor prognosis, and are potential candidates for more aggressive therapy.

Response to therapy is another possible discriminating variable to define patients with FL destined to have a poor outcome. An ECOG study of a multivariate analysis of patients with low-grade NHL, relapsing after initial CT treatment, found that those patients achieving a CR or a partial response (PR) that lasted for less than 1 yr had a 5-yr OS of only 33%; patients who had never achieved a CR, but had a PR that lasted for greater than 1 yr, had a 5-year OS rate of 40%; patients who achieved a CR that lasted longer than 1 yr had a 5-yr OS of 55% *(24)*. Median survival for those experiencing a CR of more than 1 yr was 5.9 yr, compared with 2 yr for those with a PR of more than 1 yr, and 2.5 yr with a CR or PR of less than 1 yr ($p < 0.01$). Those authors concluded that those patients with low-grade lymphomas who had a response lasting less than 1 yr were potential candidates for more aggressive therapy, including ASCT. Additionally, it has been shown that the duration of response inversely correlates with the number of courses of prior CT. By the fourth cycle of conventional CT, virtually all patients either do not respond or have a response measured in weeks *(25)*. Thus, not only is a poor response to initial CT an important prognostic variable with respect to outcome of patients with follicle-center lymphoma, but so is the number of courses of prior CT that the patient has received.

Transformation to a higher-grade histology is indicative of a poor outcome. Response to therapy may predict which patients are more likely to transform. Bastion et al. *(28)* recently reported on 220 patients with FL, with a median follow-up of 9 yr, with respect to histologic transformation. Transformation occurred in 37% of patients studied, with a median survival after transformation of only 7 mo. Patients achieving a CR to initial therapy were far less likely to transform into a higher-grade histology than were patients with a PR. The probability of transformation for patients with an initial CR was 24%, compared to 51% for those who achieved only PR ($p < 0.0001$). Thus, patients not achieving a CR have a lower survival after relapse than do those that achieve an initial CR, and are more likely to suffer histologic transformation and its resultant dismal prognosis.

The recent REAL classification of lymphomas does not segregate follicular large-cell lymphomas into the intermediate histology grouping *(27)*. Rather, it classifies FLs as grade I—III, depending on the number of large cells present. However, the classification does not precisely define a given percentage of large cells that constitutes grade I–III. Thus, whether all FLs, according to the REAL classification, are truly low-grade is an open question. Indeed, the original analysis by the Working Formulation *(28)* found median survival of follicular large-cell lymphoma to be 3.0 yr, compared with a median survival of 5.1 yr for follicular mixed-cell lymphoma, and 7.2 yr for follicular small-cleaved. A retrospective review by Martin et al. *(29)*, of the prognostic value of histologic grade in FL, found that OS was worse for follicular large-cell lymphomas, compared with other follicular histologies. However, depending on the classification used, FFS might actually be better for follicular large-cell lymphoma, with a plateau on the survival curve similar to diffuse large-cell lymphoma. Wendum et al. *(30)* compared patients with follicular large-cell lymphoma, treated with intensive CT, with patients with diffuse large-cell lymphoma. Overall 5-yr freedom from progression was identical in the two treatment groups (39 vs 43%), and it was felt that the overall results of follicular large-cell lymphoma were similar to that with diffuse large-cell lymphoma. Thus, at least some authors feel that follicular large-cell lymphoma (or FL of grade III) behave more aggressively than other indolent lymphomas, and have outcomes that may be similar to diffuse large-cell lymphoma. Additionally, a conservative approach may not be optimal in some patients, because of the potential poor OS, as originally shown by the Working Formulation analysis.

Increasing data now are available to determine subsets of patients with FLs who may have a much worse prognosis than the usual stated expected survival rate of 5–10 yr: Specifically, those patients with a high IPI score; those patients who do not achieve a CR to initial CT; patients with an initial response to CT lasting less than 1 yr; patients who have received multiple courses of prior CT; and, potentially, those patients with follicular large-cell lymphoma are candidates for more aggressive therapy, including HDCT and ASCT.

3.3. Potential Goals of Transplantation

The most commonly stated goal of transplantation is cure. It is important to remember that FLs are, in fact, curable. Stage I–II patients with FLs have long been treated with radiation therapy. A landmark article by Kaplan in 1966 *(31)* showed evidence for a tumoricidal dose level of radiotherapy of Hodgkin's disease, demonstrating that a clear dose–response curve existed. One might argue that this represented the first clinical proof of principle that dose intensity is important in cancer therapy. Stanford recently updated their experience *(32)* with radiation therapy for stage I–II Fls, and showed that patients who remained disease-free for 10 yr were very unlikely to relapse, implying that many of these patients were cured. Thus, FLs can, potentially, be cured.

The technique of HDCT and ASCT has been refined to the point that mortality rates associated with the procedure are 1–3%. This is not significantly different than the mortality risk of outpatient CT, as reported in cooperative group trials. Thus, in addition to cure, one might argue that another goal of autotransplantation is improved disease control, even if patients are destined to relapse at a later date. If OS, progression-free survival (PFS), and quality of life are found to be enhanced by HDCT and ASCT, then ABMT would clearly be worthwhile.

3.4. BMT for FL: Current Results

Small number of patients, and short follow-up, limit many reports concerning the outcome of ABMT for follicular NHL. Recently, several studies have been published with more mature data. The author et al. *(12)* recently reported the experience at the Cleveland Clinic Foundation of autotransplantation for NHL using the Cy, carmustine (BCNU), VP-16 (CBV) preparative regimen. Between 1988 and 1993, a total of 110 patients were studied, with a median follow-up of survivors of approx 4 yr *(12)*. Included in this analysis were 22 patients with low-grade NHL, and another 10 patients with follicular large-cell NHL. Two-yr PFS of follicular small-cleaved, follicular mixed, and follicular large-cell, after autotransplantation, was 67, 67, and 40%, respectively. The LDH at the time of transplant was the most important prognosis variable. Of patients in CR 24 mo after transplantation with low-grade lymphoma, 70% remained in CR with additional 2–5 yr follow-up. Overall, there was no difference in either OS or PFS among patients with low-, intermediate-, or high-grade lymphoma.

Bierman et al. *(33)* recently reported a retrospective review of 100 patients undergoing autotransplantation for follicular low-grade lymphoma from 1983 through 1993. With a median follow-up of survivors of 2.6 yr, 48% were alive and failure-free, with an OS rate of 67%. The number of CT regimens prior to transplantation was the most significant variable associated with OS and FFS. Because all patients had either refractory or relapsed disease, the fact that a significant percentage of patients were alive and failure-free, many years posttransplant, suggested that a long FFS was possible following ABMT.

Vose et al. *(34)* recently reported a retrospective review of 289 patients treated with HDCT ABMT/ASCT for large-cell lymphoma, from 1983 through 1986. With a median follow-up of 24 mo for surviving patients, 39% were alive and 28% were failure-free. In a multivariate analysis, several prognostic features were associated with a poor FFS, including a diffuse histology at the time of transplant, compared with a follicular histology of patients in the good prognosis category (normal LDH, less than three prior CT regimens, nonbulky disease, and not CT-resistant). Those with diffuse large-cell lymphoma had a 5-yr survival rate of 42%, compared with 58% for patients with follicular large-cell lymphoma ($p = 0.05$), leading to the conclusion that, among patients with favorable prognostic factors, patients with follicular large-cell lymphoma had a

Table 2
ABMT for FL

Author	Patients	Follow-up (yr)	Results
Cervantes et al., 1995 (36)	34 32% resistant	3.5	5 yr OS 37% 2 yr probability of relapse 75%. Resistant disease → ↓ prognosis
Colombat et al., 1994 (37)	42 All PR or SR	3.5	83% OS, 66% RFS
Verdonck et al., 1997 (38)	18 Autologous (SR) 10 Allogeneic (RR)	3.7	RFS 70% Allogeneic 17% Autologous Allo: 0% relapse → GVL
Weaver et al., 1998 (39)	49 27% SR	3.6	55% OS 35% RFS 54% relapse, median 9 mo

PR, partial response; SR, sensitive relapse; RR, resistant relapse; OS, overall survival; RFS, relapse-free survival; GVE, graft vs-host effect.

greater survival after ABMT than did those with diffuse large-cell lymphoma. The data suggested that the prognosis of follicular large-cell lymphomas was such that a plateau on the survival curve was apparent.

Freedman et al. (35) had reported a trial of 77 patients, age less than 55 yr, with CD20+ follicular NHL. Patients responding to CHOP were consolidated with ABMT with monoclonal antibody purging. The 3-yr PFS was 63%, with an estimated OS at 3 yr at 89%. The vast majority of patients who relapsed did so in sites of prior disease. Those patients who had successful bone marrow purging, with no detection of residual lymphoma cells by polymerase chain reaction (PCR), had a better outcome than did those who were PCR-positive.

Table 2 is a summary of other selective series reporting the results of autotransplantation for FL, with smaller series of patients. The Cervantes study (36) found that resistant disease was associated with a poor prognosis, similar to that seen with transplant outcomes for more aggressive histologies.

Taken as a whole, this data is similar to the overall clinical results of ABMT/ASCT for immediate high-grade NHLs. Five-yr OS for patients with relapsed or resistant disease is 25–45% in most series: 30–40% have extended PFS, lasting 4–5 yr and beyond (12,39,40). Whether a plateau in this survival curve is seen after autotransplantation for FL is, currently, unknown. However, it is clearly apparent that the long PFS is achievable.

3.5. Commentary: Is Autotransplantation Underutilized for Follicular NHL?

Approximately 57,000 new cases of NHL are detected annually in the United States, with 35% representing FLs, for a total of approx 20,000 new cases of FLs annually. The median age is 55 yr at diagnosis; approx 75% of patients are less than age 70 yr at the time of diagnosis. If patients have a high IPI at the time of diagnosis, their overall prognosis is dismal, and consideration of dose-intensive therapy clearly should be entertained. No more than 5% of FLs present with poor IPI scores at diagnosis, however. Patients receiving CT have a CR rate of 45–70%, and approx 12% of the patients are refractory to CT. The median duration of CR is approx 1.6 yr; thus, approx

35% of patients achieving a CR have one which lasts less than 1 yr. Approximately 35% of patients will achieve a PR to CT, and most of those will have a response lasting less than 1 yr. Therefore, approx 2500 patients will either have poor IPI scores, or have refractory disease to CT; another 2500 will have a CR lasting less than 1 yr; and another 5000 will achieve a PR, the majority of whom will have a PR lasting less than 1 yr. Thus, based on variables at presentation, as well as on response to initial CT, approx 10,000 patients annually will be less than 70 yr old, and will have poor survival predicted by several prognostic variables, and, therefore, will be candidates for dose-intensive therapy. These 10,000 patients with high-risk features at diagnosis have a survival that is clearly less than 5 yr. No prospective randomized trial exists comparing ABMT with conventional CT. Given that the results of ABMT for patients with relapsed/refractory NHL show a 5-yr chance of continuous CR of 30–50%, the author believes that such patients are clearly potential candidates for transplantation, because OS, disease-free survival (DFS), and likely quality of life will be enhanced. Since results, published to date, of transportation for FLs mimic those with intermediate-grade lymphomas, it is also likely that a subset of these patients will have a remission that lasts indefinitely.

The decision to perform a BMT/SCT on patients with FL is not necessarily an issue of the curative potential of transplantation. Rather, it involves the realistic application of prognostic features of relatively young patients diagnosed with FL; it involves the fact that the mortality of SCT is extraordinarily low; and it involves the fact that the extended PFS is attainable in patients with relapsed and refractory FLs treated with autotransplantation. There are very strong arguments in favor of dose-intensive therapy for selective patients with FL, so this option is a viable one until future, novel, and, hopefully, less-toxic therapies offer better results.

4. ASCT FOR HIGH-RISK NHL IN FIRST REMISSION

ABMT cures 25–45% of patients with relapsed/refractory NHL. Although encouraging, these results are not optimal, because most patients relapse after autotransplantation. Results of allo-BMT have shown superior efficacy when employed in first CR in patients with acute leukemia, compared to transplant at relapse or in second CR. An ability to predict patients destined to have a poor outcome might allow for a strategy of ABMT in first remission, in an attempt to optimize the potential therapeutic benefits of transplantation. Such a strategy relies on a reproducible ability to predict patients destined to have a poor prognosis. Fortunately, the IPI is such a reproducible and verifiable prognostic tool *(21)*.

The age-adjusted IPI stratifies patients into four prognostic categories, based on the presence or absence of three identifying variables: serum LDH level (normal vs high), performance status (ECOG 0–1 vs 2–4), and tumor stage (Ann Arbor staging 1–2 vs 3–4). Those with zero risk factors were classified as low-risk; those with one risk factor as low-intermediate; those with two risk factors as high-intermediate; and those with three risk factors as high-risk. Five-yr survival rates for the three groups showed that those with low-risk factors had an 83% 5-yr survival rate; low-intermediate had a 69% 5-yr survival rate; and intermediate-high and high had 46 and 32% 5-yr survival rates, respectively.

Once one identifies patients with a poor IPI risk, the next issue is testing ABMT in first remission, attempting to improve a patient's otherwise poor prognosis. Several studies have recently been published in which high-risk NHL patients were treated with ABMT as part of an initial treatment plan. Vitolo et al. *(41)* examined a group of patients with high-risk diffuse large-cell lymphoma, as defined by either an elevated LDH coupled with high tumor burden, or those with stage IV disease with bone marrow involvement. Historically, this group of patients was found to have 3-yr survival rates of 29%, when treated with conventional CT. Fifty patients with high-risk diffuse large-cell lymphoma were treated with 8 wk adriamycin-based CT regimen; intensified with a 3-d course of mitoxantrone, high-dose cytosine arabinoside, and dexamethasone; PBPCs were then collected, and the patients were treated with high-dose CT consisting of BCNU, etoposide, cytosine arabinoside, and melphalan, and ASCT. Seventy-two percent achieved a CR, and 3-yr survival rates were 66%, which compared favorably to the 29% found with similarly matched historical controlled patients.

Pettengell et al. *(42)* studied patients with high-intermediate or high IPI scores. Thirty-four patients were treated with conventional CT, and compared with 33 patients treated with conventional therapy, followed by busulfan, Cy, and ASCT. Two-yr event-free survival was 61% for the patients receiving transplantation vs 35% ($p = 0.01$), and OS was 64 vs 35% ($p = 0.01$). Two SCT patients died of veno-oclusive disease. The authors concluded that the early consolidation with autotransplantation was appropriate for patients with high-risk NHL.

Haioun et al. *(43)* reported a large randomized trial comparing HDCT and autotransplantation with a preparative regimen of CBV vs a consolidation scheme of Cy, VP-16, L-asparaginase, cytarabine, and methotrexate, in intensified but nontransplant doses for patients with intermediate- or high-grade NHL, achieving a CR to conventional therapy. Thus, this was a study comparing two different consolidative strategies, after patients had already achieved a CR. A retrospective review of those with high-intermediate or high-risk patients, based on the IPI, revealed that autotransplantation resulted in superior 5-yr DFS rates, compared with the other consolidative regimen (59 vs 39%, $p = 0.01$). Those authors *(43)* concluded that dose-intensive therapy, including ASCT, should be considered for patients at high-risk who achieve a CR after standard therapy.

The City of Hope Medical Center and Stanford transplant groups published another pilot study *(44)* of ASCT for NHL patients with high-intermediate or high-risk IPI scores. Fifty-two patients received autotransplantation: 39 transplanted in first CR, and 13 in PR, after conventional therapy. The preparative regimen was total body radiation, etoposide, and Cy. Three-yr OS rate was 84%; patients with intermediate-grade and immunoblastic lymphoma achieved 3-yr DFS rates of 89% for high-risk patients and 92% for high-intermediate-risk patients. Those authors felt that these results compared favorably to historical data in these high-risk patients, and that ASCT should be considered for such patients.

Gianni et al. *(45)* have reported a prospective, randomized trial comparing ASCT vs standard CT in patients with diffuse large-cell lymphoma or diffuse large-cell immunoblastic lymphoma. The patients were not necessarily defined as high-risk: Eligibility included bulky stage I or II disease, stage III, or stage IV. Patients were randomized to receive standard CT vs standard CT plus ASCT. The preparative regimen was either total body radiation plus melphalan, or high-dose mitoxantrone plus melphalan. The patients receiving autotransplantation had a 96% response rate vs 70% in the conventional CT group ($p = 0.001$). With 7-yr follow-up, freedom from progression was 84% for those receiving transplantation vs 49% for conventional CT ($p < 0.001$). Of 50 patients treated with conventional CT, 23 either did not respond or relapsed. Fourteen (61%) were able to receive HDCT and ASCT at a later date; of those 14, four (29%) achieved a continuous CR.

4.1. Is Autotransplantation for High-Risk Intermediate/High-Grade NHL Underutilized?

All of these studies have been published within the past 3 yr. Traditionally, the strategic approach for patients with intermediate- and high-grade NHL is to treat the patients with standard CT; should the patient subsequently relapse, attempt to salvage them with autotransplantation at that time. These new data suggest an alternative strategy, namely, identifying patients at high-risk at diagnosis, and employing autotransplantation as part of the initial treatment plan. The question is, can one clearly say that one strategy is superior to another? If one looks at 100 patients treated with each strategy, the answer, in my opinion becomes clear. No conventional-dose CT has been proven to be superior to CHOP (15), which cures 30% of all patients (low- and high-risk) with diffuse large-cell NHL (16). Thus, it is generous to say that 30 of the original 100 patients with high-risk large-cell NHL will be cured with conventional CT. The remaining 70 patients will either not respond to CHOP, or will later relapse. Not all of these patients will ever come to autotransplantation. In the Parma trial, a distinct minority of patients, failing standard CT, ever came to autotransplantation. In the Gianni trial, described above, 60% of patients, failing standard CT, later underwent autotransplantation. A realistic estimate is that approx 50% of the 70 patients might come to autotransplantation. Thus, 35 patients would later receive an autotransplant. If one assumes that 40% of such patients would be cured, then an additional 14 (35 × 40%) would be salvaged with ASCT. This means a total of 44 of the original group of 100 patients, using this treatment strategy, would be cured, and 56 patients would die of their lymphoma. Alternatively, the study from the City of Hope for high-risk patients revealed that 84% of patients treated with autotransplantation, as part of the initial treatment strategy, were alive and disease-free (44); Pettengell et al. (43) showed that 61% were alive and disease-free; and the randomized trial of Gianni et al. (45), although it did not identify high-risk patients, found a 7-yr freedom from progression rate of 84%. A conservative estimate of this treatment strategy would reveal that at least 60% of patients would likely be cured, when employing autotransplantation as part of the initial treatment strategy. Thus, 60/100 patients might be cured, compared with 44 patients, using a strategy of autotransplantation for salvage.

In the absence of prospective randomized trials beyond that of Gianni, ABMT for high-risk patients is a compelling option.

Forty-six percent of patients with intermediate- or high-grade NHL present with a high-intermediate or high-IPI risk (21). Based on the analysis discussed in Subheading 2 of this chapter, of 57,000 new cases of NHL diagnosed in 1999, this means that approx 10,000 patients will be less than 70 yr old, with either high-intermediate or high-IPI risks at presentation. A treatment strategy of early transplantation for this high-risk group increases the curative potential by approx 36%, which again demonstrates that, potentially, thousands of patients could be cured of their lymphoma, if appropriate utilization of transplantation was performed.

5. SUMMARY AND COMMENTARY

Only approx 2000 autotransplants are performed in North America for NHL patients annually, according to the statistical registry at the Autologous Blood and Marrow Transplant Registry *(46)*. Even if this registry captures only 50% of NHL transplants, the author believes there are thousands more who should be transplanted in the United States.

In the field of medical oncology, nonsurgical curative therapies are rare. Most medical oncologic therapy is palliative in nature. Autotransplantation for NHL is somewhat unique, in that it not only offers the possibility of cure for some NHL patients who would otherwise be incurable, but it also represents potential effective palliation of disease, dramatically extending OS and DFS, as well as quality of life. The controversy about autotransplantation in the United States for breast cancer, multiple myeloma, autoimmune diseases, and other disorders, has, to some extent, been clouded by social, economic, insurance, and political issues. The issue of autotransplantation for NHL is, in the author's opinion, a straightforward medical issue. Autotransplantation saves lives, cures patients, and enhances OS and DFS. Perhaps, in the years to come, many more NHL patients, who are appropriate candidates for transplantation, will be referred to transplant centers, and therefore many more patients will be cured of their disease.

REFERENCES

1. Philip T, Guglielmi C, Hagenbeek A, et al. Autologous bone marrow transplantation as compared with salvage chemotherapy in relapses of chemotherapy-sensitive non-Hodgkin's lymphoma, *N. Engl. J. Med.,* **333** (1995) 1540–1545.
2. Applebaum FR, Sullivan KM, Buckner CD, et al. Treatment of malignant lymphoma in 100 patients with chemotherapy, total body irradiation, and marrow transplantation, *J. Clin. Oncol.,* **5** (1987) 1340–1347.
3. Takvorian T, Canellos GP, Ritz J, et al. Prolonged disease-free survival after autologous bone marrow transplantation in patients with non-Hodgkin's lymphoma with a poor prognosis, *N. Engl. J. Med.,* **316** (1987) 1499–1505.
4. Vose JM, Armitage JO, Bierman PH, et al. Salvage therapy for relapsed or refractory non-Hodgkin's lymphoma utilizing autologous bone marrow transplantation, *Am. J. Med.,* **87** (1989) 285–288.
5. Vose JM, Anderson JR, Kessinger A, et al. High-Dose Chemotherapy and Autologous Hematopoietic Stem-Cell Transplantation for Aggressive Non-Hodgkin's Lymphoma, *J. Clin. Oncol.,* **11** (1993) 1846–1851.
6. Peterson FB, Appelbaum FR, Hill R, et al. Autologous Marrow Transplantation for Malignant Lymphoma: a Report of 101 Cases from Seattle, *J. Clin. Oncol.,* **8** (1990) 638–647.
7. Popat U, Przepiork D, Champlin R, et al. High-Dose Chemotherapy for Relapsed and Refractory Diffuse Large B-Cell Lymphoma: Mediastinal Localization Predicts for a Favorable Outcome, *J. Clin. Oncol.,* **16** (1998) 63–69.
8. Vaughan WP, Kris E, Vose J, et al. Phase I/II Study Incorporating Intravenous Hydroxyurea into High-Dose Chemotherapy for Patients with Primary Refractory or Relapsed and Refractory Intermediate-Grade and High-Grade Malignant Lymphoma, *J. Clin. Oncol.,* **13** (1995) 1089–1095.
9. Wheeler C, Strawderman M, Ayash L, et al. Prognostic Factors for Treatment Outcome in Autotransplantation of Immediate-Grade and High-Grade Non-Hodgkin's Lymphoma with Cyclosphosphamide, Carmustine, and Etoposide, *J. Clin. Oncol.,* **11** (1993) 1085–1091.
10. Rapoport AP, Rowe JM, Kouides PA, et al. One Hundred Autotransplants for Relapsed or Refractory Hodgkin's Disease and Lymphoma: Value of Pretransplant Disease State for Predicting Outcome, *J. Clin. Oncol.,* **11** (1993) 2351–2361.
11. Verdonck LF, Dekker AW, de Gast GC, et al. Salvage Therapy with ProMACE-MOPP Followed by Intensive Chemoradiotherapy and Autologous Bone Marrow Transplantation for Patients with Non-Hodgkin's Lymphoma Who Failed to Respond to First-Line CHOP, *J. Clin. Oncol.,* **10** (1992) 1949–1954.

12. Bolwell B, Goormastic M, and Andresen S. Durability of Remission After ABMT for NHL. The Importance of the 2-year Evaluation Point, *Bone Marrow Transplant.*, **19** (1997) 443–448.

13. Philip T, Guglielmi C, Hagenbeek A, et al. Autologous Bone Marrow Transplantation as Compared with Salvage Chemotherapy in Relapses of Chemotherapy-Sensitive Non-Hodgkin's Lymphoma, *N. Engl. J. Med.*, **333** (1995) 1540–1545.

14. Philip T, Gomez F, Guglielmi C, et al. Long-Term Outcome of Relapsed NHL Patients Included in the Parma Trial: Incidence of Late Relapses, Long-Term Toxicity and Impact of the International Prognostic Index (IPI) at Relapse, *Proc. ASCO.*, **17** (1998) 16A(Abstract).

15. Fisher RI, Gaynor ER, Dahlbert S, et al. Comparison of Standard Regimen (CHOP) with Three Intensive Chemotherapy Regimens for Advanced Non-Hodgkin's Lymphoma, *N. Engl. J. Med.*, **328** (1993) 1002–1006.

16. Coltman CA, Dahlbert S, Jones S, et al. CHOP is Curative in Thirty Percent of Patients with Diffuse Large Cell Lymphoma. A Twelve-Year Southwest Oncology Group Follow-up, *Proc. Am. Soc. Clin. Oncol.*, **5** (1986) 197(Abstract).

17. Peters WP, Rosner G, Ross M, et al. Comparative Effects of Granulocyte-Macrophage Colony-Stimulating Factor (GM-CSF) and Granulocyte Colony-Stimulating Factor (G-CSF) on Priming Peripheral Blood Progenitor Cells for Use with Autologous Bone Marrow After High-Dose Chemotherapy, *Blood*, **81** (1993) 1709–1719.

18. Chao NJ, Schriber JR, Grimes K, et al. Granulocyte Colony-Stimulating Factor "Mobilized" Peripheral Blood Progenitor Cells Accelerate Granulocyte and Platelet Recovery After High-Dose Chemotherapy, *Blood*, **81** (1993) 2031–2035.

19. Bolwell BJ, Fishleder A, Andresen SW, et al. G-CSF Primed Peripheral Blood Progenitor Cells in Autologous Bone Marrow Transplantation: Parameters Affecting Bone Marrow Engraftment, *Bone Marrow Transplant.*, **12** (1993) 609–614.

20. Bolwell B, Goormastic M, Dannley R, et al. G-CSF Post-Autologous Progenitor Cell Transplantation: A Randomized Study of 5, 10 and 16 µg/kg/day, *Bone Marrow Transplant.*, **19** (1997) 215–219.

21. International Non-Hodgkin's Lymphoma Prognostic Factors Project. Predictive Model for Aggressive Non-Hodgkin's Lymphoma, *N. Engl. J. Med.*, **329** (1993) 987–994.

22. López-Guillermo A, Montserrat E, Bosch F, et al. Applicability of the International Index for Aggressive Lymphomas to Patients with Low-Grade Lymphoma, *J. Clin. Oncol.*, **12** (1994) 1343–1348.

23. Non-Hodgkin's Lymphoma Classification Project. A Clinical Evaluation of the International Lymphoma Study Group Classification of Non-Hodgkin's Lymphoma, *Blood*, **89** (1997) 3909–3918.

24. Weisdorf DJ, Anderson JW, Glick JH, et al. Survival After Relapse of Low-Grade Non-Hodgkin's Lymphoma: Implications for Marrow Transplantation, *J. Clin. Oncol.*, **10** (1992) 942–947.

25. Gallagher CJ, Gregory WM, Jones AE, et al. Follicular Lymphoma: Prognostic Factors for Response and Survival, *J. Clin. Oncol.*, (1986) 1470–1480.

26. Bastion BY, Sebban C, Berger F, et al. Incidence, Predictive Factors, and Outcome of Lymphoma Transformation in Follicular Lymphoma Patients, *J. Clin. Oncol.*, **15** (1997) 1587–1594.

27. Harris NL, Jaffe ES, Stein H, et al. A Revised European-American Classification of Lymphoid Neoplasms: a Proposal from the International Lymphoma Study Group, *Blood*, **84** (1994) 1361–1392.

28. Non-Hodgkin's Lymphoma Pathologic Classification Project. National Cancer Institute Sponsored Study of Classifications of Non-Hodgkin's Lymphomas: Summary and Description of a Working Formulation for Clinical Usage, *Cancer*, **10** (1982) 2112–2135.

29. Martin AR, Weisenburger DD, Chan WC, et al. Prognostic Value of Cellular Proliferation and Histologic Grade in Follicular Lymphoma, *Blood*, **85** (1995) 3671–3678.

30. Wendum D, Sebban C, Gaulard P, et al. Follicular Large-Cell Lymphoma Treated with Intensive Chemotherapy: an Analysis of 89 Cases Included in the LNH87 Trial and Comparison with the Outcome of Diffuse Large B-Cell Lymphoma, *J. Clin. Oncol.*, **15** (1997) 1654–1663.

31. Kaplan HS. Evidence for a Tumoricidal Dose Level in the Radiotherapy of Hodgkin's Disease, *Cancer Res.*, **26** (1996) 1221–1224.

32. MacManus MP, Hoppe RT. Is Radiotherapy Curative for Stage I and II Low-Grade Follicular Lymphoma? Results of a Long-Term Follow-Up Study of Patients Treated at Stanford University, *J. Clin. Oncol.*, **14** (1996) 1282–1290.

33. Bierman PH, Vose JM, Anderson JR, et al. High-Dose Therapy with Autologous Hematopoietic Rescue for Follicular Low-Grade Non-Hodgkin's Lymphoma, *J. Clin. Oncol.*, **15** (1997) 445–450.

34. Vose JM, Bierman PJ, Lynch JC, et al. Effect of Follicularity on Autologous Transplantation for Large-Cell Non-Hodgkin's Lymphoma, *J. Clin. Oncol.*, **16** (1998) 884–849.

35. Freedman AS, Gribben JG, Neuberg D, et al. High-Dose Therapy and Autologous Bone Marrow Transplantation in Patients with Follicular Lymphoma During First Remission, *Blood,* **88** (1996) 2780–2786.

36. Cervantes F, Shu XO, McGlave PB, et al. Autologous Bone Marrow Transplantation for Non-Transformed Low-Grade Non-Hodgkin's Lymphoma, *Bone Marrow Transplant.,* **16** (1995) 387–392.

37. Colombat PH, Donadio D, Fouillard L, et al. Value of Autologous Bone Marrow Transplantation in Follicular Lymphoma: a France Autogreffe Retrospective Study of 42 Patients, *Bone Marrow Transplant.,* **13** (1994) 157–162.

38. Verdonck LF, Dekker AW, Lokhorst HM, et al. Allogeneic Versus Autologous Bone Marrow Transplantation for Refractory and Recurrent Low-Grade Non-Hodgkin's Lymphoma, *Blood,* **90** (1997) 4201–4205.

39. Weaver CH, Schwartzberg L, Rhinehart S, et al. High-Dose Chemotherapy with BUCY or BEAC and Unpurged Peripheral Blood Stem Cell Infusion in Patients with Low-Grade Non-Hodgkin's Lymphoma, *Bone Marrow Transplant.,* **21** (1998) 383–389.

40. Vose JM, Anderson JR, Kessinger A, et al. High-Dose Chemotherapy and Autologous Hematopoietic Stem-Cell Transplantation for Aggressive Non-Hodgkin's Lymphoma, *J. Clin. Oncol.,* **11** (1993) 1846–1851.

41. Vitolo U, Cortellazzo S, Liberati AM, et al. Intensified and High-Dose Chemotherapy with Granulocyte Colony-Stimulating Factor and Autologous Stem-Cell Transplantation Support as First-Line Therapy in High-Risk Diffuse Large-Cell Lymphoma, *J. Clin. Oncol.,* **15** (1997) 491–498.

42. Pettengel R, Radford JA, Morgenstern GR, et al. Survival Benefit from High-Dose Therapy with Autologous Blood Progenitor-Cell Transplantation in Poor-Prognosis Non-Hodgkin's Lymphoma, *J. Clin. Oncol.,* **14** (1996) 586–592.

43. Haioun C, Lepage E, Gisselbrecht C, et al. Benefit of Autologous Bone Marrow Transplantation Over Sequential Chemotherapy in Poor-Risk Aggressive Non-Hodgkin's Lymphoma: Updated Results of the Prospective Study LNH87-2, *J. Clin. Oncol.,* **15** (1997) 1131–1137.

44. Nademanee A, Molina A, O'Donnell MR, et al. Results of High-Dose Therapy and Autologous Bone Marrow/Stem Cell Transplantation During Remission in Poor-Risk Intermediate- and High-Grade Lymphoma: International Index High and High-Intermediate Risk Group, *Blood,* **90** (1997) 3844–3854.

45. Gianni AM, Bregni M, Siena S, et al. High-Dose Chemotherapy and Autologous Bone Marrow Transplantation Compared with MACOP-B in Aggressive B-Cell Lymphoma, *N. Engl. J. Med.,* **336** (1997) 1290–1297.

46. ABMTR Newsletter. IBMTR/ABMTR Statistical Center. Vol. 5, No. 1, Dec. 1998.

III TRANSPLANTATION FOR SOLID TUMORS

13

Do Patients Benefit from Autotransplants for Advanced Ovarian Cancer?

Janet Ruzich, DO, and Patrick J. Stiff, MD

1. INTRODUCTION

One of the most controversial areas in transplantation in the late 1990s has been the use of autologous stem cell transplants for the management of advanced ovarian cancer (OC). In some respects, this tumor has some of the best evidence in the solid tumor field that dose intensity is important: This was made most clear with two recent positive trials of regional high-dose chemotherapy (HDCT) by the intraperitoneal (ip) route *(1,2)*. The numbers of transplants are increasing rapidly in this country, but data demonstrating their efficacy comes only from retrospective comparisons to conventional therapy. Appropriately, this data has led to the development of a randomized national four-member cooperative group National Cancer Institute (NCI)-sponsored trial, a trial that is languishing, primarily because of a lack of support from physicians providing the initial care of these patients.

As the controversy rages, a large percentage of women continue to die of this disease. In fact, in 1999, OC will continue as the fourth leading cause of cancer death in women raged 35–74 yr. There are currently 25,400 new cases of OC in the United States per year, with an estimated 14,500 deaths *(3)*. Despite the development of new strategies for treatment, death from OC has continued at approximately the same rate over the past three decades. Although some claim an improvement in overall survival (OS),

From: *Current Controversies in Bone Marrow Transplantation*
Edited by: B. Bolwell © Humana Press Inc., Totowa, NJ

compared to the early 1970s, this is mostly the result of improvements in optimal debulking surgery at the time of diagnosis, and the successful treatment of germ cell and stromal tumors, which are now associated with a high cure rate.

Indeed, there have been no significant changes in the number of deaths in epithelial OC in the approx 60% of women presenting with advanced disease secondary to the early development of drug resistance. Because the majority of these women presenting with advanced disease will relapse and eventually succumb to their disease, innovative methods need to be developed to increase the odds of long-term survival and possible cure.

There is, however, hope for the future. All recent data from conventional therapy do suggest that improvements in survival may soon be seen. Yet, whether these treatments will only delay an ultimate death, or lead to an improvement in cure rates, remains unknown. With the introduction of paclitaxel and the use of aggressive upfront CT, the number of patients completing initial therapy with either a pathologic complete remission (CR) or with microscopic residual disease is increasing. These improvements may be an appropriate platform upon which to build. New three-drug combinations, such as topotecan, paclitaxel, and platinum (Pt), appear promising, as recently studied in a phase I trial (4), in which an overall response rate of 86.7% was seen, albeit with significant hematologic toxicity requiring growth factor support. A similar, aggressive phase I/II study (5) was conducted by the NCI, investigating combination therapy with paclitaxel, cisplatin, and cyclophosphamide (Cy). Unfortunately, although the results were encouraging, with a clinical CR of 75% and a pathologic CR of 36%, the regimen is felt by some to be too toxic, and has not been studied in a randomized trial.

Yet these and other studies strongly suggest that, like hematologic malignancies, dose and dose intensity may be the most successful way to overcome drug resistance, particularly for minimal residual disease. The rationale and evidence that dose-intensive therapy is of value in OC comes from in vitro studies, clinical trials investigating regional high-dose therapy (HDT), dose-intensive subablative CT, and systemic HDCT with stem cell rescue (1,2,6,7,7a–7g,8).

2. IN VITRO TESTING

OC is a very chemosensitive disease, and several studies have demonstrated an increased response rate with dose intensity of cisplatin and alkylating agents, both in vitro and in vivo (6–7,9–11). Behrens et al. (10) demonstrated a dose–response relationship for cisplatin in resistant cell lines, and others (11) have demonstrated synergy of alkylating agent combinations in vitro. Several agents with minimal activity in OC at conventional doses were found to have activity at high doses in vitro. In particular, mitoxantrone was shown to have an increased cell kill at increasing doses (6). Recently, paclitaxel was found to have a dose–response relationship when tested in vitro, and is now being incorporated into transplant regimens (12,13).

3. IP THERAPY

IP therapy is one of the strategies designed to overcome drug resistance by exploring Pt dose–response in patients with OC. This approach provides clinical evidence to support the use of systemic HDT with stem cell rescue. Studies have shown that using cisplatin with this modality achieves an ip concentration that is 20-fold higher than

Table 1
Optimal Initial Management of Stage III/IV Epithelial OC

	Suboptimal III/IV	Optimal III
Study	McGuire (61)	Markman (2)
Regimen	Paclitaxel (135 mg/m^2) iv over 24 h + Cisplatin (75 mg/m^2) q 3 wks × 6 cycles	Carboplatin (AUC 9) × 2 Paclitaxel (135 mg/m^2) iv + cisplatin (100 mg/m^2)ip q 3 wks × 6 cycles
PFS	18 mo	27.6 mo
OS	38 mo	52.9 mo

PFS, progression-free survival; OS, overall survival.

when given via the intravenous route (14). The modality, however, is limited to patients with previous Pt-responsive disease with optimal tumor size (0.5 cm or less), and in patients without significant adhesive disease, or extraperitoneal disease. It is estimated that only one-third of patients are eligible for this therapy, secondary to these restrictions. In a retrospective analysis conducted by Memorial Sloan-Kettering Cancer Center, evaluating patients with persistent/recurrent disease, there was a 56% overall response rate and a 33% CR rate to second-line ip cisplatin therapy in those patients who previously responded to systemic cisplatin therapy (7c). Even though patients with highly cisplatin-resistant disease received no added benefit from ip therapy, several patients in their series responded to ip cisplatin, despite evidence that their disease had not responded to systemic therapy previously. They concluded that approx 5–10% of patients will become partially sensitive to the drug with the 10–20-fold increase in concentration achieved in the ip compartment.

The benefit of using regional dose-intensive therapy as part of initial therapy was demonstrated in a study reported by Alberts et al. (1). Patients with previously untreated minimal-bulk stage III OC were randomized to ip cisplatin/iv Cy vs iv cisplatin/iv Cy. Of the 546 patients included in the trial, median survival was 49 mo for the group receiving ip cisplatin vs 41 mo for the iv cisplatin group. When a separate analysis was done for patients with residual tumor <0.5 cm, median survival was 51 mo for ip cisplatin vs 46 mo for iv cisplatin. The results of this study suggest that regional dose-intensive therapy may play an important role as initial therapy, specifically in patients with low-volume disease.

The clinical utility of using ip therapy as consolidation, in an attempt to improve progression-free survival (PFS) and OS, was investigated by Markman et al. (2) in a recent intergroup trial with the Gynecologic Oncology Group (GOG), Southwest Oncology Group (SWOG), and Eastern Cooperative Oncology Group (ECOG), which also included paclitaxel for patients with optimal stage III disease (2). This phase III trial was conducted comparing iv cisplatin/iv paclitaxel vs iv carboplatin/iv paclitaxel and ip cisplatin, in optimal residual OC. There was a total of 465 evaluable patients in the study, with the experimental arm receiving <2 courses of ip cisplatin therapy. PFS was significantly longer with ip therapy, but the OS was not. However, the median survival for ip regimen was 52 mo, the longest documented for optimal stage III disease. The results of this trial are promising, and studies are ongoing using paclitaxel for ip therapy (15).

4. SUBABLATIVE DOSE-INTENSITY STUDIES

Early attempts at dose intensity, at approximately twice the conventional dose of Pt compounds, involved patients with refractory or end-stage disease. The in vitro data predicting a higher response rate for dose-intensive therapy was validated in these trials; however, no improvement was seen in PFS or OS, as compared to other available therapies *(16,17)*. Subsequent trials evaluated dose-intensive therapy before the onset of drug resistance (i.e., at diagnosis), but most of these trials also had negative results *(18,19)*. The reasons are many, however, since the actual dose used was less than planned because of unacceptable toxicity in most of these trials, and therefore was not a true test of HDCT. Also, most of these trials included patients with bulky advanced disease. Exceptions to those studies were two trials conducted in patients with small-volume disease, which showed improvement in response rate and survival *(20,21)*.

In the Scottish Ovarian Cancer Study Group, in which patients with minimal bulk after surgery were treated, Cy was combined with cisplatin at a varying dose of 50 and 100 mg/m^2 *(20)*. The response rate for the lower-dose arm was 34% vs 64% for the high-dose arm. The high-dose arm had superior PFS and OS of 85 vs 41 wk and 114 vs 69 wk, respectively. However, these authors did not recommend HDT secondary to significant toxicity. The second trial, by the Hong Kong Ovarian Carcinoma Study Group, treated patients with Cy in combination with cisplatin, at a dose of either 60 or 120 mg/m^2, mostly in patients with small-volume disease *(21)*. Of the low-dose group, 30% had a clinical CR vs 55% in the high-dose group. The 3-yr survival rate of the high-dose arm was 60% vs 30% for the low-dose arm. Although the toxicity was significant in both studies, the higher response rate (RR) and increase in OS seen in the high-dose arms suggest a possible advantage to transplantation.

5. HDT FOR RELAPSED/REFRACTORY DISEASE

Because the majority of patients with OC relapse, and, once relapsed, are incurable with conventional CT, novel approaches such as HDCT were developed. Two groups of patients have been described, depending on their duration of remission to Pt-based therapy. Pt-resistant patients are those who progress during, or relapse within, 6 mo of Pt therapy. These patients have a median survival of 10–12 mo with best-available conventional therapy *(22–25)*. PT-sensitive patients are those responding to Pt, or those who relapse after an initial remission of 6 mo or longer. These patients have a median survival of 16–20 mo with best-available conventional therapy.

Despite the introduction of a number of newer agents, such as topotecan, paclitaxel, etoposide, and gemcitabine, used as salvage therapy for relapsed OC, the majority of phase II studies have only demonstrated a 13–30% response rate *(23)*. Although these agents have activity in OC, and perhaps in combination, their use may lead to better response rates, none have yet been shown to significantly prolong survival or, more importantly, produce long-term disease-free survival (DFS). The initial HDCT phase I trials that were conducted for a variety of tumors, including OC, did show high-response rates for this disease *(26–36)*. However, response duration was particularly short, on average, lasting approx 6 mo. In almost all trials, however, a few long-term survivors were seen, even in those with Pt-refractory disease. In such a phase I trial, the authors' group treated seven patients with OC with high-dose carboplatin (1500

Table 2
Autotransplants for Persistent/Relapsed OC at Loyola: 10/89–2/96

Number transplanted	100
Median age, yr (range)	48 (23–64)
Initial stage of disease:	
I	7
II	10
III	66
IV	16
Unknown	1
Initial surgical response	
Optimal	75
Suboptimal	25
Response to initial CT	
Clinical CR	28
Pathologic CR	18
PR	30
Induction failure	19
Unknown	5
Median time from diagnosis to transplant (range)	18 (2–132)
Median number of pretransplant regimens (range)	2 (1–4)
Pt-sensitive	34
Bulk <1 cm	39
Median PFS/OS (mo)	
All patients	7.0/13.5
Pt-resistant	5.4/9.6
Pt-sensitive	12.2/23.1
Pt-sensitive + <1 cm	18.6/29.0

mg/m^2 over 5 d), mitoxantrone (10–25 mg/m^2 × 3), and Cy (30–50 mg/m^2 × 3), and six patients who responded did so for greater than 20 mo, including one patient who failed induction CT, but who survived progression-free for greater than 2 yr (29). With a number of trials documenting long-term survivors, a survey of bone marrow transplant (BMT) programs across the country was conducted in 1992, to more carefully describe this treatment modality (37). The report described 146 patients with relapsed/refractory OC who were transplanted: 14% were disease-free at 1 yr. The survey also found that those patients who were Pt-sensitive had a CR rate of 73% vs 34% for those who were Pt-resistant. Subsequent trials would further validate the importance of having Pt-responsive disease prior to transplant (38–40).

One such phase II trial of 30 patients (40) was conducted by this institution, and included patients with both Pt-sensitive and -resistant disease. Patients received mitoxantrone (75 mg/m^2), carboplatin (1500 mg/m^2) and Cy (120 mg/m^2), followed by autotransplant. The overall response rate was 89%, with a CR of 88% in Pt-sensitive patients vs 47% in Pt-resistant patients. For all 30 patients in the trial, the median survival was 29 mo, and the PFS was 10.1 mo in the Pt-sensitive group vs 5.1 mo in the Pt-resistant group.

Holmberg et al. (39) subsequently treated 31 patients with the busulfan (12 mg/kg), melphalan (100 mg/m^2), and thiotepa (500 mg/m^2) regimen, and found 11% of Pt-resistant patients to be progression-free at 18 mo vs 46% of Pt-sensitive patients. These results suggest that Pt-resistant disease responds poorly to transplantation, and would benefit instead from alternative conventional CT; those with Pt-sensitive disease appear to do better than they would have if treated with conventional CT.

Two multivariate analyses, one conducted at Loyola University Medical Center *(41)*, and the other by the American Blood and Marrow Transplant Registry (ABMTR) *(42)*, specifically looked at pretransplant prognostic variables. At Loyola, a multivariate analysis was performed on 100 consecutively treated patients, from 1989 to 1996. The majority of patients were treated with carboplatin, mitoxantrone, and Cy, and the remaining patients were treated with either melphalan and mitoxantrone, with or without paclitaxel, or other regimens. Of the patients included in the study, 66% were Pt-resistant, and 61% had tumor bulk >1 cm. Two or more CT regimens were used in 70% of patients prior to transplant.

In the multivariate analysis, age group, disease bulk > or <1 cm, and Pt sensitivity were predictors of OS, with tumor bulk being more important than Pt sensitivity. The best predictors of PFS were tumor bulk and Pt sensitivity, with tumor bulk again being more important. The OS for Pt-sensitive patients was 23.1 mo vs 9.6 mo for Pt-resistant patients. The PFS was 12.2 mo vs 5.4 mo in Pt-sensitive and Pt-resistant patients, respectively. As stated above, tumor bulk was an important predictor of OS and PFS. Among Pt-sensitive patients, those with tumor bulk <1 cm had a OS of 29 mo, vs 18 mo for those with tumor bulk >1 cm. Differences in OS, between those patients who were debulked surgically, and those who received CT to achieve tumor bulk <1 cm, were not statistically significant. Therefore, conclusions can be made from this analysis of a large cohort that the best candidates for transplantation are those who are Pt-sensitive, with <1 cm tumor bulk. Those patients who are Pt-resistant, with tumor bulk >1 cm, clearly do not benefit from transplantation. Further follow-up of the Loyola analysis *(43)* included a total of 164 patients, and this continued to show that Pt sensitivity and tumor bulk <1 cm remained important prognostic factors.

The ABMTR also carried out a multivariate analysis of data on 421 women, collected from 57 transplant centers, transplanted from 1989 to 1996 *(42)*. PT-resistant disease was documented in 41% of patients, and 38% had bulky disease. The analysis found that age, performance status, Pt sensitivity, disease status at start of transplant, and clear cell histology were important prognostic factors for PFS. All of the factors were important, except for disease status at the time of transplant, in predicting OS. The overall 2-yr PFS and OS were 12 and 35%, respectively. Those patients with Pt-sensitive disease in first relapse, second CR, or first PR, with low tumor bulk, had a 2-yr survival of 49%. Pt-resistant patients had a PFS and OS of 7 and 21%, respectively. The survival rates seen in this study were lower than in the Loyola study, but Pt sensitivity and low tumor bulk appeared to predict which patients would benefit from transplant.

There are no phase III randomized studies comparing transplant with conventional CT for relapsed/refractory OC. This study will probably never be conducted, since women with relapsed OC are incurable, and will ultimately die with conventional CT alone. However, over the next several years, the ABMTR is planning on completing a case-controlled study comparing conventional therapy with HDCT and hematopoietic stem cell rescue. Until that time, women with relapsed OC after first remission have few options. HDCT with hematopoietic stem cell rescue is a viable option, with acceptable toxicity for women who are Pt-sensitive with low tumor burden. It is this therapy alone that provides a 15–20% 4-yr or more DFS.

6. HDCT AS CONSOLIDATION THERAPY OF AN INITIAL REMISSION

Given the encouraging results obtained with HDCT for chemosensitive low-tumor-bulk, persistent or relapsed OC, many investigators have looked at instituting transplantation earlier in the course of the disease, i.e., after an initial remission. Today, conventional therapy after initial debulking surgery involves treating the patient with a paclitaxel/Pt regimen. Although this regimen has increased PFS and OS, compared to previous Cy/Pt regimens, up to 80% of these women will relapse. Alternatives tested after initial CT is completed, such as additional debulking surgery or additional consolidation CT, have uniformly not been of value in achieving a significantly higher cure rate.

There have been several phase II trials evaluating the use of HDCT as consolidation of an initial remission *(44–49)*. However, it is important to note that, in all of these trials, Cy and cisplatin were used to induce remission. Therefore, direct comparisons cannot be made regarding outcome between present conventional CT and HDCT used as consolidation. However, given the better cytoreduction with paclitaxel/Pt regimens, one could expect a greater benefit to high-dose consolidative therapy in this group of patients. Legros et al. *(45)* was one of the largest trials that examined HDCT as part of consolidation. The trial included patients with stage III and IV disease and poor prognostic factors, such as bulky disease, initial suboptimal surgery, or positive second-look laparotomy. Of the 53 patients undergoing therapy, all patients had a second-look operation, except for five patients who had a clinical CR, and refused surgery. All patients were treated initially with surgical debulking, followed by cisplatin-combination CT. After a second-look procedure, they received either HDCT with high-dose melphalan (140 mg/m^2) or carboplatin (400 mg/m^2 d 1–4) and Cy (1.6 g/m^2 d 1–4). For those patients with no macroscopic disease at second look, the DFS at 5 yr was 26.9%, with a 5-yr OS of 71.2% and a median survival of 80.3 mo. The entire group, including both those patients with macroscopic disease and those without, had a 5-yr OS of 59.9% and a DFS of 23.6%. Given that 5-yr OS for stage III and IV disease is approx 20% for those treated with Cy and Pt as initial therapy, HDCT as consolidation appears very promising. Other smaller trials revealed similar improvements in DFS and OS, compared to conventional therapy. Dauplet et al. *(44)* administered melphalan (140 mg/m^2) to 12/14 patients who had positive findings at second-look operation, 12 of whom had minimal-to-no residual disease and two patients with macroscopic disease. The 3-yr survival rate was 64%, and the 3-yr DFS was 33%. There were no treatment-related deaths. Mulder et al. *(50)* administered Cy (7 g/m^2) with etoposide (1 g/m^2) to 11 patients with residual disease after initial tumor debulking and CT. Eight of the 11 had optimal stage III disease. Of the 11 patients, six achieved a CR, with two patients remaining in CR for 43 and 75 mo. As seen in other trials for relapsed disease, the patients who seemed to benefit were those with minimal tumor bulk. Extra et al. *(47)* treated 37 patients who had received a median number of six courses of cisplatin-based CT. All but one had a second look, with eight patients having a pathologic CR. High-dose Cy (2.2 g/m^2/d × 2), with abdominal pelvic radiation (5 Gy × 2), was given in

Table 3
Transplant as Consolidation Therapy of Initial Remission in Patients
with Advanced OC: Combined French Retrospective Analysis 1998[a]

	Optimal stage III (mo)	Suboptimal stage III/IV (mo)
Conventional therapy	40–50	20–24
Transplant	65	39

Conventional therapy outcome using conventional therapy with Pt and Cy, which was used as the induction regimen in these studies.

[a]Median survival from diagnosis.

17 patients, melphalan (140 mg/m^2) in three patients, and carboplatin (600–1500 mg/m^2) in 14 patients. The median OS was 47 mo from diagnosis. In a retrospective analysis of five French transplant centers, with patients receiving melphalan (140–240 mg/m^2), Viens et al. *(46)* studied 35 patients, 10 of whom had tumor bulk <2 cm, and nine who had pathologic CR prior to transplant. A total of 6/9 patients, with a pathologic CR prior to transplant, were alive and without evidence of disease at a median follow-up of 23 mo. Of the 10 patients with macroscopic disease, there were three alive and without evidence of disease at the same follow-up time.

A recent retrospective study of six French centers *(49)* analyzed the outcome of 181 patients who underwent transplants as consolidation therapy of an initial remission, induced by Pt/CY-based CT. The patients treated had either stage III (76%) or stage IV (24%) disease at diagnosis, with, again, the majority (164 patients) undergoing a second-look procedure prior to transplant. A total of 10 different regimens were used among the six centers, with the most-used regimen being high-dose Cy (1500 mg/m^2/d × 4) with carboplatin (400 mg/m^2/d × 4). The 5-yr projected survival was 36%, with a PFS of 23% at a median follow-up of 38 mo. Median survival for the entire group was 46 mo from diagnosis, with 43% alive at 5 yr. The 5-yr survival from diagnosis for the 55% of patients who had suboptimal disease was 25%, longer than the expected 5-yr survival of 15–20% for patients treated with the same initial conventional CT. The 5-yr survival from diagnosis for those with optimal stage III disease was 51%, again, longer than the anticipated 5-yr survival of 40–45% for conventional therapy with Cy and Pt.

These data certainly suggest a benefit to transplant for patients with stage III and IV disease. Obviously, the above studies treated a select group of typically younger women with advanced OC, compared to those seen in everyday practice. However, with the recent data of Duska et al. *(51)* demonstrating no difference in survival of women with advanced disease in the reproductive age group, once borderline tumors were excluded, there may indeed be a benefit to transplant when used as consolidation therapy.

The only way to validate these results is to conduct randomized trials. Several trials are underway worldwide, including a U.S. NCI-sponsored trial activated through the GOG, SWOG, ECOG, and Cancer and Leukemia Group B (CALGB). The trial includes patients with stage III/IV suboptimal disease, who are randomized to receive a single transplant or six cycles of conventional-dose paclitaxel and carboplatin after the documentation of a clinical CR to initial CT. Patients with optimal stage III disease are also eligible only if they have microscopic residual disease.

Unfortunately, the trial, which was expected to take 5 yr, is not currently meeting accrual goals. In discussions at the BMT committees of the major cooperative groups (SWOG, CALGB, ECOG), the universal finding is a lack of referrals by gynecologic oncologists. The reasons appear obscure, with many feeling that the therapy is either too toxic or ineffective, despite the above data. They will now probably point to the negative data from the breast cancer transplant studies, to be presented at the 1999 American Society of Clinical Oncology (ASCO) meeting, which, for early-stage disease, is being presented too early to draw firm conclusions.

In addition, OC appears to be more chemosensitive than breast cancer. One need only consider the DFS of a breast cancer patient with >10 lymph nodes found at diagnosis, who is without disease at the time of adjuvant CT, who has approximately the same 5-yr survival as a suboptimal stage III OC patient and who is left with a significant tumor burden at the completion of her initial surgical procedure.

There are, however, BMT centers transplanting these patients on local, pilot studies, with poorly described end points, patient-selection biases, and toxic deaths, which will answer no appropriate scientific questions.

7. HDCT AS INITIAL THERAPY

Attempts have been made to institute HDCT even earlier in the course of the disease, usually after a short course of conventional CT, or as multiple cycles of dose-intensive therapy with stem cell support (52–60). Benedetti-Panici et al. (53) conducted one of the largest trials to date, transplanting 35 patients after 2–4 cycles of standard dose Cy and cisplatin. Patients were treated with high-dose cisplatin (100 mg/m^2), carboplatin (1800 mg/m^2), and etoposide (1800 mg/m^2), or with carboplatin (1200 mg/m^2), etoposide (900 mg/m^2), and melphalan (100 mg/m^2). After primary cytoreduction, 79% had disease bulk <2 cm, but none had microscopic residual disease. The 24 patients who completed all of the CT cycles, and who underwent a second-look procedure, had a pathologic CR rate of 42%. In a smaller trial, Palmer et al. (55) treated 10 patients with five cycles of paclitaxel and cisplatin, followed by high-dose melphalan (140–160 mg/m^2), with or without mitoxantrone (30–60 mg/m^2). Five/7 completing all therapy, and a second-look procedure, had a pathologic CR.

Multiple cycles of dose-intensive therapy with stem cell support have been used as another strategy for initial therapy (56–60). The rationale for this strategy is the rapid development of drug resistance in this disease, and the Norton-Simon hypothesis, in which rapid alternating cycles of CT are theoretically better at eliminating chemosensitive tumors. The doses used in these trials are approximately twice the standard conventional dose used, but the dose intensity (dose/m^2 divided by time in weeks) is increased 4–5-fold. Fennelly et al. treated 27 evaluable patients with two courses of high-dose Cy (3.0 g/m^2), and then four courses of combination carboplatin (1000 mg/m^2) plus Cy (1500 mg/m^2), administered at approx 14-d intervals (56). Among the 27 patients, there were five pathologically documented CRs and 16 partial responses. The five patients in pathologic CR continued to be free of disease 15+, 15+, 16+, 16+, and 25+ mo after completion of therapy, and all had optimal stage III disease at diagnosis. Overall, 22 patients were alive at a median follow-up of 20.8 mo.

In a follow-up trial by the same group, 16 patients were treated with two cycles of escalating doses of paclitaxel, with Cy for cytoreduction and mobilization of hematopoietic stem cells, which were subsequently collected by apheresis, followed by four cycles of intensive carboplatin (1000 mg/m^2) and Cy (1500 mg/m^2) and peripheral stem cell rescue *(58)*. Of the 13 patients who were assessable for response, 38.5% had a pathologic CR, again, however, exclusively in patients with optimal stage III disease at diagnosis.

As a result of this promising single-institution pilot data, a multicenter pilot study sponsored by the GOG, was conducted, with a modification of the Fennelly regimen for patients with optimal stage III disease *(60)*. Patients received a single cycle of Cy (3000 mg/m^2) and paclitaxel (300 mg/m^2), followed by stem cell collection, and then four cycles of carboplatin (area-under-the-curve 15) and paclitaxel (250 mg/m^2), and a single course of melphalan (140 mg/m^2), with stem cell support. Unfortunately, of nine patients in this study, only one had a pathologic CR at second-look laparotomy, vs an anticipated four patients (R. Schilder, personal communication). Overall, the results of this dose-dense trial have been disappointing, although additional trials incorporating topotecan are in progress.

Given that, treating patiently initially with HDT, one would be treating patients with *de novo* Pt resistance, it is not surprising that some patients will have residual disease at completion of therapy. The logical alternative would be to treat only those patients who respond to a brief course of conventional therapy, i.e., those with a normal exam and normal CA125 after two cycles of CT.

8. CONCLUSIONS

Advanced OC presently has a 5-yr survival of approx 20–25%, despite recent advances in debulking surgery techniques and CT regimens. HDCT with stem cell rescue offers a viable option to palliative CT for women with relapsed OC. With advances in supportive care and increased experience with transplantation regimens, patients appear to tolerate HDCT with acceptable toxicity, and centers are beginning to perform these procedures on an outpatient basis. Initial trials using HDT as consolidation of an initial remission have been promising, but need to be verified by prospective, randomized phase III trials. Only patients being entered on such trials should be transplanted in the consolidation setting. Currently, multicycle HDT is not recommended as initial therapy, given the results of the recently completed GOG trial, except as part of an exploratory pilot study program with defined outcomes *(60)*. Progress will only be made in this disease through continual exploration of newer agents and combinations for first-line therapy, and actively enrolling patients in phase III studies at all stages of this disease, when available.

REFERENCES

1. Alberts DS, Liu PY, Hannigan EV, et al. Intraperitoneal cisplatin plus intravenous cyclophosphamide versus intravenous cisplatin plus intravenous cyclophosphamide for stage III ovarian cancer, *N. Engl. J. Med.*, **335** (1996) 1950–1955.
2. Markman M, Bundy B, Benda J, et al. Randomized phase III study of intravenous (IV) cisplatin (CIS)/paclitaxel (PAC) versus moderately high dose IV carboplatin (CARB) followed by IV PAC and intraperitoneal (IP) CIS in optimal residual ovarian cancer (OC): an intergroup trial (GOG, SWOG, ECOG), *Proc. Am. Soc. Clin. Oncol.*, **17** (1998) 361a(Abstract).
3. Landis SH, Murray T, Bolden S, and Wingo PA. Cancer statistics, 1998 [published errata appear in *CA Cancer J. Clin.*, **48** (1998) 192 and **48** (1998) 329], *CA Cancer J. Clin.*, **48** (1998) 6–29.

4. Herben VM, Panday VR, Richel DJ, et al. Phase I and pharmacologic study of the combination of paclitaxel, cisplatin, and topotecan administered intravenously every 21 days as first-line therapy in patients with advanced ovarian cancer, *J. Clin. Oncol.*, **17** (1999) 747–755.

5. Kohn EC, Sarosy GA, et al. A Phase I/II study of dose-intense paclitaxel with cisplatin and cyclophosphamide as initial therapy of poor-prognosis advanced-stage epithelial ovarian cancer, *Gynecol. Oncol.*, (1996) 181–191(Abstract).

6. Alberts DS, Young L, Mason N, and Salmon SE. In vitro evaluation of anticancer drugs against ovarian cancer at concentrations achievable by intraperitoneal administration, *Semin. Oncol.*, **12 (Suppl 4)** (1985) 38–42.

7. Andrews PA, Velurg S, Mann SC, et al. Cis-diamminedichloroplatinum (III) accumulation in sensitive and resistant ovarian carcinoma cells, *Cancer Res.*, (1988) 68–73.

7a. Behrens BC, Hamilton TC, Masuda H, et al. Characterization of a cis-diamminedichloroplatinum(II)-resistant human ovarian cancer cell line and its use in evaluation of platinum analogues, *Cancer Research*, **47** (1987) 414–418.

7b. Lidor YJ, Shpall EJ, Peters WP, Bast RC. Synergistic cytotoxicity of different alkylating agents for epithelial ovarian cancer. *Int J Cancer*, (1991) 704–707.

7c. Markman M, Reichman B, Hakes T, et al. Responses to second-line cisplatin-based intraperitoneal therapy in ovarian cancer: influence of a prior response to intravenous cisplatin, *J. Clin. Oncol.*, **9** (1991) 1801–1805.

7d. Kaye SB, Lewis CR, Paul J, et al. Randomised study of two doses of cisplatin with cyclophosphamide in epithelial ovarian cancer [see comments]. *Lancet*, **340** (1992) 329–333.

7e. Ngan HY, Choo YC, Cheung M, et al. A randomized study of high-dose versus low-dose cis-platinum combined with cyclophosphamide in the treatment of advanced ovarian cancer. Hong Kong Ovarian Carcinoma Study Group. *Chemotherapy*, **35** (1989) 221–227.

7f. Stiff PJ, McKenzie RS, Alberts DS, et al. Phase I clinical and pharmacokinetic study of high-dose mitoxantrone combined with carboplatin, cyclophosphamide, and autologous bone marrow rescue: high response rate for refractory ovarian carcinoma. *J. Clin. Oncol.*, **12** (1994) 176–183.

7g. Holmberg LA, Demirer T, Rowley S, et al. High-dose busulfan, melphalan and thiotepa followed by autologous peripheral blood stem cell (PBSC) rescue in patients with advanced stage III/IV ovarian cancer. *Bone Marrow Transplant.*, **22** (1998) 651–659.

8. Stiff P, Bayer R, Camarda M, et al. A phase II trial of high-dose mitoxantrone, carboplatin, and cyclophosphamide with autologous bone marrow rescue for recurrent epithelial ovarian carcinoma: analysis of risk factors for clinical outcome [see comments]. *Gynecol. Oncol.*, **57** (1995) 278–285.

9. Teicher B, Holden SA, Jones SM, Eder JP, and Herman TS. Influence of scheduling in two-day combinations of alkylating agents in vivo, *Cancer Chemother. Pharmacol.*, (1989) 161–166.

10. Behrens BC, Hamilton TC, Masuda H, et al. Characterization of a cis-diamminedichloroplatinum(II)-resistant human ovarian cancer cell line and its use in evaluation of platinum analogues, *Cancer Res.*, **47** (1987) 414–418.

11. Lidor YJ, Shpall EJ, Peters WP, and Bast RC. Synergistic cytotoxicity of different alkylating agents for epithelial ovarian cancer, *Int. J. Cancer,* (1991) 704–710.

12. Stemmer SM, Cagnoni PJ, Shpall EJ, et al. High-dose paclitaxel, cyclophosphamide, and cisplatin with autologous hematopoietic progenitor-cell support: a phase I trial, *J. Clin. Oncol.*, **14** (1996) 1463–1472.

13. Raymond E, Hanauske A, Faivre S, et al. Effects of prolonged versus short-term exposure paclitaxel (Taxol) on human tumor colony-forming units, *Anti-Cancer Drugs*, **8** (1997) 379–385.

14. Lopez JA, Krikorian JG, Reich SD, Smyth RD, Lee FH, and Issell BF. Clinical pharmacology of intraperitoneal cisplatin, *Gynecol. Oncol.*, **20** (1985) 1–9.

15. Markman M. Intraperitoneal therapy of ovarian cancer, *Semin. Oncol.*, **25** (1998) 356–360.

16. Ozols RF, Ostchega Y, Myers CE, Young RC. High-dose cisplatin in hypertonic saline in refractory ovarian cancer, *J. Clin. Oncol.*, **3** (1985) 1246–1250.

17. Ozols RF, Ostchega Y, Curt G, Young RC. High-dose carboplatin in refractory ovarian cancer patients, *J. Clin. Oncol.*, **5** (1987) 197–201.

18. Gore ME, Mainwaring PN, MacFarlane V, et al. A randomized study of high versus standard carboplatin in patients with advanced epithelial ovarian cancer, *Proc. Am. Soc. Clin. Oncol.,* (1996) A768(Abstract).

19. Piccart MJ, Nogaret JM, Marcelis L, et al. Cisplatin combined with carboplatin: a new way of intensification of platinum dose in the treatment of advanced ovarian cancer. Belgian Study Group for Ovarian Carcinoma, *J. Natl. Cancer Inst.*, **82** (1990) 703–707.

20. Kaye SB, Lewis CR, Paul J, et al. Randomised study of two doses of cisplatin with cyclophosphamide in epithelial ovarian cancer, *Lancet,* **340** (1992) 329–333.

21. Ngan HY, Choo YC, Cheung M, et al. A randomized study of high-dose versus low-dose cis-platinum combined with cyclophosphamide in the treatment of advanced ovarian cancer. Hong Kong Ovarian Carcinoma Study Group, *Chemotherapy,* **35** (1989) 221–227.

22. Seltzer V, Vogl S, and Kaplan B. Recurrent ovarian carcinoma: retreatment utilizing combination chemotherapy including cis-diamminedichloroplatinum in patients previously responding to this agent, *Gynecol. Oncol.,* **21** (1985) 167–176.

23. Sabbatini P, Spriggs D. Salvage therapy for ovarian cancer, *Oncology,* **12** (1998) 833–843.

24. Eisenhauer EA, Vermorken JB, and van Glabbeke M. Predictors of response to subsequent chemotherapy in platinum pretreated ovarian cancer: a multivariate analysis of 704 patients, *Ann. Oncol.,* **8** (1997) 963–968.

25. Markman M, Rothman R, Hakes T, et al. Second-line platinum therapy in patients with ovarian cancer previously treated with cisplatin, *J. Clin. Oncol.,* **9** (1991) 389–393.

26. Kotz KW and Schilder RJ. High-dose chemotherapy and hematopoietic progenitor cell support for patients with epithelial ovarian cancer, *Semin. Oncol.,* **22** (1995) 250–262.

27. Fennelly D. The role of high-dose chemotherapy in the management of advanced ovarian cancer, *Curr. Opin. Oncol.,* **8** (1996) 415–425.

28. Mulder PO, Sleijfer DT, Willemse PH, de Vries EG, Uges DR, and Mulder NH. High-dose cyclophosphamide or melphalan with escalating doses of mitoxantrone and autologous bone marrow transplantation for refractory solid tumors, *Cancer Res.,* **49** (1989) 4654–4658.

29. Stiff PJ, McKenzie RS, Alberts DS, et al. Phase I clinical and pharmacokinetic study of high-dose mitoxantrone combined with carboplatin, cyclophosphamide, and autologous bone marrow rescue: high response rate for refractory ovarian carcinoma, *J. Clin. Oncol.,* **12** (1994) 176–183.

30. Shea TC, Flaherty M, Elias A, et al. A phase I clinical and pharmacokinetic study of carboplatin and autologous bone marrow support [published erratum appears in *J. Clin. Oncol.,* **8** (1989) 1177], *J. Clin. Oncol.,* **7** (1989) 651–661.

31. Shpall EJ, Clarke-Pearson D, Soper JT, et al. High-dose alkylating agent chemotherapy with autologous bone marrow support in patients with stage III/IV epithelial ovarian cancer, *Gynecol. Oncol.,* **38** (1990) 386–391.

32. Wolff SN, Herzig RH, Fay JW, et al. High-dose N,N′,N″-triethylenethiophosphoramide (thiotepa) with autologous bone marrow transplantation: phase I studies, *Semin. Oncol.,* **17 (Suppl. 3)** (1990) 2–6.

33. Viens P and Maraninchi D. High dose chemotherapy and autologous marrow transplantation for common epithelial ovarian carcinoma. In Armitage J, Antman K e. (eds.), *High Dose Chemotherapy,* Williams and Wilkins, Baltimore, 1992, pp. 729–734.

34. Willemse PH, Sleijfer DT, deVries EG, et al. Ablative chemotherapy and autologous bone marrow transfusion in patients with refractory ovarian cancer, *Proc. Am. Soc. Clin. Oncol.,* (1987) 478a(Abstract).

35. Shea TC, Storniolo AM, Mason JR, et al. High dose itravenous and intraperitoneal combination chemotherapy with autologous stem cell rescue for patients with advanced ovarian cancer, *Proc. Am. Soc. Clin. Oncol.,* (1992) 756(Abstract).

36. Broun ER, Belinson JL, Berek JS, et al. Salvage therapy for recurrent and refractory ovarian cancer with high-dose chemotherapy and autologous bone marrow support: a Gynecologic Oncology Group pilot study, *Gynecol. Oncol.,* **54** (1994) 142–146.

37. Stiff P, Antman K, Broun RE, et al. Bone marrow transplantation for ovarian carcinoma in the United States: a survey of active programs, *Proceedings of Sixth International BMT Symposium,* 1992, pp. 1–9.

38. Weaver CH, Greco FA, Hainsworth JD, et al. A phase I–II study of high-dose melphalan, mitoxantrone and carboplatin with peripheral blood stem cell support in patients with advanced ovarian or breast carcinoma, *Bone Marrow Transplant.,* **20** (1997) 847–853.

39. Holmberg LA, Demirer T, Rowley S, et al. High-dose busulfan, melphalan and thiotepa followed by autologous peripheral blood stem cell (PBSC) rescue in patients with advanced stage III/IV ovarian cancer, *Bone Marrow Transplant.,* **22** (1998) 651–659.

40. Stiff P, Bayer R, Camarda M, et al. A phase II trial of high-dose mitoxantrone, carboplatin, and cyclophosphamide with autologous bone marrow rescue for recurrent epithelial ovarian carcinoma: analysis of risk factors for clinical outcome, *Gynecol. Oncol.,* **57** (1995) 278–285.

41. Stiff PJ, Bayer R, Kerger C, et al. High-dose chemotherapy with autologous transplantation for persistent/relapsed ovarian cancer: a multivariate analysis of survival for 100 consecutively treated patients, *J. Clin. Oncol.,* **15** (1997) 1309–1317.

42. Horowitz MM, Stiff PJ, Vuem-Stone, Rowlings PA. Outcome of autotransplants for advanced ovarian cancer, *Proc. Am. Soc. Clin. Oncol.*, (1997) 353a(Abstract).

43. Stiff PJ, Kerger C, and Bayer RA. High dose chemotherapy and autologous stem cell transplantation for ovarian carcinoma: comparisons to conventional therapy and future directions, in autologous marrow and blood transplantation. Proceedings of the Ninth International Symposium, Karel Dicke and Armand Keating eds, *Cancer Treatment Research and Educational Institute,* Arlington, T 1999, (in press).

44. Dauplat J, Legros M, Condat P, Ferriere JP, Ben Ahmed S, Plagne R. High-dose melphalan and autologous bone marrow support for treatment of ovarian carcinoma with positive second-look operation, *Gynecol. Oncol.*, **34** (1989) 394–298.

45. Legros M, Dauplat J, Fleury J, et al. High-dose chemotherapy with hematopoietic rescue in patients with stage III to IV ovarian cancer: long-term results, *J. Clin. Oncol.*, **15** (1997) 1302–1308.

46. Viens P, Maraninchi D, Legros M, et al. High dose melphalan and autologous marrow rescue in advanced epithelial ovarian carcinomas: a retrospective analysis of 35 patients treated in France, *Bone Marrow Transplant.*, **5** (1990) 227–233.

47. Extra JM, Giacchetti S, Bourstyn E, et al. High dose chemotherapy with autologous bone marrow reinfusion as consolidation therapy for patients with advanced ovarian adenocarcinoma, *Proc. Am. Soc. Oncol.*, (1992) 234(Abstract).

48. Barnett MJ, Swenerton KD, Hoskins PJ, et al. Intensive therapy with carboplatin, etoposide, and melphalan (CEM) and autologous stem cell transplantation (SCT) for epithelial ovarian cancer (EOC), *Proc. Am. Soc. Clin. Oncol.*, (1990) 168(Abstract).

49. Cure H, Extra JM, Viens P, et al. High dose chemotherapy with hematopoietic stem cell support as consolidation therapy for patients with platinum-sensitive advanced epithelial ovarian cancer, *Bone Marrow Transplant.* **22** (1998) 5102–5103.

50. Mulder PO, Willemse PH, Aalders JG, et al. High-dose chemotherapy with autologous bone marrow transplantation in patients with refractory ovarian cancer, *Eur. J. Cancer Clin. Oncol.*, **25** (1989) 645–649.

51. Duska L, Chang Y, Goodman A, Fuller A, Nikrui N. Epithelial ovarian tumors in the reproductive age group, *Proc. Am. Soc. Clin. Oncol.*, (1988) 335a(Abstract).

52. Rubella J, Henriquez I, Algarra MS, et al. High-dose combination of carboplatin (CBDCA) and etoposide (VP-16) followed by peripheral blood stem cell transplantation in the treatment of ovarian carcinoma, *Proc. Am. Assoc. Cancer Res.*, **32** (1991) 172(Abstract).

53. Benedetti-Panici P, Greggi S, Scambi G, et al. Very high-dose chemotherapy with autologous peripheral stem cell (APSC) as hematologic support (HS) in previously untreated advanced ovarian cancer (AOC), *Proc. Soc. Gynecol. Oncol.*, (1995) (Abstract).

54. Menichella G, Pierelli L, Foddai ML, et al. Autologous blood stem cell harvesting and transplantation in patients with advanced ovarian cancer, *Br. J. Haematol.*, **79** (1991) 444–450.

55. Palmer PA, Schwartzberg L, Birch R, West W, Weaver CH. High-dose melphalan +/– mitoxantrone with peripheral blood progenitor cell support as a comonent of initial treatment of patients with advanced ovarian cancer, *Proc. Am. Soc. Clin. Oncol.*, **14** (1995) 991(Abstract).

56. Fennelly D, Wasserheit C, Schneider J, et al. Simultaneous dose escalation and schedule intensification of carboplatin-based chemotherapy using peripheral blood progenitor cells and filgrastim: a phase I trial, *Cancer Res.*, **54** (1994) 6137–6142.

57. Shea T, Graham M, Steagall A, et al. Multiple cycles of high dose taxol plus carboplatin with G-CSF and peripheral blood progenitor cell (PBPC) support, *Proc. Am. Soc. Clin. Oncol.*, **14** (1994) 395(Abstract).

58. Fennelly D, Schneider J, Spriggs D, et al. Dose escalation of paclitaxel with high-dose cyclophosphamide, with analysis of progenitor-cell mobilization and hematologic support of advanced ovarian cancer patients receiving rapidly sequenced high-dose carboplatin/cyclophosphamide courses, *J. Clin. Oncol.*, **13** (1995) 1160–1166.

59. Wendt H, Birkmann J, Eckart-Schaefer K, et al. Sequential cycles of high-dose chemotherapy supported by G-CSF (filgastrim) mobilized peripheral progenitor cells (PBPC) in advanced ovarian cancer. A phase I/II dose escalation study for carboplatin, *Proc. Am. Soc. Clin. Oncol.*, **16** (1997) 92a(Abstract).

60. Schilder RJ and Shea TC. Multiple cycles of high dose chemotherapy for ovarian cancer, *Semin. Oncol.*, (1998) 349–355.

61. McGuire WP, Hoskins WJ, Brady MF, et al. Cyclophosphamide and cisplatin compared with paclitaxel and cisplatin in patients with stage III and stage IV ovarian cancer, *N. Engl. J. Med.,* (1996) 1–6.

14 What Is the Optimal Timing of Autologous Transplantation for Metastatic Breast Cancer?

Stephanie F. Williams, MD

CONTENTS

1. INTRODUCTION

Breast cancer (BC) remains a common life-threatening condition that has undergone extensive scientific and clinical investigation over the past two decades. Despite expanding knowledge of genetics, prognostic factors, and biology, as well as advances in surgical management, adjuvant chemotherapy (CT), and radiotherapy, many women will die from progressive, metastatic breast cancer (MBC). Over the past 10 yr, many investigators have studied the role of high-dose chemotherapy (HDCT) with hematopoietic stem cell support. Many phase II high-dose regimens have been explored, and, recently, some small randomized clinical trials have been undertaken. Despite this interest, questions remain concerning the exact role of this modality in therapy for BC. The development, rationale, and results of this modality are reviewed here, and the appropriate timing of applying this therapy in the treatment of MBC are addressed.

2. EXPERIMENTAL RATIONALE

Dose–response is the key concept underlying HDCT programs. Laboratory studies in tumor cell lines have demonstrated that the amount of tumor cell killing can be

From: *Current Controversies in Bone Marrow Transplantation*
Edited by: B. Bolwell © Humana Press Inc., Totowa, NJ

related to the dose of chemotherapeutic agent. For small increments in the dose of certain agents, logarithmic tumor cell killing can occur. This is a steep dose–response effect. Investigators have shown that alkylating agents, such as cyclophosphamide (Cy), thiotepa, and melphalan, exhibit this steep dose–response effect in cultured BC cell models (1). In addition, the combination of alkylating agents in these models has synergistic effects on tumor cell killing (2). However, other factors can influence this dose–response effect in the clinical setting. These include the type of chemotherapeutic agent utilized, the schedule of administration, and such intrinsic tumor factors as tumor cell type, tumor growth kinetics, tumor volume, and emergence of drug resistance (3).

The characteristics of antineoplastic agents that would be optimal for high-dose therapy (HDT) or dose-intensive therapy are demonstration of a steep dose–response curve, myelosuppression as major dose-limiting toxicity, lack of crossresistance, and minimal long-term toxicity. Alkylating agents fit many of these characteristics, and have emerged as the cornerstones of HDCT regimens in BC trials.

3. CLINICAL RATIONALE

Clinical studies of dose intensity with standard regimens have shown a correlation of dose with response. Retrospective and prospective clinical studies in advanced BC have shown improved response rates in patients receiving higher-dose intensity (4). However, improvement in overall survival was not satisfactorily demonstrated in this experience. These observations prompted the use of HDCT with autologous stem cell rescue (ASCR) (initially bone marrow, now primarily mobilized peripheral blood progenitor or stem cells) in the metastatic disease setting.

Early clinical experience in the mid-1980s consisted of phase I HDT with ASCR trials in solid tumors. Many of these patients had refractory BC. Both single agents, as well as combinations, were explored (5–10). The notable result was high response rates, including complete responses (CRs) in refractory patients, although these responses were of short duration. As with conventional therapy, combination therapy appeared superior. These encouraging results led to the development of the treatment strategies that are discussed below.

As this therapeutic modality has become increasingly available and safer, through the use of hematopoietic growth factors and peripheral blood stem cell rescue, many patients have been treated. Current Autologous Blood and Marrow Transplant Registry (ABMTR) data has shown the growth in utilization of this modality since 1989 (11). BC is now the leading indication for a stem cell transplant. Many of these patients are not treated on investigational protocols, limiting the ability to adequately assess this therapy in the BC armamentarium.

4. TREATMENT STRATEGIES

Over the years, based on the above results, two distinct treatment strategies emerged in MBC, to allow utilization of HDT with ASCR earlier in the disease course, before exposure to multiple CT agents (Table 1). The most-investigated strategies involved initial or upfront HDT in untreated disease, or intensification or consolidation with HDT in CT-responsive or -sensitive disease. More recently, application of HDT with ASCR, at the time of first relapse after conventional CT, has been proposed and

Table 1
Treatment Strategies in MBC

1. Initial up-front HDT in untreated patients.
2. Intensification or consolidation in CT-responsive or -sensitive disease.
3. Treatment of first relapse after conventional therapy.

examined with seemingly contradictory results. Thus, the question of optimal timing of this modality in the treatment of MBC has arisen.

These strategies are also based on models of tumor cell growth. One model proposes that, for a tumor system, a constant fraction of cells are killed per given dose of drug: This is the log cell kill hypothesis of Skipper and Schabel *(12)*. The other model postulates that tumor growth follows Gompertzian kinetics: Thus, tumor doubling time decreases with increasing tumor size *(13,14)*. This Norton-Simon hypothesis suggests that tumor cell growth slows with increasing size, but reduction in size can lead to rapid regrowth. Thus, a single treatment will not be effective. So, in order to eradicate clinically apparent metastatic disease, one needs a regimen that will produce a high initial cytoreduction, or CR rate, followed by additional therapy after CR is obtained as consolidation. This therapy should be delivered rapidly and repeatedly after a CR is obtained, to prevent the rapid regrowth predicted by the Norton-Simon hypothesis.

As mentioned previously, drug resistance can exist and/or be induced in tumor cells. The precise mechanisms for this are not fully understood, although several factors have been postulated. However, clinically, one approach utilized has been to design regimens with alternating noncrossresistant combinations. This is based on the Goldie-Coldman hypothesis *(15)*. Thus, multiple or sequential courses of therapy, either HDT or combinations of conventional and HDT, may be needed to eradicate MBC.

5. INITIAL THERAPY IN UNTREATED BC

In theory, upfront or initial HDCT with ASCR could limit the emergence of drug-resistant tumor cell clones. However, the treatment of bulky tumors may be ineffective if Gompertzian kinetics occurs. Thus, multiple sequential high-dose regimens may be necessary.

Nevertheless, clinical results of single high-dose regimens have demonstrated some effectiveness. Peters et al. *(16)*, with a combination of Cy, cisplatin, and carmustine, with autologous bone marrow rescue in 22 premenopausal, estrogen-receptor-negative patients, achieved a response rate of 77%, with 54% CRs after one cycle. Three of these 22 women remain alive and disease-free. Bezwoda et al. *(17)* demonstrated the superiority of an initial double or tandem HDT with ASCR approach, compared to conventional combination CT. This small study of 90 women with MBC randomized them to initial therapy of two cycles of high-dose Cy, mitoxantrone, and etoposide with ASCR in rapid succession, or to conventional cycles of Cy, mitoxantrone, and vincristine for 6 cycles. The CR rate was significantly higher in the double-high-dose arm, compared to conventional therapy. CRs were even obtained in patients with hepatic metastases. Duration of response and survival were also better in the double-high-dose arm. However, the median survival in the double-high-dose arm was 21 mo, which is historically similar in patients with MBC treated with conventional anthracycline-based regimens *(18)*. Bezwoda has reported that those patients who are alive and disease-free for more than 3 yr were those patients who were in CR after their first cycle of HDT, and subsequently received their second cycle *(19)*. This would favor treatment approaches that address Gompertzian tumor kinetics and the Norton-Simon hypothesis.

6. INTENSIFICATION THERAPY IN CT-SENSITIVE DISEASE

A more common approach has been to treat patients initially with a standard-induction CT regimen; then, those patients without evidence of progression, or with a partial or CR to this therapy, would undergo high-dose intensification or consolidation with ASCR. In theory, this approach cytoreduces tumor bulk, and allows treatment in a minimal disease state. If Gompertzian kinetics is in action, this will allow treatment at a time when tumor cells may be more susceptible to certain CT agents, i.e., during DNA synthesis and regrowth. The HDCT regimen, if noncrossresistant with the induction CT regimen, may reduce or eliminate drug resistance.

Numerous clinical trials, examining this approach, have been performed over the years. These have been superbly reviewed and summarized elsewhere *(20)*, and thus will not be presented in detail here. These studies have shown high response rates of between 70 and 100%, with 35–60% CRs, but the overall survivals and response durations appear no better than historical controls. Only approx 15% of patients have durable responses beyond 5 yr. In fact, the group from MD Anderson Cancer Center has shown that, if one utilizes the same selection criteria as in HDCT trials, the same long-term survival rates can be seen in women with MBC treated with conventional doxorubicin-containing regimens without HDCT consolidation *(21)*.

Several important points need to be noted. Many investigators, including the ABMTR, have examined outcome as a function of response to induction therapy. Patients with responsive disease, particularly those in CR prior to HDT, clearly have a longer disease-free survival than nonresponsive patients *(11,20)*. This further corroborates approaches that are based on the Norton-Simon hypothesis.

There has been an attempt to build on this by utilizing tandem or double-HDT with ASCR after the induction CT regimen. The agents used in these programs are primarily alkylating agents, as well as, occasionally, platinum compounds, mitoxantrone, and etoposide. Several hundred women have been treated in this fashion, and reported on in the literature *(22–25)*. The results do not appear to be superior, in terms of disease control, to a single HDT with ASCR after induction CT. In some instances, there appeared to be more toxicity. As newer noncrossresistant agents with nonoverlapping toxicities to alkylating agents, such as the taxanes, become available, further work on the rational design of these programs can continue.

7. HDCT WITH ASCR AT FIRST RELAPSE

There has been one randomized study reported in preliminary form, with intriguing results, adding to the question of when is the appropriate timing for HDT with ASCR in the course of treatment for MBC *(26)*. Over 400 women, CT-naïve and hormone-insensitive, underwent induction CT with a doxorubicin-based regimen. Ninety-eight achieved a CR, and were randomized to receive either HDCT with ASCR or observation

Table 2
Summary of Current Outcomes

Disease status prior to HDT	Survival at 5-yr after therapy
Untreated; initial	15–20%
Refractory	Rare
PR to cytoreductive therapy	5–10%
CR to cytoreductive therapy	25–40%
First relapse[a]	40%

[a]Based on one study.

with HDCT with ASCR at the time of relapse. Disease-free survival was significantly longer in the group receiving immediate HDT, but median overall survival was shorter.

This further illustrates the point that timing of therapy along the tumor cell growth curve is clinically relevant and important. As patients with metastatic disease achieve CRs with induction therapy and/or a single HDT cycle, sufficient unmeasurable tumor burden remains. Additional therapy to eradicate this tumor burden is necessary. Kinetically, further noncrossresistant CT programs can be devised, and timing of administration can be further studied.

8. REASONS FOR FAILURE

Despite the aggressive use of CT with ASCR, the majority of women with MBC eventually relapse and die (see Table 2 for summary). The reasons are primarily twofold: Minimal residual disease remains and regrows, and reinfusion of a stem cell autograft contaminated with BC cells, which can lead to tumor implants.

Eliminating minimal residual disease is a major obstacle. The studies and results discussed above show how difficult it is, despite the use of high-dose regimens. Even adding two or more high-dose regimens has not yet improved results. More is not necessarily better. Perhaps further investigations, utilizing newer, more active agents, such as the taxanes, and exploiting the kinetic considerations of the Norton-Simon hypothesis, may further improve results. An optimal high-dose regimen has not been devised. However, newer non-CT approaches may have to be added after HDT with ASCR. These may include manipulation of the patients' immune system posttransplant with activated immune effector cells, dendritic cell vaccines, or immune stimulants, such as interleukin-2 or -12. Patients with Her-2/neu-positive tumors may benefit from infusions of the monoclonal antibody, herceptin.

Additionally, there is indirect evidence that reinfused tumor cells can contribute to relapse after HDT with ASCR (27–29). This can occur in peripheral blood stem cell grafts, as well as bone marrow. To minimize or avoid this problem, investigators have studied methods of purging BC cells from these autografts, including positive selection of the CD34-positive stem cell, and negative selection processes, which involve CT or monoclonal antibodies. No technique has been shown to eliminate all contaminating tumor cells. To date, no investigator has found a survival superior to historical patients utilizing purged or selected stem cells as hematopoietic rescue after HDCT (30).

9. CONCLUSION: CAN WE DESIGN A MORE EFFECTIVE APPROACH?

Despite the above considerations, approx 15–20% of women with MBC enjoy prolonged disease-free survival after HDT with ASCR. This is particularly true for those who are in CR before HDT. More effective approaches need to be investigated. These will probably be multimodality approaches integrating newer, more active CT agents with posttransplant immune therapy. More aggressive upfront induction regimens are necessary to put a higher percentage of women in a clinical CR. Then, based on the Norton-Simon hypothesis, multiple sequential courses of HDT, administered in rapid succession, with stem cell support, can be utilized. These agents should be noncrossresistant, with nonoverlapping, nonhematologic toxicities. To eliminate or decrease tumor cell contamination, the stem cell product may need to be selected or purified. Additionally, after hematologic and immunologic recovery from this therapy, stimulation of the patient's immune system to attack residual cancer cells will be necessary to eradicate any remaining disease.

The next decade should be built on the results of the past 10 yr. This therapeutic modality can be refined and improved. Once this is accomplished, large randomized studies should be undertaken to further define the appropriate timing of HDT in MBC. Every effort must be made to ensure adequate study design and patient accrual.

REERENCES

1. Frei E III, Teicher BA, Holden SA, et al. Effect of alkylating agent dose: studies and possible clinical correlation, *Cancer Res.*, **48** (1988) 6417–6432.
2. Teicher BA, Cucci CA, Lee JB, et al. Alkylating agents: in vitro studies of cross resistance patterns in human cell lines, *Cancer Res.*, **46** (1986) 4379–4383.
3. Henderson IC, Hayes DF, and Gelman R. Dose-response in the treatment of breast cancer: a critical review, *J. Clin. Oncol.*, **6** (1988) 1501–1515.
4. Hyrniuk W and Bush H. Importance of dose intensity in chemotherapy of metastatic breast cancer, *J. Clin. Oncol.*, **2** (1984) 1281–1288.
5. Peters WP, Eder JP, Henner WP, et al. High-dose combination alkylating agents with autologous bone marrow support: a phase I study, *J. Clin. Oncol.*, **4** (1986) 646–654.
6. Antman K, Eder JP, Elias A, et al. High-dose combination alkylating agent preparative regimen with autologous bone marrow support: the Dana-Farber Institute/Beth Israel Hospital Experience, *Cancer Treat. Rep.*, **71** (1987) 119–125.
7. Williams SF, Bitran J, Kaminer L, et al. Phase I–II study of bialkylator chemotherapy, high dose thiopeta and cyclophosphamide with autologous bone marrow reinfusion in patients with refractory cancer, *J. Clin. Oncol.*, **5** (1987) 260–265.
8. Slease RB, Benear JB, Selby GB et al. High-dose combination alkylating agent therapy with autologous bone marrow rescue for refractory solid tumors, *J. Clin. Oncol.*, **6** (1988) 1314–1320.
9. Eder JP, Antman K, and Elias A. Cyclophosphamide and thiotepa with autologous bone marrow transplant in patients with solid tumors, *J. Natl. Cancer Inst.*, **80** (1988) 1221–1226.
10. Peters WP, Shpall EJ, Jones RB, et al. High-dose combination alkylating agents with bone marrow support as initial treatment for metastatic breast cancer, *J. Clin. Oncol.*, **6** (1988) 1368–1376.
11. Antman KH, Rowlings PA, Vaughan WP, et al. High-dose chemotherapy with autologous hematopoietic stem cell support for breast cancer in North America, *J. Clin. Oncol.*, **15** (1997) 1870–1879.
12. Skipper HE, Schabel FM Jr, Wilcox WS. Experimental evaluation of potential anticancer agent XIII. On the criteria and kinetics associated with "curability" of experimental leukemia, *Cancer Chemother. Rep.*, **35** (1964) 1–111.
13. Norton L and Simon R. Tumor size, sensitivity to therapy and the design of treatment schedules, *Cancer Treat. Rep.*, **61** (1977) 1307–1317.
14. Norton L. Gomperztian model of human breast cancer growth, *Cancer Res.*, **48** (1988) 7067–7071.

15. Goldie J. and Goldman AJ. A mathematical model for relating the drug sensitivity of tumors to their spontaneous mutation rate, *Cancer Treat. Rep.,* **63** (1979) 1727–1773.

16. Peters WP, Shpall EJ, Jones RB, et al. High-dose combination alkylating agents in bone marrow support as initial treatment for metastatic breast cancer, *J. Clin. Oncol.,* **6** (1988) 1368–1376.

17. Bezwoda WR, Seymour L, and Dansey RD. High-dose chemotherapy with hematopoietic rescue as primary treatment for metastatic breast cancer: a randomized trial, *J. Clin. Oncol.,* **13** (1995) 2483–2489.

18. Mick R, Begg C, Antman K, et al. Diverse prognosis in metastatic breast cancer: who should be offered alternative initial therapies? *Breast Cancer Res. Treat.,* **13** (1989) 33–38.

19. Bezwoda WR. High dose chemotherapy with hematopoietic rescue in breast cancer: from theory to practice, *Cancer Chemother. Pharmacol.,* **40 (Suppl)** (1997) S79–S87.

20. Lazarus HM. Hematopoietic progenitor cell transplantation in breast cancer: current status and future direction, *Cancer Invest.,* **16** (1998) 102–126.

21. Rahman ZU, Frye DK, Buzdar AU, et al. Impact of selection process on response rate and long-term survival of potential high-dose chemotherapy candidates treated with standard dose doxorubicin containing chemotherapy in patients with metastatic breast cancer, *J. Clin. Oncol.,* **15** (1997) 3171–3177.

22. Dunphy FR, Sptizer G, Buzdar AU, et al. Treatment of estrogen receptor-negative or hormonally refractory breast cancer with double high-dose chemotherapy intensification and bone marrow support, *J. Clin. Oncol.,* **8** (1990) 1207–1216.

23. Ayash LJ, Elias A, Wheeler C, et al. Double dose-intensive chemotherapy with autologous marrow and peripheral-blood progenitor-cell support for metastatic breast cancer: a feasibility study, *J. Clin. Oncol.,* **12** (1994) 37–44.

24. Ghalie R, Williams SF, Valentino LA, et al. Tandem peripheral blood progenitor cell transplants as initial therapy for metastatic breast cancer, *Biol. Blood Marrow Transplant.,* **1** (1995) 40–46.

25. Bitran JD, Samuels B, Klein L, et al. Tandem high-dose chemotherapy supported by hematopoietic progenitor cells yields prolonged survival in stage IV breast cancer, *Bone Marrow Transplant.,* **17** (1996) 157–162.

26. Peters WP, Jones RB, Vredenburgh J, et al. Large prospective randomized trial of high dose combination alkylating agents with autologous cellular support as consolidation for patients with metastatic breast cancer achieving complete remission after intensive doxorubicin-based induction therapy, *Proc. Am. Soc. Clin. Oncol.,* **15** (1996) 121(Abstract).

27. Rill DR, Santana VM, Roberts WM, et al. Direct demonstration that autologous bone marrow transplantation for solid tumors can return a multiplicity of tumorigenic cells, *Blood,* **84** (1994) 380–383.

28. Brenner MK, Rill DR, Moan RC, et al. Gene-marking to trace origin of relapse after autologous bone-marrow transplantation, *Lancet,* **341** (1993) 85–86.

29. Brockstein BE, Ross AA, Moss TJ, et al. Tumor cell contamination of bone marrow harvest products: Clinical consequences in a cohort of advanced-stage patients undergoing high-dose chemotherapy, *J. Hematother.,* **5** (1996) 617–624.

30. Lazarus HM, Rowe JM, and Goldstone AH. Does in vitro purging improve the outcome after autologous bone marrow transplantation? *J. Hematother.,* **2** (1994) 457–466.

15 Should All Patients with Inflammatory Breast Cancer Undergo Autologous Stem Cell Transplant?

Beth A. Overmoyer, MD

CONTENTS

1. INTRODUCTION

Modern medicine has made great strides in the advancement of treatment strategies for diseases that were once considered incurable. The treatment of the most aggressive forms of breast cancer (BC), inflammatory breast cancer (IBC), has been included in medicine's quest for cure. Unfortunately, determining the optimal treatment program for IBC is hampered by several characteristics of the disease, e.g., the rareness of the disease, the lack of consistency in diagnostic criteria, and the inclusion of other stages of BC in clinical trials involving IBC.

From: *Current Controversies in Bone Marrow Transplantation*
Edited by: B. Bolwell © Humana Press Inc., Totowa, NJ

Many studies include IBC with other locally advanced BCs (stage IIIa, and stage IV, by virtue of ipsilateral infraclavicular and supraclavicular lymph node involvement). Untreated locally advanced BC may also develop secondary inflammatory changes, which are often therapeutically grouped with primary IBC, yet are associated with a more favorable prognosis *(1)*. For the author's purpose, IBC is defined as stage IIIb disease: a T4d BC, described by Haagensen as breast enlargement, erythema, warmth, diffuse skin induration, and an erysipeloid ridge *(2,3)*.

Pathologically, IBC may be defined as any invasive adenocarcinoma, with tumor emboli present with dermal lymphatics. There are conflicting data concerning differences in prognosis, depending on the definition of IBC: clinical characteristics without pathologic findings, pathologic findings without clinical characteristics (so-called "occult" IBC), and presence of both clinical and pathologic findings concurrently. The 1975–1981 National Cancer Institute's Surveillance, Epidemiology, and End Results (SEER) data suggest a worse prognosis associated with the presence of both pathologic and clinical findings, but several studies do not confirm a difference in outcome *(4–10)*. In general, evidence suggests that either feature is associated with a poor overall survival (OS), and should be treated as a single entity.

Data from the SEER program demonstrated the rareness of this disease. The incidence of IBC is estimated to be approx 0.7–1.1 cases/100,000 persons/yr. This incidence is underestimated, because the criteria of inclusion into the 1975–1992 SEER database consisted of only those patients with the pathological manifestation of IBC, i.e., the presence of invasion of breast dermal lymphatics with tumor emboli. Patients with purely clinical manifestations of IBC (erythema, skin edema or peau d'orange, ridging of the skin) were excluded from analysis *(11)*. Even when the broadest definition of IBC is used (clinical and/or pathological), the incidence is low: Approximately 6.4% of all BC diagnoses are inflammatory *(4)*.

Although many innovative therapies have attempted to impact upon this disease's relentless course, survival statistics continue to demonstrate a worse prognosis associated with IBC. Based on SEER data, the 3-yr survival is 42%, compared with 85% for non-IBC (1988–1992 unadjusted rates) *(11)*. These survival statistics underscore the need for aggressive treatment strategies for IBC. The most promising innovative therapy appears to be the application of dose-intensive chemotherapy (CT) with autologous stem cell transplantation (ASCT). This chapter presents current data supporting a role for ASCT for IBC, with the understanding that conclusive evidence is not available, given the rarity of this disease, the difficulties in diagnosis, and the inclusion of other types of locally advanced BC in the study population.

2. HISTORICAL PERSPECTIVE

2.1. Local Therapy: Radiation Therapy

As with non-IBC, primary treatment with either a simple or modified radical mastectomy was initially used for IBC. The results were appalling: mean OS of 12–32 mo, with less than 10% 5-yr survival rates *(12,13)*. Based on these data, Haagensen deemed IBC unresectable, and the primary therapeutic modality was changed to radiation therapy (RT) *(5)*. Excellent historical reviews of these studies are documented elsewhere *(12–16)*, and will only be summarized in this text. Unfortunately, RT alone, and combined surgery and RT, offered no survival advantage, compared with surgery alone,

Table 1
RT Vs Chemoradiation Therapy

Ref.	N	Treatment[a]	Local recurrence (%)	DFS (%)	OS (%)
30[b]	60	Radiation	53	16	28
	91	Radiation/AVM	32	28	44
	79	Radiation/AVCMF	31	46	66

[a]See Chapter Appendix.
[b]4-year follow-up.
DFS, disease-free survival; OS, overall survival.

having 5-yr OS rates of 0–28%, and 0–20%, respectively *(12,13,17)*. Specific attention must be given to the techniques used during RT for this disease. Most megavoltage RT has a skin-sparing effect, which may be detrimental in the treatment of IBC, given the diffuse involvement of dermal lymphatics with tumor emboli, and some evidence that a brisk skin reaction is necessary to achieve adequate local disease control *(18)*. Several investigators *(19–22)* have also noted a dose–response phenomenon between RT to the breast and duration of local control. Disappointing outcomes associated with RT alone may be linked to compromised treatment doses using less than 60 Gy to the intact breast.

2.2. Addition of CT

In 1970, systemic CT began to be applied to the treatment of IBC *(23,24)*. In the paradigm of BC, micrometastatic disease existed at the time of diagnosis, and IBC was associated with a high incidence of developing chemoresistant clones. CT was therefore added to RT, in an attempt to eradicate micrometastatic cancer prior to the development of resistance, and utilize clinical disease response as a marker for systemic chemoresponsiveness. The reasons supporting this treatment approach are: Primary Ct (neoadjuvant) allows greater tumor penetration prior to the development of RT-induced changes in the vasculature of the tumor; CT results in downstaging of the tumor, resulting in better local disease control; and alternating CT and RT allows for the application of full doses of both treatment modalities *(25–28)*.

Several studies compared primary RT with a combination of CT and radiation. The European Organization for the Research and Treatment of Cancer used primary therapy with RT as the standard arm in a four-arm randomized study published in 1989 *(29)*, and found a statistically significant delay in tumor recurrence, when local-regional RT was given concurrently with cyclophosphamide (Cy), methotrexate, 5-fluorouracil (5-FU) (CMF), CT and hormonal ablation. The major effect was a delay in local disease recurrence among patients with locally advanced BC (13% IBC). The Institut Gustave-Roussy *(30)* and Vanderbilt University Medical Center *(21)* demonstrated a survival advantage when CT was combined with RT for IBC (Table 1). The difference in outcomes may be caused by the administration of more effective CT, i.e., the use of Adriamycin (Adr)-containing regimens, or the inclusion of larger numbers of patients with IBC, rather than a subset of locally advanced disease. Regardless, CT contributed to local disease control, and had a favorable impact on delaying metastasis, though the prognosis for IBC remains grim (Table 2).

Table 2
Neoadjuvant CT and RT Therapy

Ref.	N	Treatment[a]	OR (%)	Local Recurrence (yr)	DFS (%)	OS (%)
25,31	125	CMFAV/RT	82	27% (5)	50	38
32,33	14/43[b]	ECPF/RT	86	NA (1)	56	76
26	67	VeTMFAP/RT	80	NA (2)	80	90
34	19	VIE/RT	84	58% (3)	52	63

[a]See Chapter Appendix.
[b]IBC/locally advanced BC
OR, overall disease response; RT, radiation therapy.

Table 3
Neoadjuvant CT Followed by Mastectomy

Ref.	N	Treatment[a]	OR	Local recurrence	DFS	OS
37	25	CF/S/CF	96%	23% (5 yr)	40%	45%

[a]See Chapter Appendix.

2.3. Local Therapy: Surgery

Primary CT resulted in adequate downstaging of patients initially deemed inoperable; therefore, surgical resection was performed in an attempt to improve local disease control without the need for RT. Early studies were feasibility trials, to see if simple or modified radical mastectomy could be performed without excessive complications following neoadjuvant CT (35). Eventually, these studies demonstrated a 10–25% local recurrence rate, and a 50–70% 4-yr OS (6,27,36–38). Several large randomized trials found no difference in the disease-free survival (DFS), OS, or local disease recurrence rate, when patients received mastectomy or RT following neoadjuvant CT (17,19,39–41). However, there was a trend for fewer local recurrences in the surgical treatment arm (7,40,41) (Table 3).

Investigators from Washington University School of Medicine examined their experience with IBC from an historical perspective, and found a significant improvement in local disease control when RT and surgery were combined: 19% with surgery vs 70% with RT alone. Patients who received all three treatment modalities fared the best: 35% 5-yr DFS, and 44% 5-yr OS (9). Pierce et al. (42) confirmed an advantage to combined RT and surgery to RT alone, demonstrating a 23% local failure rate with RT vs a 5% local failure rate with combined local treatment. Breast conservation was not adequate surgical treatment, because of the multifocal character of IBC (42,43). These studies and others (8,10,28,42,44,45) supported the combined modality approach to the treatment of IBC using CT, RT, and surgery (Table 4). Future studies focused on determining the optimal systemic therapy for IBC, because local treatment makes little or no impact on survival.

2.4. Combined Modality: CT, Surgery, and RT

Beginning in the late 1970s, many different CT regimens were investigated, in an attempt to significantly improve the high incidence of metastatic disease (Table 5).

Table 4
CT and RT With or Without Surgery

Ref.	N	Treatment[a]	F/U (yr)	Local recurrence (%)	DFS (%)	OS (%)
45	72/87[a]	RT/CMFV	3	NA	12	21
		S/RT/CMFV		NA	39	(23
42	46/48[b]	CAMF/RT	5	23	42	61
		CAMF/S/RT		5	46	46
9	107	CAF/RT	5	70	NA	NA
		CAF/RT/S		19	35	44
41[b]	106	FAC/RT/FAC	5	17	35	37
		FACVP/S/FACVP/RT		13	41	48

[a]See Chapter Appendix.
[b]No. inflammatory BC/locally advanced BC.
[b]Also described in refs. 18,46,47,49,54,26.
S, mastectomy (simple or modified radical); F/U, follow-up period.

Table 5
Combined Modality Treatment

Ref.	N	Treatment[a]	OR (%)	DFS	OS
28	36	CFP/RT/S	86	24% (5 yr)	34% (5 yr)
7	21	ChMAF/S/ChMAF/RT	76	22 mo (av)	43 mo (med)
1	22/128[b]	FEC/S/RT/FEC	60	29 mo (med)	54 mo (med)
38	7/55[b]	MVeACp./S/MveACp/RT	89	51% (5 yr)	63% (5 yr)
48	14/31[b]	CACp./S/CMF/RT	76	29 mo (med)	49 mo (med)
49	43	FAC/S/FAC/RT/CMF	88	48% (5 yr)	75% (5 yr)
50	31/71[b]	A/CMF/S/RT/CMF	55	25% (5 yr)	48% (5 yr)
47	178	Four protocols: CT/RT/S/CT	74	28% (15 yr)	29% (15 yr)

[a]See Chapter Appendix.
[b]No. inflammatory BC/locally advanced BC.
med, median; av, average.

Unfortunately, no single approach or sequence of therapies has demonstrated significant superiority. However, the majority of the studies presented are composed of a mixed population of locally advanced BC, and the results may be difficult to interpret. The longest follow-up of purely IBC patients is presented by Ueno et al. of MD Anderson Cancer Center (47). Data is available on 178 patients treated on four protocols using primary CT with an Adr-containing regimen, followed by local therapy (either RT, surgery, or both), then adjuvant CT. This analysis presents 15-yr follow-up, in which 20% of the patients developed a local disease recurrence. Patients who received surgery plus RT had lower incidence of local recurrence at 7 yr follow-up, compared with those receiving RT alone: 16 vs 36% (51). The morbidity associated with RT was less when patients received prior mastectomy. Therefore, combination local therapy, surgery plus RT, is recommended, but it did not impact DFS or OS. The combined 15-yr DFS was 28%, and the OS was 29%, suggesting that improvements in systemic therapy are needed (47,51).

Although combined-modality therapy has improved the outcome of IBC, DFS and OS remain poor with the use of standard-dose CT. Some conclusions can be made after a thorough review of these studies: Anthracycline use has prolonged the survival of patients with IBC *(52–54);* the number of CT cycles does not appear to impact survival *(49);* and dose intensity of CT appears to be associated with optimal disease response *(1,22,28,30,54,55).* The best example of the benefit of anthracycline CT in the treatment of IBC comes from the Roswell Park Cancer Institute *(53).* A historical comparison of CMF and 5-FU, Adr, Cy as primary CT for IBC demonstrated a significant improvement in response rate (57 vs 100%), which translated into an improved disease-free interval with FAC (median 6 mo vs 24 mo), and an improved OS (median 18 vs 30 mo). Because the incorporation of Adr into the initial treatment of IBC has occurred at many cancer centers, there are new data suggesting that the cumulative dose of Adr may also have an important effect on disease response *(53,54).*

3. DOSE INTENSITY USING STANDARD-DOSE CT

3.1. Non-IBC

Several studies have been performed examining dose intensity of CT and its effect upon disease response among non-IBCs in both the metastatic and adjuvant setting. Preclinical data demonstrate a steep dose–response curve for alkylating agents in BC cell lines *(56–58).* These principles were applied in vivo, and assessed originally in the metastatic setting. The dose intensity (dose of CT in mg/m^2/wk) of CMF was found to be important in the response of metastatic BC *(59,60).* Superior DFS was associated with higher doses of adjuvant CMF among patients with non-IBC *(61–63).*

Initial experience with dose-intensive Adr, given with the cytoxan-Adr-5-FU (CAF) regimen, did not support a dose–response relationship *(64–66).* However, when Adr was dose-escalated in conjunction with a 16-wk dose-intensive regimen, and compared with standard CAF CT, the dose-intensive treatment arm was associated with a 4-yr DFS of 68% vs 63% with standard-dose CAF *(67,68).* The Cancer and Leukemia Group (CALG) confirmed the benefit of dose-intensive Adr administered by three dose levels of adjuvant CAF for lymph-node-positive, non-IBC *(69–71).* Their data also demonstrated improved DFS and OS with higher doses of CAF: 5-yr DFS of 66% vs 56% in the low-dose arm. Subset analysis found an interaction between the presence of erbB-2 (HER-2/neu, or ERBB2) overexpression and disease response to CT dose intensity *(72).* This finding may be important when the concept of dose intensity is applied to IBC, because some studies show that erbB-2 overexpression does not convey the same adverse prognosis as overexpression in non-IBC *(73,74).* These data may suggest that IBC responds to dose-intensive CT, regardless of erbB-2 status; non-IBC may require erbB-2 overexpression in order to exhibit a dose response.

The NSABP dose escalated Cy in conjunction with standard-dose Adr for lymph-node-positive noninflammatory early stage BC *(75,76).* These data did not demonstrate a dose-response effect. One reason may be that only Cy was dose-escalated, not Adr. Ten-yr follow-up of a study by Bonadonna et al. *(77)* supports the importance of dose-intensive Adr, rather than Cy. A superior DFS was demonstrated with sequential Adr followed by CMF, compared with alternating CMF and Adr: 42 vs 28%, respectively. This is thought to result from a higher dose intensity of Adr administered in the sequential arm. BC growth kinetics may explain these clinical results. The Norton-

Table 6
Effect of CT Dose on Survival in IBC

Ref.	N	Follow-up	%Dose	DFS	OS
22	7	3 yr	<50	43%	43%
	21		>50	71%	76%
1	26	mo (med)	60	20 mo	29 mo
	24		75	NA	54 mo
	24		100	35 mo	NA

Simon hypothesis describes subclones of micrometastatic BC that develop patterns at different rates *(78)*. Therefore, optimal adjuvant therapy would include the early institution of effective CT directed against the faster-growing clone. The early administration of dose-intensive therapy is an example of the application of this hypothesis *(79)*.

3.2. Inflammatory BC

These concepts have also been applied to IBC. Several studies, beginning in 1988, demonstrated that patients who receive compromised doses of neoadjuvant CT have a significantly worse DFS and OS *(1,22;* Table 6). These data were used to promote more intensive CT protocols administering treatment over a shorter duration, again increasing the dose intensity of the CT *(30,55,80)*. Twenty patients with IBC received treatment, with other patients diagnosed with locally advanced BC on a 16-wk dose-intensive protocol at the Johns Hopkins Oncology Center *(80)*. The overall response rate was 100%, and all patients were deemed operable after completing induction CT. The 5-yr DFS and OS were 58 and 75%, respectively.

Evidence of microscopic disease or complete pathologic remission appears to be an excellent prognostic indicator for prolonged DFS and OS *(81–83)*. The Johns Hopkins dose-intensive study *(80)* resulted in 29% of the patients without evidence of invasive disease on pathologic evaluation; 49% had only microscopic foci of disease. This excellent disease response from dose-intensive therapy is supported by Chevallier, et al. *(84)* who treated 45 patients with IBC with high-dose 5-FU, epirubicin, Cy. The 96% disease response rate translates into a 26% pathologic complete remission, and a 56% incidence of microscopic disease alone.

4. HIGH-DOSE CT AND AUTOLOGOUS BONE MARROW TRANSPLANTATION

4.1. Background

Based on preclinical data and in vivo responses with standard-dose CT, studies using myeloablative doses of CT were applied to patients with highly pretreated BC. Details describing the principles of this therapeutic approach are discussed elsewhere in this book. In general, CT agents are chosen for dose intensification, based on the following characteristics: having a steep dose–response curve, primary toxicity is hematologic (myeloablative), combinations of drugs use different mechanisms of cell kill to avoid crossresistance, and no long-term toxicity *(85,86)*. Several preparative regimens have been applied to BC (Table 7). The optimal combination CT regimen for the treatment of BC has not been determined. *(87)*.

Table 7
CT Regimens Commonly Used in ABMT for BC

CT, Cy (6000 mg/m^2) and thiotepa (800 mg/m^2)
CBP, Cy (5625 mg/m^2), carmustine (BCNU) (600 mg/m^2), and cisplatin (165 mg/m^2)
CTCb, Cy (6000 mg/m^2), thiotepa (800 mg/m^2), and carboplatin (1200 mg/m^2)
ICE, ifosfamide (12 g/m^2), carboplatin (1800 mg/m^2), and etoposide (2000 mg/m^2)
NT, mitoxantrone (50 mg/m^2) and thiotepa (800 mg/m^2)
CE, Cy (7 g/m^2) and etoposide (1.5 g/m^2)
Bu/Cy, Cy (120 mg/kg) and busulfan (16 mg/kg)
CMeN, Cy (120 mg/kg), mitoxantrone (36 mg/kg), and melphalan (140 mg/m^2)

Approximate drug doses

The source of hematopoeitic progenitor cells used to reconstitute the ablated bone marrow (BM) includes harvested BM and either CT or cytokine-mobilized peripheral progenitor cells. Peripheral blood progenitor cells (PBPCs) are less contaminated with neoplastic cells; therefore, the process of using PBPCs as the source of BM reconstitution functions as a mechanism of cancer cell purging (85). Although the concept of BM purging may not be as important to BC treatment outcome, other mechanisms of purging, i.e., using monoclonal antibodies, and CD34 selection, are currently being investigated (88–92).

The advent of supportive technologies, such as the empiric use of antibiotics and antifungal agents, and the application of hematopoeitic cytokines (granulocyte and granulocyte-macrophage colony-stimulating factor), have reduced the treatment-related mortality of autologous bone marrow transplantation (ABMT) from 22 to 1% (93,94). Supportive therapies have also reduced the common morbidity associated with nausea and vomiting, mucositis, and diarrhea. Currently, the most common treatment-related toxicity is interstitial pulmonary fibrosis, which occurs in approx 30–50% of patients, and is usually reversible with a course of steroids (88,95–98). Other nonhematologic toxicity are less common, e.g., veno-occlusive disease, hemolytic-uremic syndrome, secondary leukemia or myelodysplasia, and cardiomyopathy (99,100). The duration of hospitalization has been reduced by approx 50% with the application of PBPCs to reconstitute BM and the widespread use of cytokines after BM or peripheral stem cell infusion. The average duration of neutropenia is now 13 d, which translates to an average hospital stay of 14–21 d (85,92).

The process of ABMT has been shown to be most effective in the setting of minimal disease; therefore, patients with BC have traditionally received treatment with standard doses of CT, until maximal tumor reduction, then the disease remission is consolidated with dose-intensive CT and autologous BM rescue (88,93,101). Although this treatment strategy is the most commonly used program for BC, theoretical concerns exist about inducing drug resistance with standard-dose CT prior to undergoing ABMT. Several excellent reviews of the treatment of metastatic BC with ABMT have been published (58,85,86,98–90,92–94) and are thoroughly presented in Chapter 14. The largest analysis includes data from the Autologous Blood and Marrow Transplant Registry, which calculated a 3-yr DFS of 13–32% among 3451 women with metastatic BC, who responded to standard-dose CT prior to receiving consolidation with high-dose CT (HDCT) and ABMT (93).

Table 8
ABMT in High-risk BC: Stage II/III with Four or More Positive Lymph Nodes

Ref.	N	+LN	Induction[a]	HDCT[a]	BM/PSC	F/U (yr)	DFS (%)	OS (%)
99	85	≥10	CAF × 4	CBP	Both	2.5	72	77
97	67	≥10	None	CVMPL*	Both	5	57	70
104	19	≥7	Varied × 4	Bu/Cy	BM	4	42	50[c]
95	24	≥5	MFAVP × 6	CE or MT	Both	5	84	NA
96	54	≥4	AC × 4	CBP	PSC	4	71	84
105	11	>8	AFM	Varied	Both	5	91	NA

[a]See Chapter Appendix.
[b]Cyclophosphamide, methotrexate, melphalan, cisplatin, vincristine.
[c]2.5 yr follow-up.
BM, bone marrow; PSC, peripheral stem (progenitor) cell.

4.2. Adjuvant Therapy of High-risk BC

The provocative response rates found among highly pretreated patients, combined with the concept of increased efficacy with ABMT among patients with minimal disease, made the application of ABMT to high-risk BC therapy a logical course of action. Of course, the population of high-risk BC patients is a widely diverse group. Patients with stage II or III BC, involving four or more axillary lymph nodes, are included, as are patients with unresectable stage IIIb disease, and IBC. Because of the paucity of high-risk BC patients involved in clinical trials with ABMT, the majority of studies include all high-risk subtypes in the analysis, making conclusions about the treatment of one group, or stage, difficult to interpret.

Several studies excluded patients with locally advanced or surgically unresectable BC from participation in HDCT and ABMT clinical trials. This definition of high-risk disease was based on pathologic assessment following primary treatment with surgery: either breast conservation or modified radical mastectomy. Patients with four or more axillary lymph nodes involved were eligible for participation in ABMT trials, based on historical data giving these patients a 50–80% 5 yr relapse rate. All patients received adjuvant CT in standard doses prior to consolidation with HDCT. BM reconstitution was with either BM or PBPCs. The majority of patients also received post-ABMT RT, which was found to reduce local-regional recurrences (102,103). The results are encouraging, and lend support to the application of HDCT with ABMT to other high-risk BC groups, such as IBC (95–97,99,104–106; Table 8).

Peters et al. (99) retrospectively compared his results of ABMT for patients with 10 or more positive lymph nodes with two CALGB adjuvant therapy trials. After a median follow-up of 2.5 yr, those patients who received ABMT had a 72% event-free survival, which was significantly greater than the event-free survival of 31–52% found among those patients treated on the CALGB non-ABMT adjuvant therapy trials. These data were essentially unchanged after a 5-yr follow-up, but the 5-yr OS was found to be significantly improved with ABMT, compared with standard CALGB data: 78 vs 37–45%, respectively (107). Gianni et al. (97) and Bonadonna (77) supported these findings, again with a historical comparison of ABMT among patients with 10 or more positive lymph nodes, and their best adjuvant therapy treatment with sequential Adr

Table 9
NCI-Sponsored Randomized Trials for
ABMT in Patients with >10 Positive Lymph Nodes

Study	Induction[a]	Randomization[a]
CALGB 9082	CAF × 4	High-dose CBP vs 1/3 dose of CBP
INT 0121	CAF × 4	HDCT vs observation

[a]See Chapter Appendix.
All patients receive post-CT RT.

followed by CMF. After a follow-up of 4 yr, the relapse-free survival for those receiving ABMT was 57%, compared with 41% among those receiving sequential Adr and CMF.

One criticism of a retrospective analysis is that the populations compared are not controlled for risk factors. Gianni et al. (97) performed a subset analysis comparing all patients in the two studies who had 10–20 positive lymph nodes. The difference in outcome between ABMT and standard treatment was even more striking when the very high-risk groups were analyzed: the relapse-free survival was 65% with ABMT, compared with 42% receiving standard therapy. The benefit of ABMT translated to an increase in OS: 77% with ABMT vs 61% with standard therapy.

Although these trials are highly supportive of using ABMT in high-risk BC, randomized trials are necessary to move this therapy into the realm of standard treatment. Two National Cancer Institute-sponsored randomized clinical trials, investigating the efficacy of HDCT and ABMT in patients with high-risk BC (>10 axillary lymph nodes involved), have recently closed, and the data are not expected to be available for several years (Table 9).

4.3. Inflammatory BC

A logical extension of the data from HDCT and ABMT among stage II and III BC patients, with four or more axillary lymph nodes involved, is to apply this treatment to surgically unresectable patients with locally advanced or IBC. The problems with the ABMT trials mimic those with standard-dose regimens: Patient populations include both locally advanced and inflammatory disease, sometimes also including patients with metastatic disease (87,102,108,109). This type of grouping of several disease stages makes interpretation of results difficult. Table 10 represents a subgroup analysis

Table 10
Studies of ABMT Including IBC Patients

Ref[a]	N[b]	Regimen[c]	BM/PSC	F/U (yr)	DFS (%)	OS
100	4/42	CTCb	Both	2	80	89%
110	7/14	CE	BM	4	58	NA
109	6/23	ICE	PSC	1	50	NA
87	15/120	varied	Both	3	27	NA

[a]Populations include metastatic, high-risk stage II and III, and IBC.
[b]No. of IBC/total no. high-risk patients.
[c]See Chapter Appendix.

Table 11
ABMT for IBC

Ref.	N^a	Regimen[b]	BM/PSC	F/U	DFS (%)	OS (%)
114,115	42/50	Ax4/CTCb	Both	30 mo	64	89
116	22/114	Varied	Both	3.5 yr	50	72
74	17	CAFx4/CMeN	Both	3 yr	66	68
98	30	CBP	PSC	2 yr	70	87

[a]IBC patients/total patients.
[b]See Chapter Appendix.

of these studies focusing on the results of IBC patients. Overall, the DFS and OS appears improved when compared with results from standard treatment noted in Subheading 2.

Patients with IBC have also been enrolled in clinical trials pioneering innovative strategies of progenitor cell mobilization or novel preparative regimens, but data concerning disease response are not available from these studies (107,108,111–113). This widespread approach of incorporating IBC patients into clinical trials of novel therapies is a reflection of the frustration with the results of conventional treatment for this disease. Fortunately, some studies (74,98,114–116) have focused specifically on the efficacy with ABMT among patients with IBC. The data is not pure, again, because of the rarity of IBC, and the subsequent need to include other patients with stage III disease (Table 11).

The largest cohort of IBC patients treated with ABMT in a systematic fashion was from the Dana-Farber Cancer Institute (114). Forty-two patients received neoadjuvant CT with Adr (75 mg/m^2) for four cycles, followed by consolidation with high-dose cytoxan-thiotepa, and ABMT. Mastectomy was performed after ABMT, to assess pathologic response and prognosis following dose-intensive therapy. Pathologic complete remission occurred in 14%, and microscopic disease was present in 29%. Unfortunately, 57% had continued evidence of macroscopic invasive cancer. The pathologic response correlated with DFS and OS, with 100% of patients with a complete remission having a 30-mo DFS, compared with a 38% DFS among those patients with residual macroscopic disease.

Seventeen patients with IBC were treated in a similar fashion at the Institut Paoli-Calmettes, Marseilles, France (74). A high pathologic response was found following high-dose mitoxantrone, Cy, and melphalan with ABMT. Thirty-nine percent of patients experienced a complete pathologic remission, with an additional 17% having only microscopic residual disease: 5/7 patients with macroscopic disease relapsed within a median follow-up of 3 yr.

Conversely, the University of Colorado treated 30 patients with IBC with neoadjuvant CT, followed by mastectomy, prior to receiving consolidation with cytoxan, BCNU, cisplatin (CBP) and ABMT (98). Although there was no statistically significant difference in relapse rate, only 11% of patients with a moderate pathologic response following neoadjuvant CT relapsed after 2 yr, compared with a 45% relapse rate among those patients without a significant pathologic response. Residual macroscopic disease appears to predict a worse outcome, which may warrant investigation into sequential dose-intensive therapy, or more intensive neoadjuvant CT prior to undergoing ABMT.

5. CONCLUSIONS

IBC is a rare, aggressive form of BC that requires a multidisciplinary approach to treatment, in an attempt to optimize the chance for cure. Standard therapies using neoadjuvant CT, combined with mastectomy and RT, are associated with a 37% 5-yr DFS and a 55% 5-yr OS. Several studies have demonstrated a dose-response relationship between CT and clinical and pathologic outcome in both noninflammatory and IBCs. The grave prognosis associated with IBC warrants an investigational approach to determine other avenues of systemic treatment, specifically, the application of dose-intensive CT. Promising data exists supporting the administration of ABMT for IBC. Several small studies have demonstrated an improvement in DFS and OS: 60 and 76%, respectively.

Further research should focus on developing a multi-institutional treatment plan that would facilitate larger numbers of patients with IBC treated in the same fashion. This would avoid bias and confusion that current exists in the literature resulting from combining the treatment response of IBC patients with other disease stages. Focusing on dose intensification in the treatment of IBC is appropriate, and may extend to sequential dose-intensive therapies with ABMT, or improvement in neoadjuvant treatment prior to consolidation with ABMT. Regardless of the approach, further research in the treatment of IBC is desperately needed.

6. APPENDIX: INDEX OF STANDARD-DOSE CT

Adr, Adriamycin   V, vincristine
M, methotrexate   Cy, cytoxan
F, 5-fluorouracil   Ve, vinblastine
E, epirubicin   Cp, cisplatin
I, ifosfamide   T, thiotepa
P, Prednisone   Ch, chlorambucil

REFERENCES

1. Karlsson YA, et al. Multimodality treatment of 128 patients with locally advanced breast carcinoma in the era of mammography screening using standard polychemotherapy with 5-fluorouracil, epirubicin, and cyclophosphamide. Prognostic and therapeutic implications, *Cancer,* **83** (1998) 936–47.
2. Beahrs O, et al. Manual for Staging of Cancers, 3rd ed., Lippincott, Philadelphia, 1988, pp. 145–150.
3. Haagensen C. Diseases of the Breast, 2nd ed., Saunders, Philadelphia, 1971, pp. 576–584.
4. Levine SH, et al. Inflammatory breast cancer: the experience of the Surveillance, Epidemiology, and End Results (SEER) program, *J. Natl. Cancer Inst.,* **74** (1985) 291–297.
5. Lucas F and Perez-Mesa C. Inflammatory carcinoma of the breast, *Cancer,* **41** (1978) 1595–1605.
6. Brooks HL, et al. Inflammatory breast carcinoma: a community hospital experience, *J. Am. Coll. Surg.,* **186** (1998) 622–629.
7. Schafer P, et al. Surgery as part of a combined modality approach for inflammatory breast carcinoma, *Cancer,* **59** (1987) 1063–1067.
8. Sener SF et al. Achieving local control for inflammatory carcinoma of the breast, *Surg. Gynecol. Obstet.,* **175** (1992) 141–144.
9. Fields JN, et al. Inflammatory carcinoma of the breast: treatment results on 107 patients, *Int. J. Radiat. Oncol. Biol. Phys.,* **17** (1989) 249–255.
10. Fields JN, et al. Prognostic factors in inflammatory breast cancer, *Cancer,* **63** (1989) 1225–1232.
11. Chang S, et al. Inflammatory breast carcinoma incidence and survival. The Surveillance Epidemiology, and End Results Program of the National Cancer Institute, 1975–1992, *Cancer,* **82** (1998) 2366–2372.

12. Jaiyesimi IA, Buzdar AU, and Hortobagyi G. Inflammatory breast cancer: a review, *J. Clin. Oncol.*, **10** (1992) 1014–1024.

13. Lopez MJ and Porter KA. Inflammatory breast cancer, *Surg. Clin. North Am.*, **76** (1996) 411–429.

14. Ackland SP, Bitran JD, and Dowlatshahi K. Management of locally advanced and inflammatory carcinoma of the breast, *Surg. Gynecol. Obstet.*, **161** (1985) 399–408.

15. Honkoop AH, Wagstaff J, and Pinwso HM. Management of stage III breast cancer, *Oncology*, **55** (1998) 218–227.

16. Grace WR and Cooperman AM. Inflammatory breast cancer, *Surg. Clin. North Am.*, **65** (1985) 151–160.

17. Mourali N, et al. Ten-year results utilizing chemotherapy as primary treatment in nonmetastic, rapidly progressing breast cancer, *Cancer Invest.*, **11** (1993) 363–370.

18. Thomas J, William W, et al. Multimodal treatment for inflammatory breast cancer, *Int. J. Radiat. Oncol. Biol. Phys.*, **17** (1989) 739–745.

19. Chu A, Wood WC, and Doucette JA. Inflammatory carcinoma of the breasts treated by radical radiotherapy, *Cancer*, **45** (1980) 2730–2737.

20. Duggan D. Local therapy of locally advanced breast cancer, *Oncology*, **5** (1991) 67–74, 79–80, 82.

21. Sherry MM, et al. Inflammatory carcinoma of the breast, *Am. J. Med.*, **79** (1985) 355–364.

22. Hobar PC, et al. Multimodality treatment of locally advanced breast carcinoma, *Arch. Surg.*, **123** (1988) 951–955.

23. Hortobagyi GN, et al. Primary chemotherapy for early and advanced breast cancer, *Cancer Lett.*, **90** (1995) 103–109.

24. Ragaz J. Chemotherapy and hormonal therapy in stage III disease; inflammatory breast cancer, *Curr. Opin. Oncol.*, **2** (1990) 1068–1087.

25. Thomas F, et al. Pattern of failure in patients with inflammatory breast cancer treated by alternating radiotherapy and chemotherapy, *Cancer*, **76** (1995) 2286–2290.

26. Jacquillat C, et al. Neoadjuvant chemotherapy of breast cancer, *Drugs Under Exp. Clin Res.*, **XII** (1986) 147–152.

27. Frank JL, et al. Stage III breast cancer: is neoadjuvant chemotherapy always necessary? *J. Surg. Oncol.*, **49** (1992) 220–225.

28. Pisansky TM, et al. Inflammatory breast cancer: integration of irradiation, surgery, and chemotherapy, *Am. J. Clin. Oncol.*, **15** (1992) 376–387.

29. Rubens RD, et al. Locally advanced breast cancer: the contribution of cytotoxic and endocrine treatment to radiotherapy. An EORTC breast cancer co-operative group trial (10792)*, *Eur. J. Cancer Clin. Oncol.*, **25** (1989) 667–678.

30. Rouesse J, et al. Primary chemotherapy in the treatment of inflammatory breast carcinoma: a study of 230 cases from the Institut Gustave-Roussy, *J. Clin. Oncol.*, **4** (1986) 1765–1771.

31. Arriagada R, et al. Alternating radiotherapy and chemotherapy in non-metastatic inflammatory breast cancer, *Int. J. Radiat. Oncol. Biol. Phys.*, **19** (1990) 1207–1210.

32. Jones AL, et al. Phase II study of continuous infusion fluorouracil with epirubicin and cisplatin in patients with metastatic and locally advanced breast cancer: an active new regimen, *J. Clin. Oncol.*, **12** (1994) 1259–1265.

33. Bonnefoi H, et al. Phase II study of continuous infusional 5-fluorouracil with epirubicin and carboplatin (instead of cisplatin) in patients with metastatic/locally advanced breast cancer (infusional ECarboF): a very active and well-tolerated outpatient regimen, *Br. J. Cancer*, **73** (1996) 391–396.

34. Gurney H, et al. Inflammatory breast cancer: enhanced local control with hyperfractionated radiotherapy and infusional vincristine, ifosfamide and epirubicin, *Aust. NZ J. Med.*, **28** (1998) 400–402.

35. Danforth J, David N, et al. Effect of preoperative chemotherapy on mastectomy for locally advanced breast cancer, *Am. Surg.*, **56** (1990) 6–11.

36. Calderoli H, de Manzini N, and Keiling R. Role of chemotherapy in acute breast cancer. Analysis of 41 cases, *Int. Surg.*, **73** (1988) 112–115.

37. Israel L, Breau J-L, and Morere J-F. Two years of high-dose cyclophosphamide and 5-fluorouracil followed by surgery after 3 months for acute inflammatory breast carcinomas, *Cancer*, **57** (1986) 24–28.

38. Morrell LE, et al. A phase II trial of neoadjuvant methotrexate, vinblastine, doxorubicin, and cisplatin in the treatment of patients with locally advanced breast carcinoma, *Cancer*, **82** (1998) 503–511.

39. Mourali N, et al. Preliminary results of primary systemic chemotherapy in association with surgery or radiotherapy in rapidly progressing breast cancer, *Cancer*, **45** (1982) 367–374.

40. Perloff M, et al. Combination chemotherapy with mastectomy or radiotherapy for stage III breast carcinoma: a cancer and leukemia group B study, *J. Clin. Oncol.,* **6** (1988) 261–269.

41. Koh EH, et al. Inflammatory carcinoma of the breast: results of a combined-modality approach: M.D. Anderson Cancer Center experience, *Cancer Chemother. Pharmacol.,* **27** (1990) 94–100.

42. Pierce LJ, et al. The effect of systemic therapy on local-regional control in locally advanced breast cancer, *Int. J. Radiat. Oncol. Biol. Phys.,* **23** (1992) 949–960.

43. Brun B, et al. Treatment of inflammatory breast cancer with combination chemotherapy and mastectomy versus breast conservation, *Cancer,* **61** (1988) 1096–1103.

44. Knight J, Charles D, et al. Surgical considerations after chemotherapy and radiation therapy for inflammatory breast cancer, *Surgery,* **99** (1986) 385–391.

45. Pawlicki M, Skolyszewski J, and Brandys A. Results of combined treatment of patients with locally advanced breast cancer, *Tumori,* **69** (1983) 249–253.

46. Buzdar AU, et al. Combined modality treatment of stage III and inflammatory breast cancer, *Surg. Oncol. Clin. North Am.,* **4** (1995) 715–734.

47. Ueno NT, et al. Combined-mobility treatment of inflammatory breast carcinoma: twenty years of experience at M.D. Anderson Cancer Center, *Cancer Chemother. Pharmacol.,* **40** (1997) 321–329.

48. Colozza M, et al. Induction chemotherapy with cisplatin, doxorubicin, and cyclosphosphamide (CAP) in a combined modality approach for locally advanced and inflammatory breast cancer. Long term results, *Am. J. Clin. Oncol.,* **19(1)** (1996) 10–17.

49. Maloisel F, et al. Results of initial doxorubicin, 5-fluorouracil, and cyclophosphamide combination chemotherapy for inflammatory carcinoma of the breast, *Cancer,* **65** (1990) 851–855.

50. Pisansky TM, et al. A pilot evaluation of alternating preoperative chemotherapy in the management of patients with locoregionally advanced breast carcinoma, *Cancer,* **77** (1996) 2520–2528.

51. Fleming RYD, et al. Effectiveness of mastectomy by response to induction chemotherapy for control in inflammatory breast carcinoma, *Ann. Surg. Oncol.,* **4** (1997) 452–461.

52. Iino Y, et al. Multidisciplinary treatment with anthracyclines in inflammatory breast cancer, *Anticancer Res.,* **16** (1996) 3111–3116.

53. Bauer RL, et al. Therapy for inflammatory breast cancer: impact of doxorubicin-based therapy, *Ann. Surg. Oncol.,* **2** (1995) 288–294.

54. Attia-Sobol JF, Jean-Pierre, et al. Treatment results, survival and prognostic factors in 109 inflammatory breast cancers: univariate and multivariate analysis, *Eur. J. Cancer.,* **29A** (1993) 1081–1088.

55. Rouesse J, et al. Therapeutic strategies in inflammatory breast carcinoma based on prognostic factors, *Breast Cancer Res. Treatment,* **16** (1990) 15–22.

56. Teicher BA, et al. Preclinical studies relating to the use of thiotepa in the high-dose setting alone and in combination, *Semin. Oncol.,* **17 (Suppl 3)** (1990) 18–32.

57. Henderson IC, Hayes DF, and Gelman R. Dose-response in the treatment of breast cancer: a critical review, *J. Clin. Oncol.,* **6** (1988) 1501–1515.

58. Zujewski J, Nelson A, and Abrams J. Much ado about not . . . enough data: high-dose chemotherapy with autologous stem cell rescue for breast cancer, *J. Natl. Cancer Inst.,* **90** (1998) 200–209.

59. Hryniuk W and Bush H. The importance of dose intensity in chemotherapy of metastatic breast cancer, *J. Clin. Oncol.,* **2** (1984) 1281–1288.

60. Tannock IF, et al. A randomized trial of two dose levels of cyclophosphamide, methotrexate, and fluorouracil chemotherapy for patients with metastatic breast cancer, *J. Clin. Oncol.,* **6** (1988) 1377–1387.

61. Hryniuk W and Levine MN. Analysis of dose intensity for adjuvant chemotherapy trials in stage II breast cancer, *J. Clin. Oncol.,* **4** (1986) 1162–1170.

62. Geller NL, et al. Association of disease-free survival and percent of ideal dose in adjuvant breast chemotherapy, *Cancer,* **66** (1990) 1678–1684.

63. Bonadonna G and Valagussa P. Dose-response effect of adjuvant chemotherapy in breast cancer, *N. Engl. J. Med.,* **304** (1981) 10–15.

64. Buzdar AU, et al. Adjuvant therapy with escalating doses of doxorubicin and cyclophosphamide with or without leukocyte α-interferon for stage II or III breast cancer, *J. Clin. Oncol.,* **10** (1992) 1540–1546.

65. Hortobagyi GN, et al. Evaluation of high-dose versus standard FAC chemotherapy for advanced breast cancer in protected environment units: a prospective randomized study, *J. Clin. Oncol.,* **5** (1987) 354–364.

66. Ang P.-T. et al. Analysis of dose intensity in doxorubicin-containing adjuvant chemotherapy in stage II and III breast carcinoma, *J. Clin. Oncol.,* **7** (1989) 1677–1684.

67. Fetting JH, et al. Sixteen-week multidrug regimen versus cyclophosphamide, doxorubicin, and fluorouracil as adjuvant therapy for node-positive, receptor-negative breast cancer: an intergroup study, *J. Clin. Oncol.,* **16** (1998) 2382–2391.

68. Abeloff MD, et al. Sixteen-week dose-intense chemotherapy in the adjuvant treatment of breast cancer, *J. Natl Cancer Inst.,* **82** (1990) 570–574.

69. Budman DR, et al. Dose and dose intensity as determinants of outcome in the adjuvant treatment of breast cancer, *J. Natl. Cancer Inst.,* **90** (1998) 1205–1211.

70. Wood WC, et al. Dose and dose intensity of adjuvant chemotherapy for stage II, node-positive breast carcinoma, *N. Engl. J. Med.,* **330** (1994) 1253–1259.

71. Budman DR, et al. A feasibility study of intensive CAF as outpatient adjuvant therapy for stage II breast cancer in a cooperative group: CALGB 8443, *Cancer Invest.,* **8** (1990) 571–575.

72. Thor AD, et al. erbB-2, p53, and efficacy of adjuvant therapy in lymph node-positive breast cancer, *J. Natl. Cancer Inst.,* **90** (1998) 1346–1360.

73. Prost S, et al. Association of c-erb B2-gene amplification with poor prognosis in noninflammatory breast carcinomas but not in carcinomas of the inflammatory type, *Int. J. Cancer,* **58** (1994) 763–768.

74. Viens P, et al. High-dose chemotherapy and haematopoietic stem cell transplantation for inflammatory breast cancer: pathologic response and outcome, *Bone Marrow Transplant.,* **21** (1998) 249–254.

75. Wolmark N, Fisher B, and Anderson S. The effect of increasing dose intensity and cumulative dose of adjuvant cyclophosphamide in node positive breast cancer: results of NSABP B-25, *Breast Cancer Res. Treatment,* **46** (1997) 26.

76. Fisher B, et al. Increased intensification and total dose of cyclophosphamide in a doxorubicin-cyclophosphamide regimen for the treatment of primary breast cancer: findings from National Surgical Adjuvant Breast and Bowel Project B-22, *J. Clin. Oncol.,* **15** (1997) 1858–1869.

77. Bonadonna G, Zambetti M, and Valagussa P. Sequential or alternating doxorubicin and CMF regimens in breast cancer with more than three positive nodes, *JAMA,* **273** (1995) 542–547.

78. Hudis C. Is there an alternative to alternating adjuvant therapy for breast cancer? *Cancer Invest.,* **12** (1994) 329–335.

79. Hudis C. Sequential dose-dense adjuvant therapy with doxorubicin, paclitaxel, and cyclophosphamide, *Oncology.,* **II (Suppl. 3)** (1997) 15–18.

80. Armstrong DK, et al. Sixteen week dose intense chemotherapy for inoperable, locally advanced breast cancer, *Breast Cancer Res. Treatment,* **28** (1993) 277–284.

81. Feldman LD, et al. Pathological assessment of response to induction chemotherapy in breast cancer, *Cancer Res.,* **46** (1986) 2578–2581.

82. Palangie T, et al. Prognostic factors in inflammatory breast cancer and therapeutic implications, *Eur. J. Cancer,* **30A** (1994) 921–927.

83. Ferriere JP, et al. Primary chemotherapy in breast cancer, *Am. J. Clin. Oncol.,* **21** (1998) 117–120.

84. Chevallier B, et al. Inflammatory breast cancer. Pilot study of intensive induction chemotherapy (FEC-HD) results in a high histologic response rate, *Am. J. Clin. Oncol.,* **16** (1993) 223–228.

85. Brockstein BE and Williams SF. High-dose chemotherapy with autologous stem cell rescue for breast cancer: yesterday, today and tomorrow, *Stem Cells,* **14** (1996) 79–89.

86. Meropol NJ, Overmoyer BA, and Stadtmauer EA. High-dose chemotherapy with autologous stem cell support for breast cancer, *Oncology,* **6** (1992) 53–69.

87. Fields KK, et al. Defining the role of novel high-dose chemotherapy regimens for the treatment of high-risk breast cancer, *Semin. Oncol.,* **25 (Suppl 4)** (1998) 1–6.

88. Myers SE and Williams SF. Role of high-dose chemotherapy and autologous stem cell support in treatment of breast cancer, *Hematol. Oncol. Clin. North Am.,* **7** (1993) 631–645.

89. von Schilling C and Herrmann F. Dose-intensified treatment of breast cancer: current results, *J. Mol. Med.,* **73** (1995) 611–627.

90. Safah H and Weiner RS. The role of bone marrow transplantation in the management of advanced local disease, *Surg. Oncol. Clin. North Am.,* **4** (1995) 735–749.

91. Cooper BW, et al. Occult tumor contamination of hematopoietic stem-cell products does not affect clinical outcome of autologous transplantation in patients with metastatic breast cancer, *J. Clin. Oncol.,* **16** (1998) 3509–3517.

92. Bergh J. High-dose therapy with autologous bone marrow stem cell support in primary and metastatic human breast cancer, *Acta Oncol.,* **34** (1995) 669–674.

93. Vahdat L and Antman K. High-dose chemotherapy with autologous stem cell support for breast cancer, *Curr. Opin. Hematol.,* **4** (1997) 381–389.

94. Joensuu H. Autologous stem cell transplantation in breast cancer, *Ann. Med.,* **28** (1996) 145–149.

95. de Graaf H, et al. Intensive chemotherapy with autologous bone marrow transfusion as primary treatment in women with breast cancer and more than five involved axillary lymph nodes, *Eur. J. Cancer,* **30A** (1994) 150–153.

96. Bearman SI, et al. High-dose chemotherapy with autologous peripheral blood progenitor cell support for primary breast cancer in patients with 4–9 involved axillary lymph nodes, *Bone Marrow Transplant.,* **20** (1997) 931–937.

97. Gianni AM, et al. Efficacy, toxicity, and applicability of high-dose sequential chemotherapy as adjuvant treatment in operable breast cancer with 10 or more involved axillary nodes: five-year results, *J. Clin. Oncol.,* **15** (1997) 2312–2321.

98. Cagnoni PJ, et al. High-dose chemotherapy with autologous hematopoietic progenitor-cell support as part of combined modality therapy in patients with inflammatory breast cancer, *J. Clin. Oncol.,* **16** (1998) 1661–1668.

99. Peters WP, et al. High-dose chemotherapy and autologous bone marrow support as consolidation after standard-dose adjuvant therapy for high-risk primary breast cancer, *J. Clin. Oncol.,* **11** (1993) 1132–1143.

100. Holland HK, et al. Minimal toxicity and mortality in high-risk breast cancer patients receiving high-dose cyclophosphamide, thiotepa, and carboplating plus autologous marrow/stem-cell transplantation and comprehensive supportive care, *J. Clin. Oncol.,* **14** (1996) 1156–1164.

101. Vaughan WP. Autologous bone marrow transplantation in the treatment of breast cancer: clinical and technologic strategies, *Semin. Oncol.,* **20 (Suppl 6)** (1993) 55–58.

102. Marks LB, et al. Post-mastectomy radiotherapy following adjuvant chemotherapy and autologous bone marrow transplantation for breast cancer patients with ≥10 positive axillary lymph nodes, *Int. J. Radiat. Oncol. Biol. Phys.,* **23** (1992) 1021–1026.

103. Marks LB, et al. Impact of conventional plus high dose chemotherapy with autologous bone marrow transplantation on hematologic toxicity during subsequent local-regional radiotherapy for breast cancer, *Cancer,* **74** (1994) 2964–71.

104. Lalisang RI, et al. High-dose chemotherapy with autologous bone marrow support as consolidation after standard adjuvant therapy in primary breast cancer patients with seven or more involved axillary lymph nodes, *Bone Marrow Transplant.,* **21** (1998) 243–247.

105. Dillman RO, et al. High-dose chemotherapy with autologous stem cell rescue in breast cancer, *Breast Cancer Res. Treatment,* **37** (1996) 277–289.

106. Antman K, et al. High-dose cyclophosphamide, thiotepa, and carboplatin with autologous marrow support in women with measurable advanced breast cancer responding to standard-dose therapy: analysis by age, *Monogr. Natl. Cancer Inst.,* **16** (1994) 91–94.

107. Peters WP, et al. Five year follow-up of high-dose combination alkylating agents with ABMT as consolidation after standard-dose CAF for primary breast cancer involving ≥10 axillary lymph nodes (DUKE/CALGB 8782), *Proc. ASCO,* **14** (1995) 317.

108. Somlo G, et al. High-dose doxorubicin, etoposide, and cyclophosphamide with stem cell reinfusion in patients with metastatic or high-risk primary breast cancer, *Cancer,* **73** (1994) 1678–1685.

109. Fields KK, et al. Intensive dose ifosfamide, carboplatin, and etoposide followed by autologous stem cell rescue: results of a phase I/II study in breast cancer patients, *Surg. Oncol.,* **2** (1993) 87–95.

110. Mulder NH, et al. Induction chemotherapy and intensification with autologous bone marrow reinfusion in patients with locally advanced and disseminated breast cancer, *Eur. J. Cancer,* **29A** (1993) 668–671.

111. Ravagnani F, et al. Clinical application of growth factors for collection of circulating hematopoietic progenitors in breast cancer patients treated with high-dose cyclophosphamide, *Int. J. Artif. Organs.,* **16** (1993) 35–38.

112. Bregni M, et al. High-dose cyclophosphamide in patients with operable breast cancer: recombinant human GM-CSF ameliorates drug-induced leukopenia and thrombocytopenia, *Haematologica,* **75 (Suppl 1)** (1990) 95–98.

113. Raxis ED, et al. TMJ: a well-tolerated high-dose regimen for the adjuvant chemotherapy of high risk breast cancer, *J. Med.,* **25** (1994) 241–250.

114. Ayash LJ, et al. High-dose multimodality therapy with autologous stem-cell support for stage IIIB breast carcinoma, *J. Clin. Oncol.,* **16** (1998) 1000–1007.

115. Ayash LJ, et al. High-dose chemotherapy with autologous stem cell support for breast cancer:

a review of the Dana-Farber Cancer Institute/Beth Israel Hospital experience, *J. Hematother.,* **2** (1993) 507–511.

115. Rosti G, et al. Epirubicin + G-CSF as peripheral blood progenitor cells (PBPC) mobilising agents in breast cancer patients, *Ann. Oncol.,* **6** (1995) 1045–1047.

116. Somolo G, et al. High-dose chemotherapy and stem-cell rescue in the treatment of high-risk breast cancer: prognostic indicators of progression-free and overall survival, *J. Clin. Oncol.,* **15** (1997) 2882–2893.

16 High-Dose Chemotherapy with Stem Cell Rescue for Germ Cell Cancer

E. Randolph Broun, MD

CONTENTS

1. INTRODUCTION

Germ cell cancer (GCT) is an uncommon malignancy that occurs most often in young men, and accounts for about 1% of malignancies in men. Although highly curable, particularly when discovered early, stage at presentation is the predominant factor in determining outcome and treatment. Fortunately, even patients who present with disseminated disease can be cured with cisplatin-based combination chemotherapy (CT) and aggressive surgical extirpation of residual disease. There are, however, groups of patients who do poorly despite the best therapeutic efforts: Some of these have poor prognostic factors at diagnosis, such as far-advanced disease, choriocarcinoma, or markedly elevated serum markers; others do not achieve remission, or relapse following primary or salvage therapy; and, finally, a few patients demonstrate refractoriness to cisplatin. In each of these settings, high-dose therapy (HDT) with hematopoietic stem cell rescue (HSCR) has been attempted, with varying degrees of success. This chapter examines these various settings and the trials, which have been performed to alter the otherwise dismal course of these patients.

2. CONVENTIONAL-DOSE THERAPY

Conventional-dose cisplatin-based CT has been very successful in the treatment of patients with disseminated GCT. The most commonly employed regimens in this setting

From: *Current Controversies in Bone Marrow Transplantation*
Edited by: B. Bolwell © Humana Press Inc., Totowa, NJ

Table 1
Indiana University Staging System

Extent of disease	Characteristics
Minimal	Elevated serum markers only
	Unpalpable retroperitoneal mass
	>5 pulmonary nodules <2 cm in size per lung field
	Cervical lymph nodes
Moderate	Palpable abdominal mass w/o supradiaphragmatic disease
	Pulmonary metastases: 5–10 per lung field <3 cm or solitary metastasis >2 cm
Advanced	Primary mediastinal nonseminomatous GCT
	>10 pulmonary metastasis per lung field
	Multiple pulmonary metastasis with largest >3 cm
	Palpable abdominal mass and supradiaphragmatic disease
	Liver, bone, or central nervous system metastasis

are either bleomycin, etoposide (VP-16) and cisplatin (BEP), as developed by the Indiana University group *(1)*, or cisplatin and VP-16 (EP) without bleomycin. The development of these regimens has been presented in great detail elsewhere *(2)*, and will not be repeated here. The Indiana University (IU) Staging System (Table 1) is a useful conceptual approach to these patients. The usual approach for patients with minimal or moderate disease at presentation is three cycles of BEP or four cycles of EP; for those with advanced disease, four cycles of BEP is considered standard. More than 90% of patients presenting with minimal or moderate extent of disease can anticipate long-term disease-free survival (DFS) as a result of such treatment. Those patients presenting with advanced disease fare relatively poorly, with only about 50% doing well long-term *(2)*. In terms of salvage therapy, a few will be cured with surgery *(3)*, but most men who relapse following initial treatment of GCT will require CT. In this setting, combinations of conventional-dose cisplatin plus ifosfamide (IFX) have been somewhat effective. For patients failing BEP or EP, salvage treatment with vinblastine, IFX, and cisplatin yields approx 25% long-term DFS *(4–6)*. Those patients failing salvage CT, or those with cisplatin-refractory disease, are incurable with further conventional-dose cisplatin-based CT.

3. PROGNOSTIC FACTORS

Because treatment with conventional-dose CT and surgery has been a successful strategy, producing cures in most men presenting with GCT, it has been a challenge to identify those patients for whom the risk-to-benefit ratio of HDT with HSCR would be favorable. Several groups have attempted to develop schema for predicting poor prognosis on the basis of initial presenting factors. Among these have been the National Cancer Institute *(7)*, the European Organization for the Research and Treatment of Cancer (EORTC) *(8)*, the Memorial Sloan-Kettering Cancer Center (MSKCC) *(9)*, the Medical Research Council *(10)*, and the Danish Testicular Carcinoma Study Group *(11)*.

A more recent international effort has examined the outcome of 283 patients with relapsed or refractory GCT, treated at four centers in the United States and Europe with HDT and HSCR (12). This retrospective analysis was carried out to identify prognostic variables for response and survival in patients treated in this fashion. This study is not without flaws, because these patients had been treated in a variety of trials using differing regimens and supportive care in the four centers (IU, Institut Gustav-Roussy, Allgemeines Krankenhaus der Stadt Wien, and Virchow Klinikum) between 1984 and 1993. It is, however, the largest and most complete effort of its kind in this field. This group of investigators used a standardized questionnaire filled out by an investigator at each institution, to identify patient characteristics of potential prognostic significance. Despite differences in initial conventional treatment regimens, no differences were found in the response rate or duration following first-line treatment. As would be expected, all patients had been treated with cisplatin-based regimens prior to HDT with HSCR.

The use of HDT with HSCR was quite effective in this group of patients. Maximum response of either a complete remission (CR) or marker-negative partial remission (PRm⁻) was achieved by 157/283 patients (55%). Early deaths occurred in 8% of patients in whom response could not be evaluated. In univariate analysis, patients with disease that was not responsive to conventional-dose CT prior to HDT were less likely to achieve remission with HDT. Likewise, those with extensive metastatic disease (involving brain, lung, liver, or bone), advanced Indiana stage, or high levels of alpha-fetoprotein (AFP) or beta subunit of human chorionic gonadotrophin (βHCG) had a poor rate of response following HDT. Specifically, those who had marker-positive PR, stable disease (SD), or PD, following salvage therapy, had only a 41% CR/PRm⁻, with 22% long-term failure-free survival (FFS). Those with AFP >1000 had a 13% CR/PRm⁻, and among those ≥10,000, only 1/5 patients were long-term survivors. Similarly, elevated βHCG was of significance, with only 1/15 patients with levels ≥10,000 being a long-term survivor. Those who were absolutely cisplatin-refractory (progression within 4 wk of last dose of cisplatin) had a 30% CR/PRm⁻, and only a 2% FFS. Reviewing the prognostic factors for shortened FFS, following HDT, reveals that extragonadal primary (particularly primary mediastinal GCT) failure to achieve CR/PRm⁻ to salvage therapy, cisplatin refractoriness, and elevation of the βHCG to ≥1000 U/L, were important. Multivariate analysis revealed that, similar to the univariate analysis, primary mediastinal GCT, sensitivity to cisplatin, remission status, and level of βHCG prior to HDT were important factors in the likelihood of FFS. The authors went on to develop a scoring system to classify patients as good, intermediate, or poor risk, based on the above factors (Table 2).

There are, therefore, easily evaluable factors assessed prior to HDT, which carry strong prognostic importance in determining a patient's likelihood of benefiting from the rigors of HDT. Fortunately, those patients achieving control of their disease, and surviving free of relapse for 1 yr, had durable remissions: For the group as a whole, the actuarial FFS was 32% at 1 yr, 30% at 2 yr, and 29% at 3 yr.

4. IU EXPERIENCE: DOSE-INTENSE THERAPY WITH HSCR IN GCT

Investigations into the use of high-dose carboplatin (CBDCA) and VP-16 with autologous bone marrow (BM) support began at IU in 1986. Initial investigations used this combination in patients, who were heavily pretreated, usually multiple-relapsed or

Table 2
Prognostic Factors

Characteristic	Score
Progressive disease prior to HDT	1
Primary mediastinal GCT	1
Refractory disease prior to HDT	1
Cisplatin-refractory disease prior to HDT	2
βHCG >1000 U/L prior to HDT	2

Good risk = score 0; intermediate risk = score 1–2; poor risk = score >2.
Adapted with permission from ref *12*.

cisplatin-refractory, and for whom no other therapeutic options existed. Subsequent studies explored modifications of this regimen in refractory patients, and the efficacy of the initial regimen in patients in first relapse after conventional therapy.

The initial study was a phase I dose-escalation study, done in collaboration with Vanderbilt University *(13)* which examined the use of two courses of high-dose CBDCA and VP-16 with autologous bone marrow transplant (ABMT), in patients with GCTs that were either cisplatin-refractory (defined as progression of disease within 4 wk of previous cisplatin-based therapy) or recurrent after a minimum of two prior courses of cisplatin-based therapy. Thirty-three patients were entered on this trial: The initial 13 patients were treated with varying doses of CBDCA, to establish a maximum-tolerated dose in combination with 1200 mg/m² VP-16; the subsequent 20 patients were treated with VP-16 1200 mg/m² and the phase II dose of CBDCA 1500 mg/m² given in three divided doses on d −7, −5, and −3. Toxicities seen in the protocol were the expected severe myelosuppression, moderate enterocolitis, and stomatitis. Grade III hepatic toxicity (more than five-fold increase in liver enzymes), usually in association with massive infection, was observed in 8/33 patients. Significant ototoxicity, neurotoxicity, and nephrotoxicity were not seen, despite the heavy previous exposure to cisplatin in this group of patients. Overall, 7/33 (21%) patients died as a consequence of treatment: two died on the phase I portion of the study. Deaths were primarily caused by infection, but one patient died of veno-occlusive disease of the liver. This was a very heavily pretreated patient population, with over one-half having received three or more prior CT regimens, and 67% were cisplatin-refractory. There were eight patients who achieved a CR, and six a PR, for an overall response rate of 44% (95% confidence interval, 27–63%). Of these, eight patients remained alive and disease-free with 18 mo of follow-up. Review of the responding patients reveals that CR could be achieved despite advanced disease or cisplatin refractoriness. The use of high-dose CBDCA and VP-16 can provide long-term DFS as third- or fourth-line salvage therapy in a small percentage of patients, and overt cisplatin resistance can occasionally be overcome with this approach.

The results in this group of very heavily pretreated, unfavorable prognosis patients are reminiscent of the results reported by the BMT group in Seattle, who carried out the initial studies into the use of allo-BMT in the treatment of patients with acute myeloid leukemia *(14)*. In each case, a small number of poor-prognosis patients did well, leading to further investigations. Motzer et al. *(15)*, at Memorial Sloan Kettering Hospital (MSKCC), investigated the addition of cyclophosphamide to the CBDCA/

VP-16 backbone in a similar group of patients. They were able to safely add 150 mg/kg cyclophosphamide in divided doses, and observed a 23% long-term DFS, which was not significantly different to that seen in the IU trials.

Following the initial phase I/II trial, a larger phase II trial was carried out through the Eastern Cooperative Oncology Group, utilizing the same dose and schedule of agents as in the phase II portion of the initial study *(16)*. Again, patients had to have failed at least two prior cisplatin-based regimens, at least one of which contained IFX, or had to be cisplatin-refractory. Forty patients were entered on this multi-institution cooperative group effort between July 1988 and September 1989: 22/38 (58%) evaluable patients proceeded to the second course of HDT. Toxicity was similar to that seen in the phase I trial, with 5/38 (13%) patients dying of treatment-related causes. Infection (one), hemorrhage (two), and hepatic toxicity (two) accounted for the deaths, all of which occurred in the first course of therapy. Other extramyeloid toxicities were comparable to those seen in the initial study. Nine patients (24%) achieved a CR, including two who were rendered disease-free with post-BMT surgical resection, and eight achieved a PR, for an overall response rate of 45%. Three of the CRs occurred on first BMT, and four patients converted from PR to CR on second BMT: 5/9 are alive and free of disease with follow-up of 24 mo. Notably, all PRs recurred with a median duration of remission of 2.5 mo. The goal of this therapy is necessarily a CR. Achievement of a CR was associated with testicular, rather than extragonadal, primary ($p = 0.12$), absence of liver metastases ($p = 0.08$), and embryonal cell type ($p = 0.11$).

A striking finding in this study was the poor outcome in patients with nonseminomatous primary mediastinal germ cell tumors (PMGCTs). This parallels the reported IU institutional experience in patients with PMGCT, treated at second or greater relapse with HDT and ABMT. From 1987 to 1990, 12 patients with a diagnosis of PMGCT were treated with CBDCA (1500–1800 mg/m^2), VP-16 (1200–1350 mg/m^2), and, in two patients, IFX (10 g/m^2) was added, with ABMT. Patients were relapsed or cisplatin-refractory: They had received a median of two prior CT regimens (range 1–3), all had prior cisplatin therapy, and most had failed IFX-based therapy. Six patients were cisplatin-refractory, and, of these, only one achieved a PR, which was of short duration. It was planned that all patients would undergo two rounds of therapy, but only 5/12 patients received two courses. The remainder had only one round of therapy, either because of inadequate response (three) or excessive toxicity (four). There were four patients who died in the peritransplant period, because of sepsis (two) or bleeding (two). The median survival of the group is 107 d (range 14–>347 d). No patient achieved a CR, there were six PRs (four stable disease and 2 progressive disease) *(17)*. Unfortunately, this report mirrors the experience at other institutions.

The results with high-dose CBDCA/VP-16/ABMT, in patients with recurrent and refractory GCT, indicated that a fraction of patients could be rendered disease-free. Because of the known activity of IFX in recurrent and refractory GCT *(18–21)*, and its favorable side-effect profile for dose escalation in the setting of BMT *(22)*, high-dose IFX was then added to the preparative regimen.

A trial utilizing the same doses of CBDCA/VP-16 as in the phase II trial, and, adding to this, IFX in escalating doses, starting at 2 g/m^2 daily × 5, given by 30 min infusion with mesna uroprotection, was carried out. Seven patients with GCTs, which were either recurrent following a minimum of two regimens of platinum-based CT or cisplatin-refractory, were treated on this trial. The patients were treated with one or two courses of HDT. The doses given were 500 mg/m^2 CBDCA, qod × 3, and 400 mg/m^2, VP-16 qod × 3, plus IFX at a dose of 2 g/m^2 daily × 5 d with mesna. Because of excessive renal toxicity at the first-dose level, escalation of the IFX dose was impossible. Of the seven patients treated, four developed a marked decline in their renal function, with 3/4 requiring hemodialysis or hemofiltration; 6/7 patients treated had a decline in their serum markers, indicating a response to therapy: Unfortunately, all relapsed *(23)*. The conclusion was that, although the combination of CBDCA/VP-16/IFX with ABMT has activity in this group of patients, given in this fashion (by brief iv infusion), it was associated with excessive renal toxicity, probably as a result of underlying renal dysfunction secondary to extensive prior cisplatin-based CT.

A second phase I trial, with further dose escalation of the combination of CBDCA and VP-16, was subsequently carried out. This was possible in patients undergoing this therapy with much less pretreatment than those in the initial phase I trial. Thirty-two patients were enrolled on a careful dose-escalation schema of each of these agents. The maximum-tolerated dose level was CBDCA 700 mg/m^2 and VP-16 750 mg/m^2, given daily on d −6, −5, and −4. Dose-limiting toxicity for this regimen was mucositis. There were five treatment deaths: four caused by sepsis and multiorgan failure, and one by central nervous system hemorrhage. Significant ototoxicity was also seen. These new doses are used in the treatment of patients in first relapse, or with limited prior therapy *(24)*.

The use of HDT with ABMT in the treatment of multiple-relapsed and refractory GCT has resulted in an overall response rate of approx 50%, with a fraction of patients cured of their disease *(25)*. A logical extension of this therapy was to move it higher in the sequence of treatment for GCT. Because the overall cure rate for patients with recurrent testis cancer, treated with IFX and cisplatin-based salvage CT, is in the range of 20–25% *(18)*, a logical step to improve the outcome of these patients was the use of HDT at time of first relapse. The initial trial at IU used two rounds of conventional-dose IFX and cisplatin, with either vinblastine or VP-16 (depending on prior treatment), followed by a single round of HDT with ABMT, using CBDCA and VP-16 in the dose and schedule used in the ECOG phase II trial. Twenty-five patients were enrolled in this study between July 1989 and January 1992. There was one early death caused by sepsis during conventional-dose induction therapy, and there were no transplant-related deaths on this study. For the group as a whole, 18/25 patients completed the planned treatment, including HDT and ABMT. Reasons for not undergoing high-dose therapy and ABMT were ineligibility because CNS metastasis (one) and abdominal abcess (one), insurance refusal (two), and refusal of the high-dose portion of the protocol (one). With median follow-up of 19 mo (range 4–30 mo), 9/25 (36%) were both alive and free of disease; three had relapsed, and were alive with disease; and six had died of progressive disease *(26)*. Two of the patients who relapsed were cisplatin-refractory, and progressed shortly after HDT and ABMT. A follow-up trial examined the use of two cycles of HDT with HSCR in 25 patients in first relapse of cisplatin-sensitive testicular GCT. Patients were treated with 1–2 cycles of conventional-dose salvage CT, followed by two consecutive cycles of CBDCA 2100 mg/M^2 and VP-16 2250 mg/m^2 with HSCR. At a median follow-up of 26 mo, 13/25 (52%) were alive and free of disease, and only one had died of treatment-related causes *(27)*.

A number of conclusions can be drawn from this series of studies. It is clear that a fraction (15–20%) of patients with GCT, which is either multiple-relapsed or overtly cisplatin-refractory, can be cured with high-dose CBDCA and VP-16 with ABMT *(13,16,24,25)*. For this population of patients, this clearly is not investigational therapy, and, in fact, represents the therapy with the greatest curative potential. It is important to note that cisplatin-refractory patients represent a very small proportion of this population of survivors. For these patients, new and innovative approaches are needed. Finally, the use of HDT with ABMT in patients with gonadal GCT in first relapse, who are platinum-sensitive, is quite successful, with high response rates and low toxicity. From these trials, it would appear that there is a therapeutic advantage to the use of HDT with HSCR, compared to conventional-dose salvage therapy.

The group of MSKCC has done extensive work in identifying patients at high risk of relapse early in the course of their disease, who could benefit from HDT. Motzer et al. *(28)* treated 22 patients with reduced clearance of serum markers after two cycles of conventional-dose therapy with HDT and HSCR. Criteria were a prolonged half-life of AFP (>7 d) or βHCG (>3 d), a group, which, in their experience, did poorly with further conventional-dose therapy. They reported 13 patients (46%) alive and free of disease, with 31-mo median follow-up, which was an improvement over historical groups with similar characteristics treated with conventional-dose therapy *(28)*.

5. HDT IN GCT: EUROPEAN EXPERIENCE

A number of institutions in Europe have reported their experience in the treatment of GCT with HDT and HSCR. Among the earliest reports of this approach is that of Mulder et al. *(29)*, who treated 11 patients with VP-16 (2500 mg/m^2) and cyclophosphamide (7 g/m^2). This was a heavily pretreated group of patients, several of which were cisplatin-refractory. They observed seven responses, including 2 CRs (46 and 66 + wk). Median survival was 40 wk.

Shortly after that report, Droz et al. *(30)* reported on 17 patients treated with cisplatin (200 mg/m^2), VP-16 (1750 mg/m^2) and cyclophosphamide (6400 mg/m^2) with BM rescue. Again, this was a heavily pretreated group of patients, and they observed CRs in 9/17 (53%), with 4/17 in long-term DFS. Among the refractory patients treated on this protocol, there were no long-term survivors. This group went on to carry out a randomized trial conventional-dose therapy vs HDT with BM rescue, in patients with poor-risk characteristics. The conventional-dose arm consisted of cisplatin (200 mg/m^2), vinblastine, and bleomycin given every 3 wk for 3–4 cycles, and the high-dose arm, as described above in subheading 3. 115 patients were enrolled, of whom 114 were evaluable. The 2-yr survival was 82% in the conventional-dose arm, and 60% in the high-dose arm, statistically not significantly different. Unfortunately, this trial suffered from some deficiencies: The dose intensity and total dose of cisplatin was actually higher on the conventional-dose arm than the transplant arm, and the numbers were insufficient to draw definite conclusions. Nonetheless, this study did not show an advantage for the use of HDT with BM rescue for the initial treatment of poor-risk GCT patients *(31)*.

Rosti et al. *(32)* published the Italian multicenter experience with high-dose carboplatin, IFX and etoposide with BM rescue in the treatment of 28 patients. They observed that the five long-term disease-free survivors in this group were all cisplatin-sensitive at the time of transplant, and concluded that cisplatin refractoriness predicted for a universally poor outcome. In contrast to the IU experience, nephrotoxicity was not observed, despite the administration of 12 g/m^2 IFX. This may be the result of the administration of IFX by prolonged infusion.

Two other groups have reported a significant experience with the addition of IFX to the combination of CBDCA and VP-16. The German Testicular Cancer Cooperative Study Group published their initial phase I/II experience with this regimen in a single transplant schema, in 1994 (33). They reported on 74 patients, 20 of whom were treated on the phase II doses of CBDCA 1500 mg/m^2, VP-16 2400 mg/m^2, and IFX 10 g/m^2. IFX was again administered by prolonged infusion. Renal toxicity in this group was mild, with median maximum serum creatinine level of 1.4 mg/dL; however, with escalating doses of CBDCA, much more severe renal toxicity was observed. Of 23 patients with cisplatin-refractory disease, only one was alive, free of disease, with 7-mo follow-up. This group updated their results in 1997 (34), revealing an overall survival of 38%, with a failure free survival of 31% at 5 yr. There were no long-term survivors among cisplatin-refractory patients. Late toxicities of renal insufficiency, paresthesias, and ototoxicity were seen in 20–30% of survivors

Lotz et al. (35) carried out a phase I/II trial of this regimen, using a tandem transplant schema in 39 patients, including five with metastatic trophoblastic disease. They administered 69 cycles of HDT, with IFX (7500–12,500 mg/m^2), CBDCA (875–1225 mg/m^2), and VP-16 (1000–1250 mg/m^2), to 39 patients. IFX was infused over 6 h in this trial. Three patients developed severe nephropathy: Two required hemodialysis and later died toxic deaths. Overall, there were 13 CRs and four PRs, for an overall response rate of 46%. Thirty-three patients treated on this trial had cisplatin-refractory disease (defined as failure to respond/progression on cisplatin-based CT or relapse within 4 wk of cisplatin-based CT). In this group were 21 patients with gonadal GCT, nine of whom achieved a CR with a median duration of 29 mo (range 2–84 + mo), and no patient with refractory extragonadal GCT was a long-term survivor. The investigators concluded that cisplatin refractoriness could be overcome with dose-intense therapy.

Although most trials in this area have dosed CBDCA on a mg/m^2 basis, more recent trials have begun using an area-under-the-curve (AUC) schema for dosing. Lampe et al. (36) have published their experience with 23 patients, 12 of whom underwent tandem transplantation. Based on toxicity parameters, they recommended CBDCA dosed at an AUC of 30 mg/min/mL for further trials.

6. CONCLUSIONS

The use of HDT with HSCR has been successful and life-saving for some patients, but many questions remain. Clearly, there are groups of patients for whom this approach is much less helpful than others. In particular, those with primary mediastinal nonseminomatous GCT in relapse, and those with cisplatin-refractory disease, are helped either rarely or not at all. The cumulative information on relapsed mediastinal GCT indicates that this group of patients should be spared the rigors of HDT and autologous stem cell transplantation. New and innovative approaches are needed for these patients. For those who have cisplatin-refractory disease, the question is more difficult. There appears to be a fraction of such patients who are long-term disease-free survivors in most large series. This is a small fraction, probably no more than 5%, and yet, it is not zero. Ideally, however, such patients should be enrolled in clinical trials to develop more effective approaches. The use of allotransplantation in these two groups has yet to be explored, and may be worthy of evaluation.

For patients who are multiple-relapsed, HDT is the treatment of choice at present, although, again, the expectations should be limited. Those in first relapse following cisplatin-based CT appear to have a outcome following HDT superior to further conventional-dose therapy, and there may be an advantage of tandem HDT in this group. Finally, whether there is a benefit to the use of HDT as part of upfront therapy is the subject of an ongoing international collaborative study enrolling patients at high risk of relapse, and eligible patients should be enrolled to help answer this important question.

REFERENCES

1. Williams SW, Birch R, Einhorn LH, Irwin L, Greco FA, and Loehrer PJ. Treatment of disseminated germ cell tumors with cisplatin, bleomycin and either vinblastine or etoposide, *N. Engl. J. Med.*, **316** (1987) 1435–1440.

2. Birch R, Williams SD, Cone A, et al. Prognostic factors for favorable outcome in disseminated germ cell tumors, *J. Clin. Oncol.*, **4** (1986) 400–407.

3. Murphy B, Breeden E, Donohue J, et al. Surgical salvage of chemorefractory germ cell tumors, *J. Clin. Oncol.*, **11** (1993) 324–329.

4. Einhorn LH, Weathers T, Loehrer P, Nichols C. Second line chemotherapy with vinblastine, ifosfamide, and cisplatin after initial chemotherapy with cisplatin, VP-16, and bleomycin (PVP16B) in disseminated germ cell tumors (GCT): long-term follow-up, *Proc. ASCO*, **11** (1992) 196.

5. Loehrer PJ, Lauer R. Roth BJ, Williams SD, Kalasinski LA, Einhorn LH. Salvage therapy in recurrent germ cell cancer: ifosfamide and cisplatin plus either vinblastine or etoposide, *Ann. Int. Med.*, **109** (1988) 540–546.

6. Motzer RJ, Cooper K, Geller NL, et al. The role of ifosfamide plus cisplatin-based chemotherapy as salvage therapy for patients with refractory germ cell tumors, *Cancer*, **66** (1990) 2476–2481.

7. Ozols R, Diesseroth A, Javadpour N, et al. Treatment of poor prognosis nonseminomatous testicular cancer with a "high dose" platinum combination chemotherapy regimen, *Cancer*, **51** (1983) 1803–1807.

8. Stoter G, Kaye S, Sleyfer D, et al. Preliminary results of BEP (bleomycin, etoposide, cisplatin) versus an alternating regimen of BEP and PVB (cisplatin, vinblastine, bleomycin) in high volume metastatic testicular non-seminomas: an EORTC study, *Proc. ASCO*, **5** (1986) 106.

9. Bosl G, Geller N, Cirrincione C, et al. Multivariate analysis of prognostic variables in patients with metastatic testicular cancer, *Cancer Res.*, **43** (1983) 3403–3407.

10. Horwich A, Stenning S, Mead B, et al. Prognostic factors for survival in advanced nonseminomatous germ cell tumours, *Proc. ASCO*, **9** (1990) 132.

11. Vaeth M, Schultz H, von der Masse H, et al. Prognostic factors in testicular germ cell tumours: experiences from 1058 consecutive cases, *Acta. Radiol. Oncol.*, **23** (1984) 271–285.

12. Beyer J, Kramar A, Mandanas R, et al. High-dose chemotherapy as salvage treatment in germ cell tumors: a multivariate analysis of prognostic variables, *J. Clin. Oncol.*, **14** (1996) 2638–2645.

13. Nichols CR, Tricot G, Williams SD, et al. Dose-intensive chemotherapy in refractory germ cell cancers: a phase I-II trial of high dose carboplatin and etoposide with autologous bone marrow transplantation, *J. Clin. Oncol.*, **7** (1989) 932–939.

14. Thomas ED, Storb R, Clift RA, et al. Bone marrow transplantation, *N. Engl. J. Med.*, **92** (1975) 832–843; 895–902.

15. Motzer RJ, Gulati SC, Tong WP, et al. Phase I trial with pharmacokinetic analyses of high dose carboplatin, etoposide, and cyclophosphamide with autologous bone marrow transplantation in patients with refractory germ cell tumors, *Cancer Res.*, **53** (1993) 3730–3735.

16. Nichols CR, Andersen J, Wolff SN, et al. High-dose carboplatin and etoposide with autologous bone marrow transplantation in refractory germ cell cancer: an Eastern Cooperative Group protocol, *J. Clin. Oncol.*, **10** (1992) 558–563.

17. Broun ER, Nichols CR, Einhorn LH, Tricot GJK. Salvage therapy with high-dose chemotherapy and autologous bone marrow support in the treatment of primary nonseminomatous mediastinal germ cell tumors, *Cancer*, **68** (1991) 1513–1515.

18. Loehrer PJ Sr, Gonin R, Nichols CR, Weathers T, Einhorn LH. Vinblastine plus ifosfamide plus cisplatin as initial salvage therapy in recurrent germ cell tumor, *J. Clin. Oncol.*, **16** (1998) 2500–2504.

19. Loehrer PJ, Einhorn LH, Williams SD. Salvage therapy for refractory germ cell tumors with VP-16 plus ifosfamide plus cisplatin, *J. Clin. Oncol.*, **4** (1986) 528–546.

20. Loehrer PJ, Lauer R, Roth BJ, et al. Salvage therapy in recurrent germ cell cancer: ifosfamide and cisplatin plus either vinblastine or etoposide, *Ann. Int. Med.*, **109** (1988) 540–546.

21. Motzer RJ, Cooper K, Geller NL, et al. The role of ifosfamide plus cisplatin-based chemotherapy as salvage therapy for patients with refractory germ cell tumors, *Cancer*, **66** (1990) 2476–2481.

22. Elias AD, Ayash LJ, Eder JP, et al. Phase I study of high dose ifosfamide and escalating doses of carboplatin with autologous bone marrow support, *J. Clin. Oncol.*, **9** (1991) 320–327.

23. Broun ER, Nichols C, Tricot G, Loehrer PJ, Williams SD, Einhorn LH. High-dose carboplatin/VP-16 plus ifosfamide with autologous bone marrow support in the treatment of refractory germ cell tumors, *Bone Marrow Transplant.*, **7** (1991) 53–56.

24. Broun ER, Nichols CR, Mandanas R, et al. Dose escalation study of high-dose carboplatin and etoposide with autologous bone marrow support in patients with recurrent and refractory germ cell tumors, *Bone Marrow Transplant.*, **16** (1995) 353–358.

25. Broun ER, Nichols CR, Kneebone P, et al. Long-term outcome of patients with relapsed and refractory germ cell tumors treated with high-dose chemotherapy and autologous bone marrow rescue, *Ann. Int. Med.*, **117** (1992) 124–120.

26. Broun ER, Nichols CR, Turns M, et al. Early salvage therapy for germ cell cancer using high-dose chemotherapy with autologous bone marrow support, *Cancer*, **73** (1994) 1716–1720.

27. Broun ER, Nichols CR, Gize G, et al.Tandem high-dose chemotherapy with autologous bone marrow transplantation for initial relapse of testicular germ cell cancer, *Cancer*, **79** (1997) 1605–1610.

28. Motzer RJ, Mazumdar M, Gulati SC, et al. Phase II trial of high-dose carboplatin and etoposide with autologous bone marrow transplantation in first line therapy for patients with poor risk germ cell tumors, *J. Natl. Cancer Inst.*, **85** (1993) 1828–1835.

29. Mulder POM, DeVries EGE, Koops HS, et al. Chemotherapy with maximally tolerable doses of VP16-213 and cyclophosphamide followed by autologous bone marrow transplantation for the treatment of relapsed or refractory germ cell tumors, *Eur. J. Cancer Clin. Oncol.*, **24** (1988) 675–679.

30. Droz JP, Pico JL, Ghosn M, et al. Long-term survivors after salvage high-dose chemotherapy with bone marrow rescue in refractory germ cell cancer, *Eur. J. Cancer*, **27** (1991) 831–835.

31. Chevreau C, Droz JP, Pico JL, et al. Early intensified chemotherapy with autologous bone marrow transplantation in first line treatment of poor risk non-seminomatous germ cell tumors. Preliminary results of a French randomized trial, *Eur. Urol.*, **23** (1993) 213–218.

32. Rosti G, Albertazzi L, Salvioni R, et al. High-dose chemotherapy with autologous bone marrow transplantation in germ cell tumors: a phase II study, *Ann. Oncol.*, **3** (1992) 809–812.

33. Siegert W, Beyer J, Strohscheer I, et al. High-dose treatment with carboplatin, etoposide and ifosfamide followed by autologous stem cell transplantation in relapsed or refractory germ cell cancer: a phase I/II study, *J. Clin. Oncol.*, **12** (1994) 1223–1231.

34. Beyer J, Kingreen D, Krause M, et al. Long-term survival of patients with recurrent or refractory germ cell tumors after high-dose chemotherapy, *Cancer*, **79** (1997) 161–168.

35. Lotz JP, Andre T, Donsimone R, et al. High-dose chemotherapy with ifosfamide, carboplatin, and etoposide combined with autologous bone marrow transplantation for the treatment of poor prognosis germ cell tumors and metastatic trophoblastic disease in adults, *Cancer*, **75** (1995) 874–885.

36. Lampe H, Dearnaley DP, Price A, et al. High-dose carboplatin and etoposide for salvage chemotherapy of germ cell tumors, *Eur. J. Cancer*, **31A** (1995) 717–723.

IV COMPLICATIONS OF TRANSPLANTATION

17 Graft-vs-Host Disease

Has Any Progress Been Made in the Past Decade?

Thomas R. Spitzer, MD, and Robert Sackstein, MD, PhD

CONTENTS

1. INTRODUCTION

The transplantation of healthy hematopoietic stem cells into a patient with aplastic anemia or leukemia is potentially curative therapy, but the development of acute graft-vs-host disease (GVHD), which often occurs even when the donor and recipient are siblings fully matched at the human leukocyte antigen (HLA) loci, significantly limits survival. The first descriptions of acute GVHD, following allogeneic bone marrow transplant (allo-BMT) in humans, were made in the 1960s. Significant strides in prophylaxis of acute GVHD have been made over the past four decades by the use of pharmacologic agents such as methotrexate (MTX) and cyclosporine (CSP), and by manipulation of the donor cell inoculum, to limit the infusion of effector donor lymphocytes. However, given the extensive clinical observations and investigations on the nature of this complication, it is remarkable that the diagnosis of acute GVHD is still clinically challenging, and that this complication continues to pose a formidable obstacle to successful allogeneic hematopoietic stem cell transplantation (allo-HSCT). On the other hand, patients with GVHD have improved leukemia-free survival (the graft-vs-leukemia effect [GVL]) and this graft-vs-malignancy effect, a beneficial byproduct of the alloreactivity of the donor cells, may extend to lymphomas, myeloma, and even solid tumors *(1–4)*. Thus, a major question in HSCT biology is how to preserve a

From: *Current Controversies in Bone Marrow Transplantation*
Edited by: B. Bolwell © Humana Press Inc., Totowa, NJ

graft-vs-malignancy effect, while eliminating GVHD. This chapter reviews some of the critical issues in the clinical manifestations and pathobiology of GVHD, including the results of recent investigations using an in vitro lymphocyte–skin adhesion assay to better define the mechanisms of GVHD. Advances during the past decade, in the prevention and treatment of GVHD, including recent evidence for a role of cellular modulation of GVHD, are also reviewed.

2. CLINICAL PRESENTATION AND PATHOBIOLOGY OF ACUTE GVHD

Acute GVHD, by classical definition, is GVHD that occurs within 100 d of HSCT, usually around the time of leukocyte engraftment, or shortly thereafter. Although this operational term is useful in distinguishing GVHD occurring immediately posttransplant from the more indolent and progressive changes of chronic GVHD, acute GVHD can occur beyond 100 d posttransplant, particularly in the setting of donor lymphocyte infusions (DLIs), used in the prevention or treatment of disease relapse. There are three principal target tissues in GVHD: the skin, liver, and gut. Although the clinical staging and overall grading of GVHD is based on the relative level of involvement of these three tissues, other organs, especially the lymphoid tissues and the bone marrow (BM), are targets of GVHD.

The most common tissue affected in acute GVHD is the skin, with over 80% of patients with GVHD manifesting skin eruptions (5). The typical skin presentation consists of a maculopapular rash, which can resemble a sunburn, initially involving the ears, neck, shoulders, upper chest and back, and the palms and soles of the extremities. The extent of skin surface involved, and the presence of bullae of desquamation, define the different stages of skin involvement. The clinical findings of cutaneous GVHD are corroborated by histologic analysis of skin biopsy material, and, therefore, discrete pathologic criteria contribute to the diagnosis of cutaneous GVHD (Table 1) (6). However, the characteristic pathologic changes of acute cutaneous GVHD are not specific for GVHD alone, and can occur in a variety of other cutaneous diseases and reactions. Many skin eruptions occur posttransplant, in response to the preparative regimen, hypersensitivity to drugs (e.g., antibiotics), infections, and even the recovery of leukocytes, and, therefore, there is no standard for accurate pathologic diagnosis of GVHD (7). Moreover, there is no correlation between the numbers of infiltrating mononuclear cells or of dyskeratotic cells in skin specimens and the clinical outcome (7). The diagnosis of cutaneous GVHD is based on exclusion of other confounding contributors, such as drugs and viral exanthems, and depends on clinicopathologic correlation, i.e., clinical history and manifestations supported by characteristic pathologic changes. Indeed, the timing of the clinical manifestations is an important component of the diagnosis, because some pathologists will consider GVHD in the differential only if characteristic histopathologic changes occur during or after engraftment.

Involvement of the gut and liver in GVHD is usually accompanied by skin changes, but, rarely, these tissues can be involved separately or together, without skin manifestations. The primary clinical manifestation of gut GVHD is diarrhea and abdominal pain. The diarrhea is initially watery in nature, but, commonly, becomes bloody, requiring transfusion support with platelets and red cells. The volume of diarrhea defines the different stages of gut involvement. Rectal biopsy is helpful in the diagnosis of gut

Table 1
Histologic Grading for Acute Cutaneous GVHD

Grade 0	Grade I	Grade II	Grade III	Grade IV
Normal skin	Perivascular MNC infiltrates	Perivascular MNC infiltrate	Grade II changes plus epidermolysis and bulla formation (from fusion of basilar vacuoles)	Denudation of epidermis (separation of epidermis from dermis)
	Vacuolar degradation of epidermal–dermal junction	Vacuolar degradation		
		Dyskeratotic cells or eosinophilic bodies in the epidermis		

231

GVHD, particularly when diarrhea occurs in the absence of cutaneous eruptions. The early finding of lymphocytic infiltrates at the crypts, accompanied by necrosis and dropout of crypt cells, is characteristic of the diagnosis, but, again, is not pathognomonic for GVHD. Like the skin, different pathologic stages are recognized, culminating in mucosal denudation (grade IV), and the differential includes drug reactions and infection (particularly cytomegalovirus infection).

Hepatic GVHD is manifested by a rise in the conjugated bilirubin, and the level of total bilirubin elevation defines the clinical stages of liver disease. Lymphocytic infiltrates in the interlobular and marginal bile ducts are characteristic histopathologic findings, which lead to the clinically identifiable cholestatic picture. The differential of liver disease occurring posttransplant includes drug toxicity, viral hepatitis, and hepatic veno-occlusive disease, an entity that is pathologically distinguishable from GVHD, and consists of damage to endothelial cells in zone 3 of the acinus, with occlusion of the hepatic venules *(8)*. Though helpful in the diagnosis, liver biopsy is not routinely performed, because of the risk of hepatic injury and bleeding. In some cases, a transjugular approach can provide enough tissue to allow histopathologic analysis, but inflammatory changes may be patchy and not evident on biopsy material.

As mentioned, the timing of skin, gut, and liver changes is a critical component to the diagnosis of GVHD. Although a hyperacute form of GVHD can occur, typically in HLA-mismatched donor–recipient pairs, manifested by fever and markedly accelerating skin changes, with diarrhea and hyperbilirubinemia before engraftment, most acute GVHD will initially present about the time of engraftment or thereafter. Within the past several years, characteristic clinical findings of an engraftment syndrome have been described in recipients of both autologous SCTs and allo-SCTs *(9–11)*. This syndrome typically consists of noninfectious fever, a maculopapular skin eruption resembling GVHD, capillary leak with resultant weight gain and pulmonary infiltrates/effusions, and, not uncommonly, hyperbilirubinemia and diarrhea. The fact that these changes occur in autotransplant recipients indicates that the pathophysiology of this entity does not depend on alloreactivity *per se*. The skin biopsy findings are consistent with GVHD *(9)*. Treatment of this syndrome requires prompt administration of corticosteroids, to prevent complications of capillary leak, including renal dysfunction and pulmonary failure.

The pathophysiology of the engraftment syndrome may overlap with that of acute GVHD. The common feature in these entities maybe primary endothelial damage as a consequence of inflammatory mediators, such as interleukin-2 (IL-2), tumor necrosis factor (TNF-α), and interferon (IFN-γ), released locally by infiltrating perivascular lymphocytes *(9,12–14)*. In GVHD, however, there is also evidence of direct cell-mediated immunologic reactivity, resulting in microvascular injury *(15)*. Studies in severe combined-immunodeficiency mice receiving partial-thickness human skin grafts, then, following anastomosis, administered allogeneic human lymphocytes, reveal upregulation of vascular cell adhesion molecules (such as VCAM-1) promoting lymphocyte migration in the human dermal vessels *(16)*. The dermal microvascular injury is confined to the human vessels, with no injury evident in mouse microvessels that have invaded the human skin. This endothelial damage is mediated by infiltrating T-cells expressing a cytolytic phenotype, containing granules laden with perforin *(16)*. In this model, co-administration of CSP A and rapamycin markedly reduces the extent of microvascular injury. Of note, CSP A or rapamycin, each given alone, does not reduce lymphocyte infiltration of the graft or vascular injury, but, when given together, markedly decrease the perivascular infiltration of perforin-laden lymphocytes. These data suggest that one effect of combining these agents is to modify the migration capabilities of lymphocytes, by altering lymphocyte and/or endothelial adhesive structures mediating lymphocyte recruitment from the vasculature and into the tissue. Corticosteroids, the first-line pharmacologic agents in the treatment of acute GVHD, also profoundly affect lymphocyte migration to lymphoid and extralymphoid tissues (17,18), and decreased lymphocyte infiltrates in affected tissues are a prognostic sign for steroid-responsiveness in GVHD therapy (19).

In Billingham's classic description of the elements required for the development GVHD (20), three requirements were emphasized: The host must be incapable of rejecting the graft, the graft must contain immunocompetent cells, and there must be incompatibilities in transplantation antigens between donor and host. Although this description needs to be modified somewhat, because of evidence of GVHD occurring in the setting of blood transfusions, solid organ transplants and, in the case of CSP-induced autologous GVHD (caused by induction of autoreactive T-cells [21]), Billingham's tenets reflect important basic principles in the biology of GVHD. However, given the data reviewed above, and the pathologic evidence of lymphocytic infiltrates consistently accompanying GVHD-induced tissue injury, a fourth requirement to Billingham's criteria must be proposed: Effector lymphocytes must migrate to the target tissues in GVHD.

The pathologic hallmark of acute GVHD is mononuclear cell (MNC) infiltrates in the involved tissues (22,23). The pathogenesis of acute GVHD involves the migration of both alloreactive lymphocytes and of natural killer (NK) cells into target tissues (24–27). A central role for alloreactive T-cells in the development of GVHD is indicated by the fact that T-cell depletion of donor marrow significantly abrogates the incidence of GVHD (28). Indeed, the lymphocytic infiltrates of dermal GVHD are composed of donor-derived cells (29). Infiltrating NK cells may contribute to tissue damage in GVHD by their local release of inflammatory cytokines, such as TNF-α and IFN-γ (30,31). The NK cell infiltrates are also donor-derived (32), indicating that their localization in tissues is likewise caused by recruitment from the circulation. The fact that phenotypically and functionally discrete subpopulations of peripheral blood mononuclear cells (PBMCs) are found within inflammatory sites of GVHD suggests that there are specific PBMC–endothelial adhesive mechanisms that promote site-directed migration of effector cells. Furthermore, the adhesive system mediating this recruitment is highly effective and efficient, because MNC infiltrates are developing during periods of profound lymphopenia in the periengraftment period. Given this fact, it is surprising that essentially nothing is known about the molecular basis of this adhesive system. A role for cytokines, such as TNF-α, in the induction of GVHD has been inferred by immunohistochemical analysis and measurements of cytokine mRNA in involved skin of cutaneous GVHD by polymerase chain reaction (31,33). This cytokine induces expression of adhesion molecules on endothelium, such as E-selectin and VCAM-1, which mediate recruitment of leukocytes (34), and immunohistochemical studies have shown an increase in E-selectin expression on endothelium of acute cutaneous GVHD (35), but whether this change reflects a prophenomenon or epiphenomenon of the inflammatory response is unknown. As noted above, VCAM-1, an endothelial adhesion molecule that serves as a ligand for VLA-4 ($\alpha_4\beta_1$-integrin expressed on lymphocytes and NK cells), similarly appears to be upregulated in perivascular areas in cutaneous

GVHD *(35)*, but, again, identification of its presence is not evidence of its role in mediating the MNC emigration.

The first step in the selective migration of circulating leukocytes into inflammatory sites is the attachment of the cells to the endothelium within the given affected tissue, a process that anchors the bloodborne, flowing cells for subsequent transmigration into the tissue parenchyma *(34,36)*. In an effort to better understand the pathophysiologic mechanisms of GVHD, the authors have undertaken a series of investigations evaluating the skin as a source tissue (because of the feasibility of obtaining samples for analysis). The authors' hypothesis is that inflammatory changes within the major target organs of GVHD (the skin, liver, and gut) result in part from specific endothelial changes that promote entry of lymphocytes and NK cells to these sites, and the resultant increased trafficking of effector cells to these organs leaves them susceptible to pathologic damage. Utilizing an in vitro lymphocyte–skin adherence assay, evidence has been obtained that endothelium of skin involved in GVHD reactions is specialized to support lymphocyte adhesion. The in vitro lymphocyte–endothelial adherence assay employed was adapted from the conventional Stamper-Woodruff assay *(37)*, which, performed under conditions of shear that mimic blood flow, allows for an in vitro approximation of physiologic, functional interaction(s) of adhesion molecules on interacting cells. A major advantage of this assay, compared to studies utilizing purified molecules, is that it tests cell–cell adherence mediated by membrane molecules in their native states, and, more importantly, as expressed by exactly those cells that are biologically relevant. This adhesion assay was fundamental in identifying the lymphocyte and endothelial membrane molecules involved in mediating lymphocyte migration into lymph nodes *(18,38)*: The authors previously utilized it to investigate the lymphocyte and endothelial membrane structures that mediate lymphocyte migration to chronic inflammatory sites, such as the dermis in psoriasis *(39)*.

The authors obtained punch biopsies from skin lesions developing within 100 d of SCT in 41 patients (20 autologous, 21 allogeneic); all autologous SCT patients were biopsied once, but 11 of the allogeneic patients underwent repeat biopsies, either because of worsening of the skin eruption or following initiation of steroid therapy for GVHD (total of 37 evaluable allogeneic biopsies). All skin biopsy specimens were divided: One portion was snap-frozen in liquid nitrogen for adherence assays, and other portions were submitted for routine histologic and microbiologic studies. For the adhesion assay, suspensions of PBMCs, prepared from blood of healthy donors, were overlaid onto 8-µ frozen sections of skin, and incubated under shear conditions at 4°C. After 30 min, sections were rinsed to remove nonadherent cells, fixed, and stained, and PBMC binding to sections was analyzed by light microscopy. PBMCs bound specifically to papillary dermal endothelium (identified by CD34 and factor VIII staining of sequential sections) in frozen sections of skin biopsies from allo-SCT patients with clinicohistologic evidence of GVHD not receiving steroids (11 patients), but not to that of non-GVHD skin eruptions in the allo-SCT population (six patients). In four allo-SCT patients, lymphocyte adherence to skin vessels was demonstrated on biopsies, without histologic changes consistent with GVHD, but, in each case, skin eruptions worsened, and subsequent biopsies adjacent to the initial biopsy site showed histologic changes typical of GVHD (and adherence assays again showed lymphocyte binding to vessels). In three patients with GVHD who responded to steroid therapy, PBMC adherence to dermal vessels was abrogated prior to clinical and histologic resolution of skin changes; PBMC adherence was persistent among biopsies from two patients who developed worsening GVHD, despite steroid therapy. Of the skin biopsies obtained from autologous SCT patients, only two demonstrated PBMC binding to dermal vessels.

These data provide evidence of a papillary dermal endothelium recognition system that regulates lymphocyte homing into skin following SCT. Moreover, the data indicate that skin eruptions following SCT can be stratified by their capacity to support PBMC binding, and the results suggest that this in vitro assay may be of value in the diagnosis and management of acute cutaneous GVHD. Studies are currently being performed to further characterize candidate PBMC and endothelial adhesion molecules mediating PBMC migration to skin in cutaneous GVHD. The authors' overall objective in these studies is to identify the molecular basis of lymphocyte migration to target tissues in GVHD, in order to develop therapeutic agents to treat GVHD by disrupting the migration of effector cells into affected tissues. In so doing, the authors hope to achieve preservation of beneficial immune reactivity, such as GVL with elimination of GVHD. Clinical studies to be described in subheading 6. also utilize novel preparative regimens to minimize GVH by achieving initial mixed hematopoietic chimerism, followed by donor lymphocyte infusions to deliver a potent graft-vs-malignancy effect.

3. PREVENTION OF GVHD

The pathophysiologic complexity of GVHD requires a multifaceted approach to its prevention. That same complexity underscores why prevention of GVHD, while still preserving a desired graft-vs-malignancy effect of the transplant, is so difficult to achieve. Three general strategies have been attempted for the prevention of GVHD (Fig. 1): pharmacologic intervention, ex vivo T-cell (or T-cell subset) depletion, and manipulation of the donor–host cellular environment posttransplant (either by cytokines or preservation [or addition] of host cells). The three strategies will be discussed separately, realizing, however, that a combination of approaches are sometimes employed, and that the donor–host cellular environment may be influenced (albeit unintentionally) by any effort aimed at providing GVHD protection.

4. PHARMACOLOGIC INTERVENTION

Single-agent MTX was shown to have potent activity in preventing GVHD in dog models, but its efficacy for GVHD protection, clinically, was limited (40). Although GVHD incidence and severity were probably diminished with MTX, overall survival (OS), as determined by several retrospective comparisons with patients not receiving GVHD prophylaxis, was not appreciably affected (41–43). The advent of combination CSP-based pharmacoprophylaxis, in the early to mid-1980s, represented a major advance in the field of clinical BMT. Prospective randomized trials evaluating the combination of CSP and MTX, compared with MTX alone, for hematologic malignancies or severe aplastic anemia, were conducted (44,45). Significant reductions in incidence of acute GVHD were seen in each case. In the case of transplantation for hematologic malignancies (acute myeloid leukemia in first complete remission or chronic-phase chronic myeloid leukemia [CML]), an OS benefit was realized. However, for severe aplastic anemia, a survival difference did not reach statistical significance. CSP in combination with MTX or corticosteroids has been shown to be considerably less effective in the

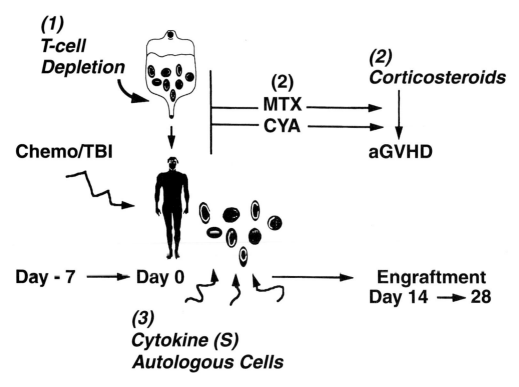

Fig. 1. Methods of GVHD prophylaxis: (1) ex vivo T-cell depletion; (2) pharmacologic intervention (e.g., MTX/CSP with corticosteroids for the treatment of GVHD); (3) Cellular modulation of GVHD (e.g., posttransplant IL-2 or IL-12, and/or the addition of host MNCs).

prevention of GVHD following HLA-mismatched donor BMT *(46,47)*. For recipients of HLA-2 or -3 antigen mismatched donor transplants, acute GVHD incidence exceeds 70–80%, and transplant related mortality (TRM) is very high *(46)*. The limitations of CSP drug combinations in the prevention of GVHD notwithstanding, these pharmaco-prophylactic strategies have had a major impact on the practice of clinical BMT. The reductions in acute GVHD-related morbidity and mortality have allowed for the transplantation of considerably older patients, and of patients without HLA genotypically identical sibling donors. In the early 1980s, the upper age limit for allo-BMT in most centers was 40–45 yr; many transplant centers are now considering patients as old as 60–65 yr for allo-BMT.

During the past decade, there have been several advances in the pharmacologic prevention of GVHD. Triple-drug immunoprophylaxis (CSP, MTX, and corticosteroids) has been shown to be superior to CSP and corticosteroids alone for the prevention of GVHD following HLA-matched donor BMT for hematologic malignancies *(48)*. In a prospective randomized trial by Chao et al. *(48)*, a 9% incidence of acute GVHD with triple-drug prophylaxis was seen, compared with a 23% incidence with CSP and corticosteroids. OS was not significantly different between the treatment groups, how-ever. Other investigators have suggested that triple-drug pharmacoprophylaxis may also be of benefit in preventing GVHD following HLA nongenotypically identical donor transplants. The primary risk of additional pharmacologic immunosuppression is infection. These infection risks, moreover, are likely to be higher following HLA nonidentical donor transplants *(49)*. If, in fact, acute GVHD incidence is reduced, but OS is not improved, it is likely that the additional immunosuppression impairs the graft-vs-malignancy effect of the transplant.

The introduction of tacrolimus has represented a potential advance in clinical BMT. Tacrolimus prevents T-cell activation in a manner similar to CSP, however, it is considerably more potent on an equimolar basis. Two multicenter prospective randomized trials *(50,51)*, comparing tacrolimus and MTX with CSP and MTX for GVHD prophylaxis following BMT for hematologic malignancies, have been conducted. In the first trial, involving HLA genotypically identical sibling donors, a significant reduction in the incidence of GVHD in the tacrolimus-treated patients was observed *(50)*. The second trial involved patients receiving transplants from HLA-matched unrelated donors: Once again, GVHD incidence was reduced in the tacrolimus-treated group *(51)*. In both trials, however, no significant difference was observed in OS between two treatment groups. The toxicity profiles of tacrolimus were somewhat different than those of CSP: More neurotoxicity was observed with tacrolimus, but, there was less renal impairment and hypertension in tacrolimus-treated patients.

Newer agents are presently being evaluated for GVHD prophylaxis. Rapamycin, deoxyspergualin, and its analog, tresperimus, are currently being evaluated in clinical trials. Borrowing from the experience of combination chemotherapy in the treatment of neoplastic diseases, in which potent drugs with different mechanisms of action and nonoverlapping toxicities are employed, the optimal pharmacoprophylactic strategy for GVHD might consist of combination drug regimens with different mechanisms of action and toxicities. Optimal drug combinations and the scheduling of the drugs, however, remain to be determined.

5. EX VIVO T-CELL DEPLETION

A series of experimental and clinical observations have shown that GVHD can be effectively prevented by infusing less than 1–5×10^5 T-cells/kg of recipient body wt *(52,53)*. Early enthusiasm for the ex vivo removal of immunocompetent T-cells from the marrow graft, however, was tempered by an increased risk of engraftment failure and relapse of the underlying malignancy *(54–56)*. This increased relapse risk was somewhat disease-specific. In CML, for example, an increase in relapse risk, from approx 10–20% following HLA-matched donor non-T-cell-depleted (TCD) transplantation, to 60–80% following TCD transplantation, was observed *(57)*. In acute lymphoblastic leukemia, on the other hand, an effect of TCD on probability of relapse is less apparent *(57)*.

Given the shortcomings of ex vivo TCD, this strategy has not reached widespread acceptance for the prevention of GVHD following HLA-genotypically identical donor BMT for hematologic malignancies, particularly CML. However, given the more profound impact of GVHD on mortality risk following HLA nongenotypically identical donor transplantation, TCD strategies are being more vigorously evaluated. A multicenter randomized trial evaluating the effect of ex vivo TCD on GVHD risk and survival, compared with pharmacologic prophylaxis, is currently in progress.

In an effort to diminish the problems of engraftment failure and relapse probability risks of ex vivo TCD, recent investigations have focused on the depletion of selective T-cell subsets. Ex vivo depletion of CD8 T-cells has been shown to result in an apparent reduction of GVHD, with no increase in relapse probability following HLA-matched sibling donor BMT for CML *(58)*. An increased risk of engraftment failure, however, has further demonstrated the importance of T-cells in overcoming host alloresistance to engraftment. Less-vigorous TCD (i.e., depletion of 1–1.5 logs of T-cells), using an antibody specific for the αβ-chain of the T-cell receptor (TCR) has been shown in several clinical trials (when combined with in vivo pharmacoprophylaxis) to be associated with impressively low acute GVHD risks in the setting of HLA-matched unrelated donor and HLA-mismatched related donor transplants *(59,60)*.

Although efforts have been made to overcome the problems of nonengraftment and increased relapse probability following ex vivo depleted BMTs by intensifying the conditioning therapy for BMT, OS has not appreciably improved, probably because of increased TRM and morbidity. Another approach to the problem of nonengraftment has been to infuse an increased number of hematopoietic progenitors. Within the past several years, there has been an increasing use of recombinant myeloid growth-factor-stimulated peripheral blood progenitor cells (PBPCs) for allotransplantation *(61)*. These growth-factor-mobilized PBMCs are enriched for CD-34-positive progenitor cells, and considerably increased numbers of CD34-positive cell progenitors are usually infused, compared with the number of infused progenitors collected from BM *(62–64)*. Despite an approximately 1-log increase in the number of T-cells in growth-factor-mobilized PBPC products, there has been no apparent increase in risk of acute GVHD, compared with BMTs (a significant increase in the risk of chronic GVHD may, however, exist with the use of PBMC) *(65,66)*. With the use of intensive total body irradiation-based conditioning therapy and TCD growth-factor-mobilized PBPC, engraftment is achievable in most cases, even following full haplotype mismatched donor transplants *(67)*. These preliminary results are encouraging, but further evaluation of immune reconstitution, and the preservation of a graft-vs-malignancy effect, will be required before this strategy becomes widely accepted.

Perhaps the most direct evidence of a cell-mediated graft-vs-malignancy effect comes from the DLI experience for treatment of relapsed CML following BMT *(68,69)*. In the majority of cases, a cytogenetic and molecular remission is achieved with these DLIs, demonstrating that a potent antitumor effect, with at least a several-log tumor cell cytoreduction, is achievable. In a nonrandomized comparison of non-TCD transplants and CD6 TCD transplants for CML (followed by DLI at time of relapse), similar survival probabilities were realized *(70)*. Although an increased probability of relapse occurred in the TCD transplant recipients, most of these patients could achieve a second remission with DLI, which in most cases appeared to be durable. This suggests that, for at least selected patients who are at high risk for TRM or morbidity, an ex vivo TCD BMT, followed by DLI for posttransplant relapse, may be an appropriate treatment strategy. DLIs are not, however, without their own risk: Substantial GVHD and aplasia risks are associated with DLI *(68,69)*. Preliminary experience with CD8[+] TCD DLI suggests that these risks may be reduced without affecting the antitumor response *(71)*.

Given the potent antitumor potential of DLI, and experimental evidence suggesting that delayed DLI may be associated with a substantially lower risk of GVHD than with early T-cell infusion(s), clinical trials evaluating ex vivo TCD BM (or PBPC) transplants, followed by delayed T-cell addback, are underway *(72,73)*. This strategy relies on achieving early alloengraftment without GVHD, followed by T-cell addback, in an effort to reduce the posttransplant relapse risk by capturing the graft-vs-malignancy potential of the transplant. Preliminary results suggest that this strategy is feasible, and that addback can be performed without a prohibitive risk of GVHD *(73)*. The optimal dosing and timing of delayed T-cell infusions remain to be determined. This strategy might obviate many of the problems associated with conventional BMT, while retaining the potent immunologically mediated antitumor effect of the transplant. However, it is probably only applicable for malignancies that are not at high risk for recurrence within the first 50–100 d posttransplant.

6. CELLULAR MODULATION OF GVHD

Experimental and clinical experiences have suggested that host cells surviving the transplant conditioning regimen may be instrumental in the regulation of GVHD *(74– 77)*. The availability of sensitive methods for detecting the presence of residual host cells (e.g., microsatellite analyses evaluating variable numbers of tandem repeat sequences) have demonstrated that at least the transient presence of host cells in many patients can be seen following BMT *(78,79)*. An increased incidence of acute GVHD, with increasing intensity of the preparative regimen, possibly because of the lack of survival of host elements following these aggressive preparative regimens, has been observed *(80)*. A relationship between the presence of mixed lymphohematopoietic chimerism and a reduced incidence of acute GVHD has also been seen in some series *(81–83)*.

In several animal models, the intentional induction of mixed lymphohematopoietic chimerism has been associated with a reduction in the incidence of acute GVHD. These mixed chimeric states are achievable following myeloablative preparative regimens, in which a combination of mixed TCD syngeneic and TCD allogeneic marrow is transplanted (mixed BMT), or following nonablative preparative regimens with peritransplant anti-T-cell therapy *(84,86)*. In a murine model established by Pelot et al. *(86a)*, mixed lymphohematopoietic chimerism was reliably induced following a nonablative preparative regimen that included cyclophosphamide, monoclonal anti-T-cell antibody therapy, and thymic irradiation. These mixed chimeras were resistant to the induction of acute GVHD followed by delayed donor leukocyte infusions, despite a potent lymphohematopoietic graft-vs-host reaction, which converted their mixed chimeric state to a state of full donor hematopoiesis. These results raised the possibility that a potent GVL effect could occur without GVHD, by initially inducing a state of mixed chimerism followed by the delayed DLI.

Based on these experimental considerations, a clinical trial at the Massachusetts General Hospital has been initiated involving a similar nonablative preparative regimen for the induction of mixed chimerism followed by DLI in patients with refractory hematologic malignancies *(87;* Spitzer et al., manuscript submitted). In a preliminary experience involving 25 patients, eight of whom received transplants from HLA 1–2 antigen-mismatched donors, stable mixed chimerism was reliably induced in most patients. In patients without GVHD, DLI were administered, stating at 5 wk posttransplant, for conversion of their mixed chimeric state to a fully donor one. Grade II GVHD has been seen in the majority of patients, but therapy with corticosteroids has been successful in most of these patients. In seven patients with HLA 2 antigen mismatched donor transplants, GVHD has also been manageable. Striking antitumor responses have been seen in the majority of cases, suggesting that a myeloablative preparative regimen is not necessary for optimal tumor cytoreduction. Rather, a potent immunologically mediated graft-vs-malignancy effect, which may be potentiated by subsequent DLI, is achievable in the presence of a mixed lymphohematopoietic chimeric state. Several other centers have had pilot experiences with nonmyeloablative preparative strategies for allo-BMT (88–90). Although no apparent reduction in GVHD incidence or severity has been reported, most of these transplants involved HLA-genotypically identical donors (thus, not evaluating whether GVHD protection was afforded following transplants from HLA mismatched donors), and, in most of the situations, mixed chimerism was not intentionally induced (or observed).

Another approach to the cellular modulation of GVHD has consisted of exogenous cytokine administration posttransplant. In a murine model, striking protection from acute GVHD mortality and preservation of a GVL effect were observed with the use of high-dose, short-course IL-2 following major histocompatibility complex (MHC)-mismatched donor transplants. The mechanism of this GVHD protection was shown to be IL-2 inhibition of donor CD4 T-cell function. However, IL-2 treatment was also shown to expand $\alpha\beta TCR^+$ $CD4^-CD8^-$ cells of both host and donor origin. It is the same host cell population that has been hypothesized to be important in the GVHD protection afforded by mixed TCD syngeneic (or autologous) and MHC-mismatched allo-BMT in small (murine) and large (miniature swine) animal models (91,92).

Murine studies using IL-2 for GVHD protection also demonstrated the potential to separate GVHD from GVL with this strategy (93,94). In two different leukemia models, GVL effects were mediated by allogeneic $CD8^+$ T-cells in a CD4-independent fashion. Because IL-2 does not affect CD4-independent CD8 cell functions, CD8-mediated GVL is completely preserved in these IL-2-treated mice. In a promonocytic leukemia model, moreover, IL-2 was shown to inhibit CD4-mediated GVHD, while not inhibiting CD4-mediated GVL effects, suggesting that IL-2 may affect some CD4-mediated function, while not affecting others.

Short-course (single-dose) high-dose IL-12 has also been shown to provide striking acute GVHD protection in an MHC-mismatched murine model (95). This seemingly paradoxical effect appears also to be mediated by a transient inhibition of donor CD4 cell function.

Given the complexity of the cellular and cytokine interactions that mediate GVHD, only rudimentary understanding exists of the manipulations of the donor–host cellular environment that occurs following BMT. Which host cells are important in the regulation of GVHD, for example, remain to be determined. Several cell populations, including $\alpha\beta TCR^+$ $CD4^-CD8^-$ cells with natural suppressor activity and lymphokine-activated killer cells exhibiting both veto and natural suppressor activity, have been postulated as having a regulatory role in the suppression of the graft-vs-host reaction (91,92,96–98). It is considerably less clear, however, how these cells inhibit alloresponsiveness, both in vitro and in vivo. Given the compelling experimental and clinical evidence for a protective effect of cytokine-modulated residual (or exogenously added) host cells, future efforts should be made to discern the mechanism of this effect, and, hopefully, to optimize its clinical benefit.

7. TREATMENT OF ACUTE GVHD

Substantial progress in the treatment of acute GVHD has not been made in the past decade. Corticosteroids remain the mainstay of therapy for acute GVHD, particularly if they were not utilized as prophylaxis (99,100). Several studies have established the response rates for treatment of GVHD with corticosteroids (101,102). The highest response rates are uniformly observed for cutaneous GVHD (66%); response rates of only 20–40% are seen for visceral (gut and liver) GVHD. Long-term survival has been correlated with grade of GVHD and response to medical therapy. Patients with grade III or IV GVHD, who do not achieve a complete remission of their GVHD with medical therapy, have a less than 50% probability of long-term survival (5). Most patients who receive corticosteroids for grades II–IV GVHD require long-term corticosteroid administration, which is usually accompanied by substantial morbidity. A heightened infection risk, hypertension, diabetes mellitus, osteoporosis, and aseptic necrosis of the hip and other bones are commonly observed (100).

Despite the longstanding experience with corticosteroids as the standard of care for the treatment of acute GVHD, several questions remain regarding the proper dose and scheduling of these agents. An uncontrolled observation suggests that a dose–response relationship exists for corticosteroids. Oblon et al. (103) showed that corticosteroid responses were possible in patients who had not achieved a response with methylprednisolone at a dose of 2 mg/kg/d, by increasing the dose to 5, and, subsequently, 10 mg/kg/d. Higher doses (particularly 10–20 mg/kg/d) were associated with increased steroid-related complications and TRM. Other investigators are unconvinced that such a dose–response relationship exists. In a recent prospective randomized trial (104), duration of corticosteroid therapy was evaluated. Shorter-course corticosteroids for the treatment of grades II–IV GVHD was associated with similar response rates and survival probabilities as longer-course steroid therapy

The past decade has seen the introduction of multiple new therapies for acute GVHD. A listing of a number of these therapies is included in Table 2. For the most part, these therapies have targeted one specific aspect of the pathophysiologic mechanism of GVHD. Monoclonal antibodies directed against effector cells (e.g., T-cells or NK cells) or cytokines (e.g., TNF-α) have generally been associated with favorable response rates (105,106); however, the responses have been only transient, which is not surprising, given the multifactorial effect or mechanisms of GVHD.

Manipulation of the host cellular environment may also have a role in the treatment of established GVHD. The most direct evidence of host cellular modulation of GVHD has perhaps been demonstrated in preliminary miniature swine experiments showing that life-threatening GVHD can be reversed following the infusion of host PBMCs (107). In this miniature swine model, host PMNC infusions, following allo-BMT across a major MHC barrier, resulted in the striking resolution of progressive, and otherwise uniformly fatal, acute GVHD. The infusion of PBMCs in these experiments resulted in a transiently mixed chimeric state, but, as demonstrated in one case of successful reversal of GVHD, fully allogeneic hematopoiesis was restored.

A beneficial effect of host MNC infusions has also been demonstrated in several case reports of successful reversal of life-threatening GVHD. In one case, successful resolution of GVHD was reported following syngeneic marrow infusion; however, the

Table 2
Therapeutic Modalities for GVHD

Acute GVHD	Chronic GVHD
Pharmacologic immunosuppression 　Corticosteroids 　CSP 　Tacrolimus 　Other 　　Deoxyspergualin 　　Tresperimus 　　Rapamycin Antibody therapy 　Polyclonal 　　Antithymocyte globulin 　Monoclonal 　　Anti-T-cell 　　Anti-IL-2 receptor 　　Anti-NK cell 　　Anti-TNF-α 　　Anti-adhesion molecule(s) 　Immunoconjugate 　　Anti-CD5-ricin Receptor blockade 　IL-1 receptor antagonist Gene therapy 　Thymidine kinase suicide gene 　　transduction/gancyclovir Cellular Modulation of GVHD 　Infusion of host MNC 　Exogenous cytokines (IL-2, IL-12)	Pharmacologic immunosuppression 　Corticosteroids 　CSP 　Tacrolimus 　Azathioprine 　Mycophenolate mofetil 　Thalidomide 　Other pharmacologic agents 　　Desferrioxamine 　　Ursodeoxycholic acid 　　Clofazimine 　　Etedrinate Total lymphoid irradiation Extracorporeal photopheresis

patient died of transplant-related complications before chimerism studies could be performed (108). In another case, grade III GVHD occurred following a combined liver–BM transplantation. Autologous marrow was infused on d 42 posttransplant, with resolution of cutaneous GVHD by d 54 (109). In a third case, successful reversal of progressive life-threatening GVHD followed infusion of autologous BM (110). Chimerism studies showed durable preservation of the allograft. Identification of the relevant cell types responsible for this anti-GVHD effect will be crucial, given the need to avoid infusion of cells that are contaminated by malignancy.

Gene therapy may offer another avenue for the reversal of severe acute GVHD. T-cells transduced with a herpes viral thymidase kinase gene have been infused in animal transplant experiments and in preliminary clinical trials. Gancyclovir was administered in the event of GVHD, resulting in T-cell death and, in some instances, reversal of the GVHD (111,112). Improving the methods of gene transduction and preservation of the cells that mediate a graft-vs-malignancy effect are important future goals of this strategy.

Advances in the treatment of chronic GVHD have similarly been modest. Treatment of severe chronic GVHD still relies on aggressive long-term immunosuppression. An alternate-day corticosteroid and CSP regimen has been shown to be reasonably well-tolerated and effective in the management of chronic GVHD *(113)*. Multiple new drugs have been evaluated for the treatment of chronic GVHD. Thalidomide and mycophenolate mofetil have been shown to have significant activity in chronic GVHD, by inhibiting T-cell function *(114,115)*. Other modalities that have shown some efficacy have been total lymphoid irradiation and extracorporeal photopheresis *(116,117)*. Clofazimine may be effective in the treatment of the connective tissue variant of chronic GVHD *(118)*. Improved supportive care, including intravenous immunoglobulin therapy for patients with severe hypogammaglobulinemia and suppressive antibiotic therapy, may reduce infectious complications of chronic GVHD.

REFERENCES

1. Weiden P, Flournoy N, Sanders J, et al. Antileukemic effect of graft-versus-host disease contributes to improved survival after allogeneic marrow transplantation, *Transplant. Proc.*, **13** (1981) 248–251.
2. Jones R, Ambinder R, Piantodosi S, and Santos G. Evidence of a graft-versus-lymphoma effect associated with allogeneic bone marrow transplantation, *Blood*, **77** (1996) 649–653.
3. Tricot G, Vesole D, Jagannath S, et al. Graft-versus-myeloma effect: proof of principle, *Blood*, **87** (1996) 1196–1198.
4. Eibl B, Schwaighofer H, Nachbaur D, et al. Evidence of a graft-versus-tumor effect in a patient treated with marrow ablative chemotherapy and allogeneic bone marrow transplantation for breast cancer, *Blood*, **88** (1996) 1501–1508.
5. Martin P, Schoch G, Fisher L, et al. A retrospective analysis of therapy for acute graft-versus-host disease: initial treatment, *Blood*, **76** (1990) 1464–1472.
6. Lerner K, Kao G, Storb R, et al. Histopathology of graft-versus-host reaction (GVHR) in human recipients of marrow from HLA matched sibling donors, *Transplant. Proc.*, **6** (1974) 367–371.
7. Horn TD. Acute cutaneous eruptions after marrow ablation: roses by other names? *J. Cutan. Pathol.*, **21** (1994) 385–392.
8. Sackstein R, Chao N. Veno-occlusive disease of the liver following bone marrow transplantation. In Epstein M. (ed.), *The Kidney in Liver Disease*. Hanley and Belfus, Philadelphia, 1996, pp. 167–178.
9. Lee C-K, Gingrich R, Hohl R, Ajram K. Engraftment syndrome in autologous bone marrow and peripheral stem cell transplantation, *Bone Marrow Transplant.*, **16** (1995) 175–182.
10. Cahill RA, Spitzer TR, Mazumder A. Marrow engraftment and clinical manifestations of capillary leak syndrome, *Bone Marrow Transplant.*, **18** (1996) 177–184.
11. Ravoet C, Feremans W, Husson B, et al. Clinical evidence for an engraftment syndrome associated with early and steep neutrophil recovery after autologous blood stem cell transplantation, *Bone Marrow Transplant.*, **18** (1996) 943–947.
12. Dickinson A, Sviland L, Dunn J, et al. Demonstration of direct involvement of cytokines in graft-versus-host reaction using an in vitro human skin explant model, *Bone Marrow Transplant.*, **7** (1991) 209–216.
13. Antin JH, Ferrara JLM. Cytokine dysregulation and acute graft-versus-host disease, *Blood*, **80** (1992) 2964–2968.
14. Carayol G, Bourhis J-H, Guillard M, et al. Quantitative analysis of T helper 1, T helper 2, and inflammatory cytokine expression in patients after allogeneic bone marrow transplantation, *Transplantation*, **63** (1997) 1307–1313.
15. Dumler J, Beschorner W, Farmer E, et al. Endothelial-cell injury in cutaneous acute graft-versus-host disease, *Am. J. Pathol.*, **135** (1989) 1097–1103.
16. Murray A, Schechner J, Epperson D, et al. Dermal microvascular injury in the human peripheral blood lymphocyte reconstituted-severe combined immunodeficient (HuPBL-SCID) mouse/skin allograft model is T cell mediated and inhibited by a combination of cyclosporine and rapamycin, *Am. J. Pathol.*, **153** (1998) 627–638.
17. Sackstein R. Lymphocyte migration following bone marrow transplantation, *Ann. NY Acad. Sci.*, **770** (1995) 177–188.
18. Sackstein R and Borenstein M. The effects of corticosteroids on lymphocyte recirculation in humans:

analysis of the mechanism of impaired lymphocyte migration to lymph node following methylprednis-olone administration, *J. Invest. Med.*, **43** (1995) 68–77.

19. Sviland L, Pearson A, Green M, et al. Prognostic importance of histological and immunopathological assessment of skin and rectal biopsies in patients with GVHD, *Bone Marrow Transplant.*, **11** (1993) 215–218.

20. Billingham R. The biology of graft-versus-host reaction, *Harvey Lect.*, **62** (1966) 21–78.

21. Fischer A, Beschorner W, Hess A. Syngeneic graft-versus-host disease: failure of autoregulation in self/non-self discrimination, **20** (1988) 493–500.

22. Woodruff J, Hansen J, Good R, et al. The pathology of the graft-versus-host reaction (GVHR) in adults receiving bone marrow transplants, *Transplant. Proc.*, **8** (1976) 675–684.

23. Horn T, Bauer D, Vogelsang G, Hess A. Reappraisal of histological features of the acute cutaneous graft-versus-host reaction based on an allogeneic rodent model, *J. Invest. Dermatol.*, **103** (1994) 206–210.

24. Lampert I, Janossy G, Suitters A, et al. Immunological analysis of the skin in graft-versus-host disease, *Clin. Exp. Immunol.*, **50** (1982) 123–131.

25. Kaye V, Neumann P, Kersey J, et al. Identity of immune cells in graft-versus-host disease of the skin, *Am. J. Pathol.*, **116** (1984) 436–440.

26. Takata M, Imai T, Hirone T. Immunoelectron microscopy of acute graft-versus-host disease of the skin after allogeneic bone marrow transplantation, *J. Clin. Pathol.*, **46** (1993) 801–805.

27. Rhoades J, Cibull M, Thompson J, et al. Role of natural killer cells in the pathogenesis of human acute graft-versus-host disease, *Transplantation*, **56** (1993) 113–120.

28. Korngold R and Sprent J. Lethal graft-versus-host disease after bone marrow transplantation across minor histocompatibility barriers in mice, *J. Exp. Med.*, **148** (1978) 1687–1698.

29. Thomas J, Wakeling W, Imrie S, et al. Chimerism in skin of bone marrow transplant recipients, *Transplantation*, **38** (1984) 475–478.

30. Chong A-F, Scuderi P, Grimes W, Hersh E. Tumor targets stimulate IL-2 activated killer cells to produce interferon-γ and tumor necrosis factor, *J. Immunol.*, **142** (1989) 2133–2138.

31. Xun C, Brown S, Jennings C, et al. Acute graft-versus-host-like disease induced by transplantation of human activated natural killer cells into SCID mice, *Transplantation*, **56** (1993) 409–417.

32. Ferrara J, Guillen F, van Dijken P, et al. Evidence that large granular lymphocytes of donor origin mediate acute graft-versus-host disease, *Transplantation*, **47** (1989) 50–54.

33. Rowbottom A, Norton J, Riches P, et al. Cytokine gene expression in skin and lymphoid organs in graft-versus-host disease, *J. Clin. Pathol.*, **46** (1993) 341–345.

34. Carlos T and Harlan J. Leukocyte–endothelial adhesion molecules, *Blood*, **84** (1994) 2068–2101.

35. Norton J, Sloane J, Al-Saffar N, Haskard D. Vessel associated adhesion molecules in normal skin and acute graft-versus-host disease, *J. Clin. Pathol.*, **44** (1991) 586–591.

36. Chin Y-H, Sackstein R, Cai J-P. Lymphocyte-homing receptors and preferential migration pathways, *Proc. Soc. Exp. Biol. Med.*, **196** (1991) 374–380.

37. Stamper H and Woodruff J. Lymphocyte homing into lymph nodes: in vitro demonstration of the selective affinity of recirculating lymphocytes for high endothelial venules, *J. Exp. Med.*, **144** (1976) 828–833.

38. Sackstein R. Physiologic migration of lymphocytes to lymph nodes following bone marrow transplant-ation: role in immune recovery, *Semin. Oncol.*, **20** (1993) 34–39.

39. Sackstein R, Falanga V, Streilein J, Chin Y. Lymphocyte adhesion to psoriatic dermal endothelium is mediated by a tissue-specific receptor/ligand interaction, *J. Invest. Dermatol.*, **91** (1988) 423–428.

40. Thomas E, Buckner C, Banaji M, et al. One hundred patients with acute leukemia treated by chemotherapy, total body irradiation, and allogeneic marrow transplantation, *Blood*, **49** (1977) 511–533.

41. Lazarus H, Coccia P, Herzig R, et al. Incidence of acute graft-versus-host disease with and without methotrexate prophylaxis in bone marrow transplant patients, *Blood*, **64** (1984) 215–220.

42. Elfenbein G, Goedert T, Graham-Pole J, et al. Is prophylaxis against acute graft-versus-host disease necessary if treatment is effective and survival not impaired, *Proc. Am. Soc. Clin. Oncol.*, **5** (1986) 643a.

43. Sullivan K, Deeg H, Sanders J, et al. Hyperacute graft-versus-host disease in patients not given immunosuppression after allogeneic marrow transplant, *Blood*, **67** (1986) 1172–1175.

44. Storb R, Deeg H, Farewell V, et al. Marrow transplantation for severe aplastic anemia: methotrexate

alone compared with a combination of methotrexate and cyclosporine for prevention of acute graft-versus-host disease, *Blood*, **68** (1986) 119–125.

45. Storb R, Deeg HF, Farewell V, et al. Methotrexate and cyclosporine compared with cyclosporine alone for prophylaxis of acute graft-versus-host disease after marrow transplantation for leukemia, *N. Eng. J. Med.*, **314** (1986) 729–735.

46. Beatty PG, Clift FM, Mickelson BB, et al. Marrow transplantation from related donors other than HLA-identical siblings, *N. Engl. J. Med.*, **313** (1985) 765–771.

47. Kernan N, Bartsch G, Ash R, et al. Analysis of 462 transplantations from unrelated donors facilitated by the National Marrow Donor Program, *N. Engl. J. Med.*, **328** (1993) 593–602.

48. Chao N, Schmidt C, Nilan J, et al. Cyclosporine, methotrexate and prednisone compare with cyclosporine and prednisone for prophylaxis of acute graft-versus-host disease, *N. Engl. J. Med.*, **329** (1993) 1225–1230.

49. Hebart H, Ehninger G, Schmidt H, et al. Treatment of steroid-resistant graft-versus-host disease after allogeneic bone marrow transplantation with anti-CD3/TCR monoclonal antibodies, *Bone Marrow Transplant.*, **6** (1995) 891–894.

50. Ratanatharathorn V, Nash R, Przepiorka D, et al. Phase III study comparing methotrexate and tracrolimus (Prograf FK506) with methotrexate and cyclosporine for graft-versus-host disease prophylaxis after HLA-identical sibling bone marrow transplantation, *Blood*, **7** (1998) 2303–2314.

51. Nash R, Antin J, Karanes C, et al. Phase III study comparing tacrolimus (FK506) with cyclosporine (CSP) for prophylaxis of acute graft-versus-host disease (GVHD) after marrow transplantation from unrelated donors, *Blood*, **90** (1997) 561a.

52. Verdonck L, de Gast G, van Heugten H, Dekker A. A fixed low number of T cells in HLA-identical allogeneic bone marrow transplantation, *Blood*, **75** (1990) 776–780.

53. Verdonck L, Dekker A, deGast G, et al. Allogeneic bone marrow transplantation with a fixed low number of T cells in the marrow graft, *Blood*, **83** (1994) 3090–3096.

54. Martin P, Hansen J, Torok-Storb B, et al. Graft-failure in patients receiving T-cell-depleted HLA-identical allogeneic bone marrow transplants, *Bone Marrow Transplant.*, **3** (1988) 445–456.

55. Butturini A, Gale R. T-cell depletion in bone marrow transplants for leukemia: current results and future directions, *Bone Marrow Transplant.*, **3** (1988) 185–192.

56. Marmont A, Horowitz M, Gale R, et al. T-cell depletion of HLA-identical transplants in leukemia, *Blood*, **78** (1991) 2120–2130.

57. Passweg J, Tiberghien P, Cahn J, et al. Graft-versus-leukemia effects in T lineage and B lineage acute lymphoblastic leukemia, *Bone Marrow Transplant.*, **21** (1998) 153–158.

58. Champlin R, Ho W, Gajewski J, et al. Selective depletion of CD8[+] T lymphocytes for prevention of graft-versus-host disease after allogeneic bone marrow transplantation, *Blood*, **76** (1990) 418–423.

59. Ash RC, Casper J, Menitove J, et al. Successful allogeneic marrow transplants utilizing HLA-closely matched unrelated donors, *N. Engl. J. Med.*, **322** (1990) 487–494.

60. Henslee-Downey PJ, Abhyankar SH, Parrish RS, et al. Use of partially mismatched related donors extends access to allogeneic marrow transplant, *Blood*, **89** (1997) 3864–3872.

61. Spitzer T. Allogeneic peripheral blood stem cell transplantation, *J. Infusion Chemother.*, **6** (1996) 33–37.

62. Dreger P, Haferlach T, Eckstein V, et al. G-CSF-mobilized peripheral blood progenitor cells for allogeneic transplantation: safety, kinetics of mobilization, and composition of the graft, *Br. J. Haematol.*, **87** (1994) 609–613.

63. Tjonnfjord G, Steen R, Evensen S, et al. Characterization of CD34[+] peripheral blood cells from healthy adults mobilized by recombinant human granulocyte colony-stimulating factor, *Blood*, **84** (1994) 2795–2801.

64. Bensinger W, Weaver C, Appelbaum F, et al. Transplantation of allogeneic peripheral blood stem cells mobilized by recombinant human granulocyte colony-stimulating factor, *Blood*, **85** (1995) 1655–1658.

65. Storek F, Gooley T, Siadak M, et al. Allogeneic peripheral blood stem cell transplantation may be associated with a high risk of chronic graft-versus-host disease, *Blood*, **90** (1997) 4705–4709.

66. Scott M, Gandhi M, Jestice H, et al. A trend towards an increased incidence of chronic graft-versus-host disease following allogeneic peripheral blood progenitor cell transplantation: a case controlled study, *Bone Marrow Transplant.*, **22** (1998) 273–276.

67. Aversa F, Tabilio A, Terenzi A, et al. Successful engraftment of T-cell depleted haploidentical "three loci" incompatible transplants in leukemia patients by addition of recombinant human granulocyte

colony-stimulating factor-mobilized peripheral blood progenitor cells to bone marrow inoculum, *Blood*, **84** (1994) 3948–3955.

68. Porter DL, Roth MS, McGarigle C, et al. Induction of graft-versus-host disease as immunotherapy for relapsed chronic myeloid leukemia, *N. Engl. J. Med.*, **330** (1994) 100–106.

69. Baurmann H, Nagel S, Binder T, et al. Kinetics of the graft-versus-leukemia response after donor leukocyte infusions for relapsed chronic myeloid leukemia after allogeneic bone marrow transplantation, *Blood*, **92** (1998) 3582–3590.

70. Schn L, JII A, Weller E, et al. Outcome following T-cell depleted (TCD) versus non-T-cell depleted (non TCD) allogeneic bone marrow transplantation (allo-BMT) for chronic myelogenous leukemia (CML): impact of donor lymphocyte infusions (DLI), *Blood*, **90** (1997) 228a.

71. Alyea E, Soiffer R, Canning C, et al. Toxicity and efficacy of defined doses of CD4(+) donor lymphocytes for treatment of relapse after allogeneic bone marrow transplant, *Blood*, **91** (1998) 3671–3680.

72. Van Rhee F, Feng L, Cullis J, et al. Relapse of chronic myeloid leukemia after allogeneic bone marrow transplantation: the case for giving donor leukocyte infusions before the onset of hematologic relapse, *Blood*, **83** (1994) 3377–3383.

73. Barrett A, Mavroudis D, Tisdale J, et al. T-cell-depleted bone marrow transplantation and delayed T cell add back to control acute GVHD and conserve a graft-versus-leukemia effect, *Bone Marrow Transplant.*, **21** (1998) 543–541.

74. Petz LD, Yam P, Wallace BR, et al. Mixed hematopoietic chimerism following bone marrow transplantation for hematologic malignancies, *Blood*, **70** (1987) 1331–1337.

75. Sykes N, Sharabi Y, Sachs D. Achieving alloengraftment without graft-versus-host disease: approaches using mixed allogeneic bone marrow transplantation, *Bone Marrow Transplant.*, **3** (1988) 379–386.

76. Sharabi Y, Abraham VS, Sykes M, Sachs DH. Mixed allogeneic chimeras prepared by a nonmyeloablative regimen: requirement for chimerism to maintain tolerance, *Bone Marrow Transplant.*, **9** (1992) 191–197.

77. Huss R, Deeg JH, Gooley T, et al. Effect of mixed chimerism on graft-versus-host disease, disease recurrence and survival after HLA-identical marrow transplantation for aplastic anemia or chronic myelogenous leukemia, *Bone Marrow Transplant.*, **18** (1996) 767–776.

78. Suttorp M, Schmitz N, Dreger P, et al. Monitoring of chimerism after allogeneic bone marrow transplantation with unmanipulated marrow by use of DNA polymophisms, *Leukemia*, **7** (1993) 679–687.

79. Socie G, Lawler M, Gluckman E, et al. Studies on hemopoietic chimerism following allogeneic bone marrow transplantation in the molecular biology era, *Leukemia Res.*, **19** (1995) 467–504.

80. Hagglund L, Bostom L, Remberger M, et al. Risk factors for acute graft-versus-host disease in 291 consecutive HLA-identical bone marrow transplant recipients, *Bone Marrow Transplant.*, **16** (1995) 747–755.

81. Hill RS, Pertersen FB, Storb R, et al. Mixed hematologic chimerism allogeneic marrow transplantation for severe aplastic anemia is associated with a higher risk of graft rejection and a lessened incidence of acute graft-versus-host disease, *Blood*, **67** (1986) 811–816.

82. Roy DC, Tantravaho R, Murray C, et al. Natural history of mixed chimerism after bone marrow transplantation with CD6-depleted allogeneic marrow: a stable equilibrium, *Blood*, **75** (1990) 296–304.

83. Bertheas MF, Lafage P, Levy M, et al. Influence of mixed chimerism on the results of allogeneic bone marrow transplantation for leukemia, *Blood*, **78** (1991) 3103–3106.

84. Sykes M, Sheard MA, Sachs DH. Graft-versus-host-related immunosuppression induced in mixed chimeras by alloresponses against either host or donor lymphohematopoietic cells, *J. Exp. Med.*, **168** (1988) 2391–2397.

85. Ildstad ST, Wren SM, Bluestone JA, et al. Effect of selective T-cell depletion of host and/or donor bone marrow lymphopoietic repopulation, tolerance, and graft-versus-host disease in mixed allogeneic chimeras (B10 + B10.D2-B10), *J. Immunol.*, **136** (1986) 28–33.

86. Sykes M, Szot GL, Swenson K, Pearson DA. Induction of high levels of allogeneic hematopoietic reconstitution and donor specific tolerance without myelosuppressive conditioning, *Nature Med.*, **3** (1997) 783–788.

86a. Pelot MR, Pearson D, Swenson K, et al. Lymphohematopoietic graft-vs.-host reactions can be induced without graft-vs.-host disease in murine mixed chimeras established with a cyclophosphamide-based nonmyeloablative conditioning regimen, *Biol. Blood Marrow Transplant.* **5** (1999) 133–143.

87. Sykes M, Preffer F, Saidman SL, et al. Mixed Lymphohematopoietic chimerism is achievable following non-myeloablative therapy and HLA-mismatched donor marrow transplantation, *Lancet,* **353** (1999) 1755–1759.

88. Giralt SE, E., Albitar M, Van Besien K, et al. Engraftment of allogeneic hematopoietic progenitor cells with purine analog-containing chemotherapy: Harnessing graft-versus-leukemia without myeloablative therapy, *Blood,* **89** (1997) 4531–4536.

89. Slavin S, Nagler A, Naparstek E, et al. Nonmyeloablative stem cell transplantation and cell therapy as an alternative to conventional bone marrow transplantation with lethal cytoreduction for the treatment of malignant and nonmalignant hematologic diseases, *Blood,* **91** (1998) 756–763.

90. Khouri IF, Keating M, Korbling M, et al. Transplant-Lite: Induction of graft-versus-malignancy using fludarabine-based nonablative chemotherapy and allogeneic blood progenitor-cell transplantation as treatment for lymphoid malignancies, *J. Clin. Oncol.,* **16** (1998) 2817–2824.

91. Ildstad ST and Sachs DH. Reconstitution with syngeneic plus allogeneic or xenogeneic bone marrow leads to specific acceptance of allografts or xenografts, *Nature,* **30** (1984) 168–170.

92. Suzuki T, Sundt M, Kortz E, et al. Bone marrow transplantation across an MHC barrier in miniature swine, *Transplant. Proc.,* **21** (1989) 3076–3078.

93. Sykes M, Abraham V, Harty W, Pearson D. IL-2 reduces graft-versus-host disease and preserves a graft-versus-leukemia effect by selectively inhibiting CD4+ T cell activity, *J. Immunol.,* **150** (1993) 197–205.

94. Sykes M, Harty W, Szot G, Pearson D. Interleukin-2 inhibits graft-versus-host disease promoting activity of CD4+ cells while preserving CD4 and CD8-mediated graft-versus-leukemia effects, *Blood,* **83** (1994) 2560–2569.

95. Sykes M, Szot G, Nguyen P, Pearson D. Interleukin-12 inhibits murine graft-versus-host disease, *Blood,* **86** (1995) 2429–2438.

96. Muraoka S, Miller R. Cells in bone marrow and in T cell colonies grown from bone marrow can suppress generation of cytotoxic T-lymphocytes directed against their self antigens, *J. Exp. Med.,* **1152** (1980) 54–71.

97. Uberti J, Martillotti F, Chou T, Kaplan J. Human lymphokine activated killer (LAK) cells suppress generation of allospecific cytotoxic T cells: implications for use of LAK cells to prevent graft-versus-host disease in allogeneic bone marrow transplantation, *Blood,* **79** (1992) 261–268.

98. Schmidt-Wolfe I, Dejbakhsh-Jones J, Ginzton N, et al. T-cell subsets and suppressor cells in human bone marrow, *Blood,* **80** (1992) 3242–3250.

99. Deeg H, Henslee-Downey P. Management of acute graft-versus-host disease, *Bone Marrow Transplant.,* **6** (1990) 1–8.

100. Lazarus H, Vogelsang G, Rowe J. Prevention and treatment of acute graft-versus-host disease: the old and new. A report from the Eastern Cooperative Oncology Group (ECOG), *Bone Marrow Transplant.,* **19** (1997) 577–600.

101. Doney K, Weiden P, Storb R, Thomas E. Treatment of graft-versus-host disease in human allogeneic marrow graft recipients: a randomized trial comparing antithymocyte globulin and corticosteroids, *Am. J. Hematol.,* **11** (1981) 1–8.

102. Kennedy M, Deeg J, Strob R, et al. Treatment of acute graft-versus-host disease after allogeneic marrow transplantation, *Am. J. Med.,* **78** (1985) 978–983.

103. Oblon D, Elfenbein G, Goedert M, et al. Successful therapy of acute graft-versus-host disease (aGVHD) with high dose methyl-prednisolone (MP), *Proc. Am. Assoc. Cancer Res.,* **29** (1988) 182a.

104. Hings I, Filipovich A, Miller W, et al. Prednisone therapy for acute graft-versus-host disease: short- versus long-term treatment. A prospective randomized trial, *Transplantation,* **56** (1993) 577–580

105. Przepiorka D, Phillips G, Ratanatharathorn V, et al. Phase II study of BT1-322, a monoclonal anti-CD2 antibody, for treatment of steroid-resistant acute graft-versus-host disease, *Blood,* **92** (1998) 4066–4071.

106. Holler E, Kolb H, Mittermuller J, et al. Modulation of acute graft-versus-host disease after bone marrow transplantation by tumor necrosis factor alpha (TNF-alpha) release in the course of pretransplant conditioning: role of conditioning regimens and prophylactic application of a monoclonal antibody neutralizing human TNF-alpha (MAK 195F), *Blood,* **86** (1995) 890–899.

107. Colby C, Sykes M, Sachs DH, Spitzer TR. Cellular modulation of acute graft-versus-host disease, *Biol. Blood Bone Marrow Transplant.,* **3** (1997) 287–293.

108. Mehta J, Powles R, Singhal S, Horton C, Treleaven J. Outcome of autologous rescue after failed engraftment of allogeneic marrow, *Bone Marrow Transplant.*, **17** (1996) 213–217.
109. Ricordi C, Tzakis AG, Zeevi A, et al. Reversal of graft-versus-host disease with infusion of autologous bone marrow, *Cell Transplant.*, **3** (1994) 187–192.
110. Mehta J, Sighal S, Fassas A, et al. Autologous marrow infusion without further conditioning for life threatening GVHD: resolution of GVHD with persistent donor-type chimerism, *Blood*, **90(Suppl 1)** (1997) 372a.
111. Cohen J, Boyer O, Salomon B, et al. Prevention of graft-versus-host disease in mice using a suicide gene expressed in T lymphocytes, *Blood*, **89** (1997) 4636–4645.
112. Bonini C, Ciceri F, Marktel S, Bordignon C. Suicide-gene transduced T-cells for the regulation of the graft-versus-leukemia effect, *Vox Sang.*, **74** (1998) 341–343.
113. Sullivan K, Witherspoon R, Storb R. Alternating-day cyclosporine and prednisone for treatment of high-risk chronic graft-versus-host disease, *Blood*, **72** (1988) 555–561.
114. Vogelsang G, Hess A, Santos G. Thalidomide for treatment of graft-versus-host disease, *Bone Marrow Transplant.*, **3** (1988) 393–398.
115. Basara N, Blau W, Romer E, et al. Mycophenolate mofetil for the treatment of acute and chronic GVHD in bone marrow transplant patients, *Bone Marrow Transplant.*, **22** (1998) 61–65.
116. Bullorsky E, Shanley C, Stemmelin G, et al. Total lymphoid irradiation for treatment of drug resistant chronic GVHD, *Bone Marrow Transplant.*, **11** (1993) 75–76.
117. Owsianowski M, Gollnick H, Siegert W, et al. Successful treatment of chronic graft-versus-host disease with extracorporeal photopheresis, *Bone Marrow Transplant.*, **14** (1994) 845–848.
118. Lee S, Wegner S, McGarigle C, et al. Treatment of chronic graft-versus-host disease with clofazimine, *Blood*, **89** (1997) 2298–2302.

18 Veno-occlusive Disease of the Liver

Does Anything Really Work?

Scott I. Bearman, MD

CONTENTS

1. INTRODUCTION

Veno-occlusive disease (VOD) of the liver is the most common and serious regimen-related toxicity following stem cell transplantation (SCT). Injury to zone 3 structures of the liver acinus by high-dose chemotherapy or chemoradiotherapy produces a clinical syndrome of jaundice, right upper quadrant pain or hepatomegaly, and fluid retention *(1,2)*. There is considerable variability in the incidence of VOD, but most reports agree that 25–50% of patients who develop VOD die within 100 d of transplant. This chapter reviews strategies for prevention and treatment of this syndrome.

2. CLINICAL FEATURES OF VOD

Hepatomegaly and/or right upper quadrant pain and fluid retention are the first signs of VOD, and occur on or around d 0 *(3)*. Jaundice usually develops 5–6 d

From: *Current Controversies in Bone Marrow Transplantation*
Edited by: B. Bolwell © Humana Press Inc., Totowa, NJ

posttransplant. Ascites and encephalopathy, which are more common in patients with severe disease, usually develop 12–14 d after transplant *(3)*. The mean maximal bilirubin (Bil) and percent weight gain are significantly greater in patients who develop severe VOD, compared with mild or moderate illness *(3)*. The rate of rise in weight and Bil can discriminate patients with severe disease from those with self-limited illness *(4)*.

Significant fluid retention appears to distinguish patients likely to develop multiorgan failure from those with mild or moderate VOD. For example, ascites occurs in fewer than 20% of patients with mild or moderate VOD, compared with 48% of patients with severe VOD *(3)*. Sodium retention, followed by peripheral edema, pulmonary infiltrates, hypoxemia, and congestive heart failure, are common and early manifestations in patients who go on to develop multiorgan failure. Blostein et al. *(5)* reported that patients who met the Baltimore criteria for VOD (jaundice, hepatomegaly, and fluid retention) had a 75% case-fatality rate, compared to a 28% case-fatality rate for patients who met Seattle criteria for VOD (jaundice, hepatomegaly or fluid retention). The author et al. *(4)* developed a model to predict which patients would die of VOD, based on the rate of rise in their Bil and weight. The probability of developing fatal VOD can be estimated by the following equation:

$$p = 1/(1 + e^{-z})$$

where $z = b_0 + b_1$ (in total serum Bil) $+ b_2$ (percent weight gain). Thus, the probability of dying, at least in the early posttransplant period, is sensitive to small changes in weight *(4)*.

The incidence of VOD in large published series is variable, ranging from 1 to 54% *(6)*. Recently, Carreras et al. *(7)* reported an incidence of 5.3% among 1652 transplants performed in 72 centers of the European Group for Blood and Marrow Transplantation. The broad range of reported incidence reflects disparity in the definition of VOD, differences in preparative regimens, and the patient selection. Risk factors for VOD include allotransplantation *(7)*, particularly mismatched grafts *(3)*, elevated aspartate aminotransferase (AST) *(1,2,7)*, high-dose cytoreductive therapy *(1,2,7)*, previous abdominal radiotherapy *(6–8)*, liver metastases *(8,9)*, and a Karnofsky performance score of <90% *(7)*.

3. PATHOLOGIC FEATURES

There is a spectrum of histopathologic changes in patients with VOD. These changes are centered in zone 3 of the liver acinus, and are characterized by hepatic venular occlusion or eccentric venular luminal narrowing, phlebosclerosis, sinusoidal fibrosis, and necrosis of hepatocytes *(10)*. Although hepatic venular occlusion is not necessary for the clinical diagnosis of VOD, most tissue samples exhibit this finding. The number of zone 3 changes strongly correlates with the severity of illness *(10)*.

Immunohistochemical staining shows deposition of fibrinogen and factor VIII in vessel walls, at the interface of hepatic sinusoids and terminal hepatic venules *(10,11)*. This observation is the basis for prophylaxis with heparin, and for treatment with recombinant human tissue plasminogen activator (TPA) or antithrombin III.

Table 1
Agents Studied to Prevent VOD of Liver

Agent (refs.)	Author's conclusions
Heparin (12–15)	Not effective, certainly not in high-risk patients.
Prostaglandin E₁ (16,17)	Possibly effective, but too toxic to use.
Pentoxifylline (18–23)	Not effective.
Ursodeoxycholic acid (25)	Possibly effective, definitely needs to be studied further.

4. PROPHYLAXIS OF VOD

A number of agents have been studied to prevent VOD after SCT, including heparin *(12–15)*, prostaglandin E_1 (PGE₁) *(16,17)*, pentoxifylline *(18–23)*, and ursodeoxycholic acid *(24)*. There is considerable disagreement about the efficacy of these agents or, at least, their mechanism of action (Table 1).

4.1. Heparin

Heparin was the first agent to be studied for prevention of VOD. The rationale for its use was the observation by Shulman et al. *(10)* that clotting material was deposited in subendothelial zones of affected venules and sinusoids. The author et al. conducted a dose-escalation study of heparin in 28 patients considered to be at high risk for VOD. Heparin was dosed to produce varying degrees of prolongation in the activated partial thromboplastin time (APTT). In this study, the degree of prolongation of the APTT ranged from <1.2 to 2 × the upper limit of normal. The overall incidence of VOD was 70%; 14% of patients developed severe VOD. There were no differences between groups of patients treated at doses to produce different degrees of APTT prolongation, or among patients treated for different periods of time. Two patients who were treated to produce an APTT of 1.5–2 × the upper limit of normal developed significant hemorrhagic complications, but survived treatment. The author et al. concluded that heparin was ineffective prophylaxis for high-risk patients. In the recent prospective study of Carreras et al. *(7)*, 335 patients received heparin prophylaxis. The incidence of VOD in those patients was 7.5%; the incidence of VOD in 660 patients who did not receive VOD prophylaxis was 4.7%. This difference was not statistically significant.

Attal et al. *(13)* performed a prospective randomized trial of heparin in 161 patients undergoing SCT. There was no differences in death caused by VOD, although nonfatal VOD occurred in 2.5% of heparin-treated patients, compared with 13.7% of untreated patients. Few patients in that trial were at high risk for VOD.

Marsa-Vila et al. *(14)* randomized a subset of patients within a larger prospective trial. In their randomized cohort, those who received heparin actually developed more VOD (7.7%) than patients randomized not to receive heparin (2.2%). More recently, Or et al. *(15)* randomized 61 patients to receive low-mol-wt heparin or placebo, from before conditioning until d 40 posttransplant. Hemorrhagic events occurred less frequently, and platelet transfusion requirements were lower in the low-mol-wt heparin-treated patients. The incidence of VOD manifestations (hyperbilirubinemia, hepatomegaly, right upper quadrant pain, weight gain, ascites) were not different between the two groups, although the duration of hyperbilirubinemia and hepatomegaly was greater in the placebo-treated group.

Does heparin prevent VOD? Unlikely.

4.2. Prostaglandin E_1

PGE_1 produces vasodilatation, inhibits platelet aggregation, and activates thrombolysis, making it an appealing drug to prevent VOD. Two studies have evaluated PGE_1 for VOD prophylaxis, one of which concluded that it was effective (16), and the other concluded that it was probably ineffective, and very toxic (17). Gluckman et al. (16) treated 50 leukemic patients with 250 mg/d (children) or 500 mg/d (adults) from the start of preparative therapy (cyclophosphamide plus 10 Gy total body irradiation) until d 30 posttransplant. They compared the results in these 50 patients with a control group treated at the same time, who did not receive PGE_1. This was not a randomized trial. Mild or moderate VOD occurred in 12.2% of PGE_1-treated patients and 25.5% of control patients. In high-risk patients, i.e., those with previous hepatitis, VOD occurred in 15.5% of treated patients and 62.5% of controls. No significant toxicities were reported.

The author et al. (17) studied PGE_1 in a group of 24 high-risk patients, starting at a dose of 10 ng/kg/min, roughly double the dose used by Gluckman et al. for an 80 kg patient. Significant toxicity, manifesting as hypotension, edema, bullae, and pain in dependent extremities, was observed, which required serial reductions in dose, to a final dose of 1.25 ng/kg/min. The author et al. concluded that PGE_1 was too toxic to use, but we did observe several patients whose PGE_1 was stopped because of toxicity, and whose signs of VOD worsened when the drug was discontinued. Twenty-two patients in the series of Carreras et al. (7) received PGE_1-prophylaxis. Their incidence of VOD was 9.1%, compared to 4.7% in unprophylaxed patients.

Does PGE_1 work? Maybe, but it is too toxic to use.

4.3. Pentoxifylline

Pentoxifylline is a methylxanthine analog that inhibits transcription of tumor necrosis factor α (TNF-α) (18). Several investigators (19,20) had implicated TNF-α in the pathogenesis of VOD and other toxicities. Pentoxifylline, therefore, seemed a logical choice. After the initial publication (21), it was thought pentoxifylline would revolutionize the practice of marrow transplantation, because it would eliminate serious regimen-related toxicities (RRTs). This enthusiasm soon wore off after two randomized trials conducted in the United States and Europe (22,23) demonstrated that pentoxifylline was ineffective in preventing RRTs.

Does pentoxifylline work? No.

4.5. Ursodeoxycholic Acid

The mechanism of action of ursodeoxycholic acid (ursodiol) in preventing VOD is unclear. Ursodiol is a hydrophilic bile acid that comprises about 1% of the total bile acid pool (25). In primary biliary cirrhosis, it is believed to protect hepatocytes from the more prevalent and more toxic, naturally occurring hydrophobic bile acids. It also increases biliary flow because of its hydrophilic composition. Essell et al. (24) conducted a placebo-controlled, prospective randomized trial of ursodiol in 67 patients prepared for transplant with busulfan and cyclophosphamide, who received cyclosporine plus methotrexate as graft-vs-host disease prophylaxis. VOD occurred in 40% of placebo-

Table 2
Use of Recombinant TPA to Treat VOD

Author (refs.)	N	No. responding (%)	Bleeding (%)	Life-threatening hemorrhage (%)
Bearman et al. (27)	42	12 (29)	37 (88)	10 (24)
Leahey and Bunin (28)	9	5 (56)	3 (33)	0
Hagglund et al. (29)	7	1 (14)	7 (100)	4 (57)
Schriber et al. (30)	45	16 (59)[a]	10 (22)	1 (2)
Total	103	34 (33)	57 (55)	15 (15)

[a]Response rate of 27 patients with established VOD.

treated patients, and in 15% of patients who received ursodiol. One-hundred-d survival was superior for ursodiol-treated patients, although this was not statistically significant. Death caused by VOD was also not statistically different between the two groups.

Does ursodiol work? Maybe. It is unclear whether its effect is physiologic or cosmetic. It needs to be studied further, particularly in patients who receive regimens other than busulfan and cyclophosphamide.

5. TREATMENT OF ESTABLISHED VOD

5.1. Tissue Plasminogen Activator

Baglin et al. (26) first reported, in 1990, using recombinant human tPA for the treatment of an autotransplant recipient with VOD. Since that time, more than 100 patients treated with tPA have been reported in the literature: Most reports have been small series. Table 2 shows the results of tPA treatment in published series with five or more patients (27–30). The response rate to tPA is approx 30%. Most patients bleed during or after treatment with tPA, although it is difficult to distinguish this from the usual amount of minor bleeding after transplant. However, treatment with tPA does pose a risk of life-threatening hemorrhage. In the series by the author et al. (27), of 42 patients, 10 developed significant bleeding, which was fatal in three and may have contributed to death in three more.

Patients with established VOD who have already developed multiorgan dysfunction do not respond to tPA (27). Schriber et al. (30) are studying early treatment with tPA, i.e., when patients are suspected of having VOD, but have not yet met the clinical criteria for VOD. They treated 38 patients with suspected VOD using tPA plus heparin. Twenty patients ultimately met the clinical criteria for VOD; the remainder never developed clinical VOD. The response rate for the 20 patients who were treated prior to meeting the clinical criteria for VOD, but who eventually developed VOD, was 80%. What is unknown is whether tPA was at all responsible for the resolution of VOD in those patients.

Does tPA work? Not for patients with multiorgan dysfunction. Possibly for patients with early disease, although it is unclear whether such patients would have self-limited illness.

5.2. Corticosteroids

Because of the potential role of cytokines in the pathogenesis of VOD, Khoury et al. (31) treated 28 patients with liver dysfunction after SCT using high-dose corticosteroids.

Patients received 500 mg/kg of methylprednisolone every 12 h for six doses after their Bil reached or exceeded 4 mg/dL. Sixty-one percent of patients with VOD or liver dysfunction of unknown etiology responded, as defined by a 50% reduction in Bil within 10 d. There were no differences in the probability of death caused by VOD *(4)* between responders and nonresponders: 16.5 and 23%, respectively. The only factor distinguishing responders from nonresponders was a lower pretransplant diffusion capacity of carbon monoxide (DLCO) in nonresponders. One-hundred-d survival for responding patients was 76%.

Do corticosteroids work? Possibly. A randomized trial is warranted.

5.3. Transjugular Intrahepatic Portosystemic Shunt

In a transjugular intrahepatic portosystemic shunt (TIPS) procedure, a percutaneously inserted catheter creates a channel between the hepatic and portal veins, and is kept patent using a metal stent *(32)*. TIPS has been used successfully in patients with cirrhosis and bleeding esophageal varices, intractable ascites, and the Budd-Chiari syndrome. Nine patients with VOD, who were treated with TIPS, have been described in the literature *(32–36)*.

In responding patients, TIPS results in a prompt reduction in ascites, jaundice, and coagulopathy *(32–36)*. Fried et al. *(34)* reported a fall in the mean portal pressure gradient from 20.2 ± 4.6 mmHg, prior to TIPS, to 6.7 ± 1.9 mmHg after the procedure *(34)*. The mean Bil prior to TIPS was 31.4 mg/dL in three nonresponding patients, and 10.7 mg/dL in three responders *(34)*. Two responding patients subsequently died, and tissue was available to compare histologic findings before and after TIPS. Significant improvement in sinusoidal congestion and hepatocyte necrosis was seen in both patients. In one, there was also resolution of venular occlusion *(34)*. TIPS has great appeal for patients with VOD: It does not require an open surgical procedure, and any bleeding that results (except capsular perforation) is intravascular.

Does TIPS work? Possibly. For patients without significant fluid retention and ascites, TIPS probably has no value. Chronic encephalopathy after TIPS is problematic.

5.4. Other Surgical Procedures

Several patients have undergone surgical portosystemic shunts to treat VOD. No large series have been reported. A patient who developed VOD after azathioprine therapy of renal graft rejection was treated using an end-to-side portacaval shunt. She was alive 8 mo after surgery *(37)*. Two additional patients, who were successfully treated with splenorenal or side-to-side portacaval shunts, have been reported *(38,39)*. Given that patients with severe VOD are profoundly thrombocytopenic, and usually have evidence of coagulopathy, the risk of such an approach is enormous.

Nine patients have undergone orthotopic liver transplantation for VOD *(40–46)* (Table 3). Acute rejection occurred in four patients, and progressed to chronic rejection in two. Seven patients have died. Three patients survived more than 9 mo after liver transplant, two of whom were still alive at the time of publication. Difficulties include finding a suitable liver graft, management of multiorgan dysfunction, and prevention of rejection of the liver graft. One patient developed acute graft-vs-host disease caused by cells from the donor liver.

Are surgical procedures worthwhile? Surgical shunting is frought with technical difficulty, and is probably not worthwhile. Orthotopic liver transplantation may be

Table 3
Orthotopic Liver Transplantation for VOD

Author (refs.)	N	Type	Bilirubin (mg/dL)	Day of liver transplant	Rejection	Survival from liver transplant	Comments
Nimer et al. (40)	1	Allo	>50	38	No	>1 yr	Died of recurrent leukemia 16 mo after marrow transplant.
Rapaport et al. (41)	1	Allo	>20	35	Yes	42 d	Died of idiopathic pneumonia.
Schlitt et al. (42)	1	Allo	58.8	23	No	>40 mo	Developed GVHD caused by lymphocytes from donor liver.
Dowlati et al. (43)	1	Allo	58.7	22, 44	Yes	70 d	Underwent second liver transplant after rejection of first liver graft. Died of acute respiration distress syndrome with normally functioning second liver graft.
Bunin et al. (44)	1	Allo	35.6	33	No	>9 mo	Partial liver transplant from mother.
Hägglund et al. (45)	3	Allo	NR	25,36,39	1 of 3	3–213 d	Causes of death: cerebral edema, idiopathic pneumonia, chronic rejection.
Norris et al. (46)	1	Auto	20.7	32	Yes	6 mo	Acute →chronic rejection, died of pneumocystis.

worthwhile from a family donor. Given the enormous costs of such procedures, they should probably be reserved for patients whose underlying disease has a high probability of being cured. There is no data regarding optimal timing.

5.5. Defibrotide

Defibrotide (DF) is the newest agent to be studied for the treatment of VOD. DF is a polydeoxyribonucleotide derived from porcine tissue by controlled depolymerization. It is an A1 and A2 adenosine receptor agonist with antithrombotic, anti-ischemic, anti-inflammatory, and thrombolytic properties (47–49). DF is well-tolerated, with flushing, transient hypotension, abdominal discomfort, and nausea being reported in 1–9% of patients. DF lacks systemic anticoagulant activity.

Richardson et al. (49) treated 19 patients with DF at doses ranging from 10 to 60 mg/kg/d. All patients had multiorgan dysfunction, and seven had failed tPA. The median serum Bil was 22.3 mg/dL at the start of treatment with DF. Patients were started a median of 6 (range 0–47) d after the diagnosis of VOD and 25 (range 10–58) d posttransplant. Eight patients achieved complete responses, as defined by improvement in signs or symptoms of VOD and a decrease in Bil to less than 2 mg/dL. Five of the eight responding patients are alive 138–976 d after the discontinuation of DF. Plasminogen activator inhibitor-1 levels, which are increased in patients with VOD (50), decrease in patients responding to DF (51).

Does DF work? Quite possibly. Further study is needed. Given its minimal toxicity, a prophylaxis study is essential.

6. NEW HORIZONS

The pathogenesis of VOD is complex, and is not only concerned with endothelial injury and hepatocyte necrosis, but also with perturbations in systems modulating tissue injury and fibrosis. Heikinheimo et al. (52) measured levels of the aminoterminal fragment of procollagen type III (PIIINP) levels in 28 children undergoing BMT, seven of whom developed VOD. Levels of PIIINP were significantly higher in the patients with VOD (52). PIIINP levels may rise in VOD patients as early as d 0 (53). In addition, Schuppan et al. (54) have recently reported that levels of tenascin, a marker of lobular fibrogenesis, and tissue inhibitor of metalloproteinases-1, an inhibitor of fibrolysis, became elevated in VOD patients within 1 wk of clinical onset. There have been no clinical trials that have targeted fibrogenesis or fibrolysis to prevent or treat VOD.

7. CONCLUSION

VOD remains the single most important RRT after SCT. It remains disputed whether effective prophylaxis exists. Strategies to treat established disease are effective in less than one-third of patients. Prospective randomized trials of DF for prevention, and corticosteroids for treatment, are needed.

REFERENCES

1. Jones RJ, Lee KSK, Beschorner WE, et al. Venocclusive disease of the liver following bone marrow transplantation, *Transplantation*, **44** (1987) 778–783.
2. Donald GB, Sharma P, Matthews DE, Shulman HM, and Thomas ED. Venocclusive disease of the

liver after bone marrow transplantation: diagnosis, incidence and predisposing factors, *Hepatology*, **4** (1984) 116–22.

3. McDonald GB, Hinds MS, Fisher LD, et al. Veno-occlusive disease of the liver and multiorgan failure after bone marrow transplantation: a cohort study of 355 patients, *Ann. Int. Med.*, **118** (1993) 255–267.

4. Bearman SI, Anderson G, Mori M, Hinds MS, Shulman HM, McDonald GB. Venocclusive disease of the liver. Development of a model for predicting fatal outcome after marrow transplantation, *J. Clin. Oncol.*, **11** (1993) 1729–1736.

5. Blostein MD, Paltiel OB, Thibault A, Rybka WB. A comparison of clinical criteria for the diagnosis of veno-occlusive disease of the liver after bone marrow transplantation, *Bone Marrow Transplant.*, **10** (1992) 439–443.

6. Bearman SI. The syndrome of hepatic veno-occlusive disease after bone marrow transplantation, *Blood*, **85** (1995) 3005–3020.

7. Carreras E, Bertz H, Arcese W, et al. Incidence and outcome of hepatic veno-occlusive disease after blood or marrow transplantation: a prospective cohort study of the European Group for Blood and Marrow Transplantation, *Blood*, **92** (1998) 3599–3604.

8. Lee JL, Gooley T, Bensinger W, Schiffman K, McDonald GB. Venocclusive disease of the liver after high-dose chemotherapy with alkylating agents: incidence, outcome and risk factors, *Hepatology*, **26** (1997) 149A.

9. Ayash LJ, Hunt MN, Antman K, et al. Hepatic venocclusive disease in autologous bone marrow transplantation of solid tumors and lymphomas, *J. Clin. Oncol.*, **8** (1990) 1699–1706.

10. Shulman HM, Fisher LB, Schoch HG, Kenne KW, McDonald GW. Venocclusive disease of the liver after marrow transplantation: histological correlates of clinical signs and symptoms, *Hepatology*, **19** (1994) 1171–1181.

11. Ganem G, Saint-Marc Giradin M-F, Keuntz M, et al. Venocclusive disease of the liver after allogeneic bone marrow transplantation in man, *Int. J. Radiat. Oncol. Biol. Phys.*, **14** (1988) 879–884.

12. Bearman SI, Hinds MS, Wolford JL, et al. A pilot study of continuous infusion heparin for the prevention of hepatic venocclusive disease after bone marrow transplantation, *Bone Marrow Transplant.*, **5** (1990) 407–411.

13. Attal M, Huguet F, Rubie H, et al. Prevention of hepatic veno-occlusive disease after bone marrow transplantation by continuous infusion of low-dose heparin: a prospective, randomized trial, *Blood*, **79** (1992) 2834–2840.

14. Marsa-Vila L, Gorin NC, Laport JP, et al. Prophylactic heparin does not prevent liver veno-occlusive disease following autologous bone marrow transplantation, *Eur. J. Haematol.*, **47** (1991) 346–354.

15. Or R, Nagler A, Shpilberg O, et al. Low molecular weight heparin for the prevention of veno-occlusive disease of the liver in bone marrow transplant patients, *Transplantation*, **61** (1996) 1067–1071.

16. Gluckman E, Jolivet I, Scrobohaci ML, et al. Use of prostaglandin E1 for prevention of liver veno-occlusive disease in leukaemic patients treated by allogeneic bone marrow transplantation, *Br. J. Haematol.*, **74** (1990) 277–281.

17. Bearman SI, Shen DD, Hinds MS, Hill HA, McDonald GB. A phase I/II study of prostaglandin E1 for the prevention of hepatic venocclusive disease after bone marrow transplantation, *Br. J. Haematol.*, **84** (1993) 724–730.

18. Han J, Thompson P, and Beutler B. Dexamethasone and pentoxifylline inhibit endotoxin-induced cachetin/tumor necrosis factor synthesis at separate points in the signaling pathway, *J. Exp. Med.*, **172** (1990) 391–394.

19. Holler E, Kolb HJ, Moller A, et al. Increased serum levels of tumor necrosis factor a precede major complications of bone marrow transplantation, *Blood*, **75** (1990) 1011–1016.

20. Tanaka J, Imamura M, Kasai M, et al. Rapid analysis of tumor necrosis factor-alpha mRNA expression during venoclusive disease of the liver after allogeneic bone marrow transplantation, *Transplantation*, **55** (1993) 430–432.

21. Bianco JA, Appelbaum FR, Nemunitis J, et al. Phase I–II trial of pentoxifylline for the prevention of transplant-related toxicities following bone marrow transplantation, *Blood*, **78** (1991) 1205–1211.

22. Attal M, Huguet F, Rubie H, et al. Prevention of regimen-related toxicities after bone marrow transplantation by pentoxifylline: a prospective, randomized trial, *Blood*, **82** (1993) 732–736.

23. Clift RA, Bianco JA, Appelbaum FR, et al. Randomized controlled trial of pentoxifylline for the prevention of regimen-related toxicities in patients undergoing allogeneic marrow transplantation, *Blood*, **82** (1993) 2025–2030.

24. Essell JH, Schroeder MT, Harman GS, et al. Ursodiol prophylaxis against hepatic complications of

allogeneic bone marrow transplantation. A randomized, double-blind, placebo-controlled trial, *Ann. Intern. Med.*, **128** (1998) 975–981.

25. Ward A, Brogden RN, Heel RC, Speight TM, Avery GS. Ursodeoxycholic acid: a review of its pharmacological properties and therapeutic efficacy, *Drugs*, **27** (1984) 95–131.

26. Baglin TP, Harper P, and Marcus RE. Veno-occlusive disease of the liver complicating ABMT successfully treated with recombinant tissue plasminogen activator, *Bone Marrow Transplant.*, **5** (1990) 439–441.

27. Bearman SI, Lee JL, Baron AE, and McDonald GB. Treatment of hepatic venocclusive disease with recombinant human tissue plasminogen activator and heparin in 42 marrow transplant patients, *Blood*, **89** (1997) 1501–1506.

28. Leahey AM and Bunin NJ. Recombinant human tissue plasminogen activator for the treatment of severe hepatic veno-occlusive disease in pediatric bone marrow transplant patients, *Bone Marrow Transplant.*, **17** (1996) 1101–1104.

29. Hägglund H, Ringdén O, Ljungman P, Winiarski J, Ericzon B, Tydén G. No beneficial effects, but severe side effects caused by recombinant human tissue plasminogen activator for treatment of hepatic veno-occlusive disease after allogeneic bone marrow transplantation, *Transplant. Proc.*, **27** (1995) 3535.

30. Schriber J, Christiansen N, Baer MR, Slack J, Wetzler M, Herzig G. Tissue plasminogen activator as therapy for hepatotoxicity following bone marrow transplantation, *Blood*, **86(Suppl 1)** (1995) 160.

31. Khoury H, Adkins D, Trinkaus K, et al. Treatment of hepatic veno-occlusive disease with high-dose corticosteroids: an update on 28 stem cell transplant recipients, *Blood*, **92 (Suppl 1)** (1998) 276a.

32. Smith FO, Johnson MS, Scherer LR, et al. Transjugular intrahepatic portosystemic shunting (TIPS) for treatment of severe hepatic veno-occlusive disease, *Bone Marrow Transplant.*, **18** (1996) 643–646.

33. Michielsen PP, Pelckmans PA, d'Archambeau OC, et al. Transjugular intrahepatic portosystemic shunt improves liver function in veno-occlusive disease, *J. Hepatol.*, **21** (1995) 685–686.

34. Fried MW, Connaghan DG, Sharma S, et al. Transjugular intrahepatic portosystemic shunt for the management of severe venocclusive disease following bone marrow transplantation, *Hepatology*, **24** (1996) 588–591.

35. Levy V, Azoulay D, Rio B, et al. Successful treatment of severe hepatic veno-occlusive disease after allogeneic bone marrow transplantation by transjugular intrahepatic portosystemic stent-shunt (TIPS), *Bone Marrow Transplant.*, **18** (1996) 443–445.

36. de la Rubia J, Carral A, Montes H, Urquijo JJ, Sanz GF, Sanz MA. Successful treatment of hepatic veno-occlusive disease in a peripheral blood progenitor cell transplant patient with a transjugular intrahepatic portosystemic stent-shunt (TIPS), *Haematologica*, **81** (1996) 536–539.

37. Eizenhauer T, Hartmann H, Rumpf KW, Helmchen U, Scheler F, and Creutzfeldt W. Favourable outcome of hepatic veno-occlusive disease in a renal transplant patient receiving azathioprine, treated by portacaval shunt, *Digestion*, **30** (1984) 185–190.

38. Jacobson BK and Kalayoglu M. Effective early treatment of hepatic venocclusive disease with a central splenorenal shunt in an infant, *J. Ped. Surg.*, **27** (1992) 531–533.

39. Murray JA, LaBrecque DR, Gingrich RD, Pringle KC, and Mitros KA. Successful treatment of hepatic venocclusive disease in a bone marrow transplant patient with side-to-side portacaval shunt, *Gastroenterology*, **92** (1987) 1073–1077.

40. Nimer SD, Milewicz AL, Champlin RE, and Busuttil RW. Successful treatment of hepatic venocclusive disease in a bone marrow transplant patient with orthotopic liver transplantation, *Transplantation*, **49** (1990) 819–821.

41. Rapoport AP, Doyle HR, Starzl T, Rowe JM, Doeblin T, and DiPersio JF. Orthotopic liver transplantation for life-threatening venocclusive disease of the liver after allogeneic bone marrow transplantation, *Bone Marrow Transplant.*, **8** (1991) 421–424.

42. Schlitt HJ, Tischler JH, Binge B, et al. Allogeneic liver transplantation for hepatic veno-occlusive disease after bone marrow transplantation: clinical and immunological considerations, *Bone Marrow Transplant.*, **16** (1995) 473–478.

43. Dowlati A, Honore P, Damas P, et al. Hepatic rejection after orthotopic liver transplantation for hepatic veno-occlusive disease or graft-versus-host disease following bone marrow transplantation, *Transplantation*, **60** (1995) 106–109.

44. Bunin N, Leahey A, and Dunn S. Related donor liver transplant for veno-occlusive disease following T-depleted unrelated donor bone marrow transplantation, *Transplantation*, **61** (1996) 664.

45. Hägglund H, Ringdén O, Ericzon BG, et al. Treatment of hepatic venocclusive disease with recombinant

human tissue plasminogen activator or orthotopic liver transplantation after allogeneic bone marrow transplantation, *Transplantation*, **62** (1996) 1076–1080.

46. Norris S, Crosbie O, McEntee G, et al. Orthotopic liver transplantation for veno-occlusive disease complicating autologous bone marrow transplantation, *Transplantation*, **63** (1997) 1521–1524.

47. Bianchi G, Barone D, Lanzarotti E, et al. Defibrotide, a single-stranded polydeoxyribonucleotide acting as an adrenergic receptor agonist, *Eur. J. Pharmacol.*, **238** (1993) 327–334.

48. Zhou Q, Chu X, and Ruan C. Defibrotide stimulates expression of thrombomodulin in human endothelial cells, *Thromb. Haemostasis*, **71** (1994) 507–510.

49. Richardson PG, Elias AD, Krishnan A, et al. Treatment of severe veno-occlusive disease with defibrotide: compassionate use results in response without significant toxicity in a high-risk population, *Blood*, **92** (1998) 734–737.

50. Salat C, Holler E, Kolb H-J, et al. Plasminogen activator inhibitor-1 confirms the diagnosis of hepatic veno-occlusive disease in patients with hyperbilirubinemia after bone marrow transplantation, *Blood*, **89** (1997) 2184–2188.

51. Richardson P, Hoppensteadt D, Elias A, et al. Elevation of tissue factor pathway inhibitor, thrombomodulin and plasminogen activator inhibitor-1 levels in stem cell transplant-associated veno-occlusive disease and changes seen with the use of defibrotide, *Blood*, **90(Suppl 1)** (1997) 219a.

52. Heikinheimo M, Halili R, and Fasth A. Serum procollagen type III is an early and sensitive marker for veno-occlusive disease of the liver in children undergoing bone marrow transplantation, *Blood*, **83** (1994) 3036–3040.

53. Rio B, Bauduer F, Arrago JP, and Zittoun R. N-terminal peptide of type III procollagen: a marker for the development of hepatic veno-occlusive disease after BMT and a basis for determining the timing of prophylactic heparin, *Bone Marrow Transplant.*, **11** (1993) 471–472.

54. Schuppan D, Farrand A, Oesterling C, Gehrmann M, and McDonald GB. Circulating markers of hepatic fibrosis predict evolution of venocclusive disease after marrow transplantation, *Hepatol.*, **26** (1997) 452A.

19 Myelodysplasia and Acute Leukemia Following High-Dose Chemotherapy

Dean S. McGaughey, MD,
and James J. Vredenburgh, MD

CONTENTS

1. INTRODUCTION

The widespread and increasing use of high-dose chemotherapy (HDCT) with autologous and allogeneic stem cell support, for an increasing number of malignancies, has

From: *Current Controversies in Bone Marrow Transplantation*
Edited by: B. Bolwell © Humana Press Inc., Totowa, NJ

Table 1
sMDS/sAML Following HDCT and ASCT for Hodgkin's Disease

Ref.	No. patients transplanted	No. patients with sMDS/sAML	Actuarial incidence	Median latency from BMT
2	4998[a]	66[a]	4.6 ± 1.5% (95% CI, 3.2–6.8%) (5 yr)	NA
3	68	3	15.2 ± 18% (5 yr)	34 mo
4	467	8	4.3% (95% CI, 1.9–9.3%) (5 yr)	21 mo
5	52	2	1.1% (95% CI, 0.02–5%) (5 yr)	19 mo
6	249	6	4% (5 yr) 10% (7 yr)	44 mo
7	108	4	9 ± 4.7% (3 yr)	0.85 yr

[a]Number of patients with HD vs NHL not available.

BMT, bone marrow transplant; NA, not available; sMDS, secondary myelodysplasia; sAML, secondary acute myeloid leukemia.

resulted in improved long-term survival for large numbers of cancer patients who previously would have succumbed to their disease within a few years. Furthermore, there is a trend to offer this therapy to a wider group of patients, as a result of decreasing transplant-related mortality. As the number of patients who have undergone this therapy increases, there has been further opportunity to evaluate the long-term effects of HDCT. Two of the most devastating complications that may arise from this treatment, particularly autologous stem cell transplantation (ASCT), are the development of secondary myelodysplastic syndrome (sMDS) and/or acute myeloid leukemia (sAML) (1). This discussion focuses primarily on sMDS/sAML arising after ASCT, because sMDS/sAML is rare in the allogeneic setting, perhaps because the conditioning regimen typically ablates the host marrow and/or a graft-vs-damaged-cell effect exists.

2. INCIDENCE

The incidence of sMDS and sAML varies, depending on a number of factors, including the underlying disease, previous therapy, and transplant center reporting results.

2.1. Lymphoma

Table 1 sets forth results regarding the incidence of sMDS/sAML for patients undergoing HDCT and ASCT for Hodgkin's disease (HD). As described therein, the actuarial incidence at 5 yr posttransplant ranges from 1.1 to 15.2%, with the largest series recently reporting a 5-yr actuarial incidence of 4.6% (2). Most series have found a similar

Table 2
sMDS/sAML Following HDCT and ASCT for NHL

Ref.	No. patients transplanted	No. patients with sMDS/sAML	Actuarial incidence	Median latency from BMT
2	4998[a]	66[a]	3.0% (95% C1, 2.0–4.3%) (5 yr)	NA
3	138	4	14 ± 14.7% (5 yr)	34 mo
5	62	0	0	0
6	262	6	4% (5 yr) 8% (7 yr)	44 mo
7	167	6	9% (3 yr)	1.75 yr
8	262	20	18 ± 9% (6 yr)	31 mo

[a]Number of patients with HD vs NHL not available.

BMT, bone marrow transplant; NA, not available; sMDS, secondary myelodysplasia; sAML, secondary acute myeloid leukemia.

incidence of sMDS/sAML in non-Hodgkin's lymphoma (NHL) patients, compared to those patients with HD. However, the European Bone Marrow Transplant Group (EBMT) noted *(2)* in their data regarding 4998 patients undergoing HDCT with ASCT, that patients with HD had an increased risk ratio of 2.78, compared to NHL patients, of developing sMDS/sAML. In all of these series, the risk of secondary disease increases with time post-HDCT. In the standard-dose setting for HD patients, the risk of sMDS/sAML begins to rise with 2 yr of treatment, reaches a maximum at 5–9 yr, and begins to decrease thereafter *(1)*. Longer follow-up is needed in the high-dose setting, to determine whether the risk similarly decreases after a number of years have passed posttransplant.

Only one group has compared the incidence of sMDS/sAML in HD patients undergoing HDCT with ASCT with HD patients receiving standard therapy *(4)*. In this study, Andre et al. *(4)* compared 467 HD patients receiving HDCT with ASCT with a group of historical controls. They noted a trend of borderline significance for an increased incidence of sMDS/sAML in patients receiving HDCT ($p = 0.056$).

Table 2 sets forth results regarding the incidence of sMDS/sAML for patients with NHL undergoing HDCT with ASCT. The actuarial incidence ranges from 3 to 18% at 5–6 yr posttransplant, with the largest series reporting a 5-yr incidence of 3% *(2)*. This incidence is not markedly different than that found in series for HD, although, as previously described, one series did find an increased risk for the development of sMDS/sAML in HD patients, compared to patients with NHL *(2)*. Although no direct comparisons exist between the incidence of sMDS/sAML in the transplant setting vs standard therapy, standard therapies for the treatment of aggressive NHL are thought to carry little risk for the development of sMDS/sAML *(9)*. The risk factors for development of sMDS/sAML described in these series are discussed below.

2.2. Breast Cancer

Compared to lymphoma, data regarding the incidence of sMDS/sAML after HDCT and ASCT for breast cancer (BC) is relatively scarce, because there has only been one large series of patients reported *(10)*. In a series of 864 BC patients receiving the same conditioning regimen of cyclophosphamide, cisplatin, and carmustine, the 4-yr actuarial incidence of sMDS/sAML was found to be only 1.6% (five patients developed sMDS/sAML), lower than noted in most of the lymphoma series described above *(10)*. However, this rate of sMDS/sAML is higher than the 0.44% incidence found in a large series of nontransplant BC patients by the National Surgical Adjuvant Breast and Bowel Project (NSABP) *(11)*. The median time to MDS in the Duke series was 28 mo posttransplant, similar to that described in lymphoma patients above.

2.3. Multiple Myeloma

There are two large series describing the incidence of sMDS/sAML in multiple myeloma patients undergoing HDCT with ASCT *(12,13)*. In the largest series of 360 patients, from the Royal Marsden Hospital, undergoing HDCT with ASCT, six patients developed sMDS/sAML, for a 10-yr actuarial incidence of 5.7%. In comparing this rate to 312 patients treated at the same institution with standard-dose chemotherapy (CT) (four of whom developed sMDS/sAML), no significant difference was found. In an effort to elucidate whether pretransplant myeloma therapy vs HDCT was the more significant factor in development of sMDS/sAML, Govindarajan et al. *(13)*, at the University of Arkansas, separated 188 patients undergoing HDCT with ASCT for multiple myeloma into two groups. Group 1 (71 patients) had received, at most, one regimen of standard CT prior to undergoing HDCT with ASCT (median duration 8 mo); group 2 (117 patients) had received more than one regimen of standard CT prior to undergoing HDCT with ASCT (median duration 24 mo). No patients in group 1 developed MDS, but seven in group 2 developed karyotypes consistent with sMDS/sAML ($p = 0.02$). The actuarial risk of developing sMDS/sAML for group 2 patients was 12% at 48 mo. All patients developing sMDS/sAML were exposed to melphalan ± carmustine prior to HDCT. Based on the different incidence of sMDS/sAML in the two groups, the authors concluded that the standard therapy was more of a factor in the development of sMDS/sAML than the HDCT; however, this difference may well be a result of cumulative treatment differences in the two groups, and therefore the HDCT may be a contributing factor.

2.4. Germ Cell Tumors

With germ cell tumors (GCTs) the focus of more recent concern regarding the incidence of sMDS/sAML posttransplant has been on the use of etoposide. As discussed below, the addition of etoposide to standard therapy for GCTs was noted by some to be associated with an increased incidence of sMDS/sAML *(14–16)*. In the largest series to date *(17)*, involving 302 patients with GCTs undergoing HDCT with ASCT, six cases of sMDS/sAML were found, for a crude cumulative incidence of 2.0% at 52 mo median follow-up. This crude incidence is somewhat higher than the approx 0.6% noted in nontransplant series *(14–16)*. Data regarding actuarial incidence of presumed epipodophyllotoxins (such as etoposide) induced sMDS/sAML was recently published

(18), and found a 2.2% (95% upper CI, 4.6%) 6-yr risk for patients receiving high-dose epipodophyllotoxins (defined as ≥ 3.0 g/m^2), compared to 3.3% risk (95% upper CI, 5.9%; $p = 0.012$) for patients receiving low-dose epipodophyllotoxins.

2.5. *Incremental Risk from Transplant*

As described above (Subheadings 2.1.–2.4.), there is a dearth of studies directly comparing the incidence of sMDS/sAML in patients undergoing HDCT and ASCT vs standard therapy. The timing of most cases of sMDS/sAML in transplant patients is approx 6 yr from the commencement of standard therapy (i.e., the typical time frame for the development of sMDS/sAML) *(3,7–9)*; data from the University of Arkansas in multiple myeloma patients undergoing HDCT with ASCT indicate that only heavily pretreated patients are developing sMDS/sAML *(13)*; and a recent study of 12 patients who developed sMDS/sAML post-HDCT with ASCT found that, in nine of the cases, the cytogenetic abnormality observed at the time of the sMDS/sAML diagnosis was detectable by fluorescence *in situ* hybridization (FISH) in pre-HDCT specimens *(19)*. Based on these facts, many authors have concluded that sMDS/sAML arising after HDCT primarily results from prior conventional-dose CT rather than for HDCT *(9,13,19,20)*. However, data show that, in NHL patients undergoing HDCT, there appears to be a substantially increased incidence of sMDS/sAML, compared to patients receiving standard-dose CT *(2,3,5–8)*; data in HD patients indicates a trend toward an increased incidence of sMDS/sAML in HDCT *(4)*; and, in four BC patients undergoing HDCT with ASCT, pretransplant cytogenetics were normal, but, postdevelopment of sMDS/sAMLs, they were abnormal *(10)*. These facts indicate that, at least in some cases of sMDS/sAML, HDCT is a likely contributing factor.

3. TIMING OF sMDS/sAML

There appear to be two separate time frames for the development of sMDS/sAML, depending on the underlying etiology. For the classic sMDS/sAML, which is typically associated with the use of alkylating agents, time to development of sMDS/sAML is 5–9 yr after treatment *(1)*. It appears that this risk then decreases after 10 yr, and eventually reaches that of the normal population *(1,21)*. As described above (Subheadings 2.1.–2.4.), the timing of sMDS/sAML does not appear to have changed with the addition of HDCT and ASCT: It still occurs 5–9 yr after initial therapy.

More recently, a second type of sMDS/sAML has been described, with the use of topoisomerase II agents. It has a much shorter latency period, occurring 1–4 yr after initial therapy *(1)*.

4. RISK FACTORS

Much of the data regarding risk factors for the development of sMDS/sAML are from series regarding patients undergoing standard-dose therapy; however, much of this is probably applicable to the setting of HDCT. Depending on the series, a number of potential risk factors exist, including CT agent, use and extent of radiation therapy (RT), cumulative dose of CT agent(s), source of stem cells (i.e., peripheral blood stem cells [PBSC] vs bone marrow [BM]), patient age, underlying disease, timing of transplant, and splenectomy.

4.1. Chemotherapy

Particular classes of CT agents are known to be associated with an increased risk of sMDS/sAML, including alkylating agents, epipodophyllotoxins, and topoisomerase II agents *(1,3,6,11,18)*. Data regarding dose intensification of these agents as a further risk factor are variable, depending on the CT agent. Alkylating agents, such as cyclophosphamide, carmustine, and melphalan, have been shown to have a clear dose–response effect in relation to sMDS/sAML (1,9,22–25). This is illustrated by the increase in relative risk of 5.7% for sMDS/sAML, found by Curtis et al. *(25)* in BC patients who received a cumulative dose of cyclophosphamide of more than 20 g, compared to patients not receiving alkylating agents, and a minimal increase in risk found in patients receiving less than 10 g. In the transplant setting, Laughlin et al. *(10)* at Duke University, found a slightly increased 4-yr cumulative risk of 1.6% of sMDS/sAML in BC patients transplanted with the cyclophosphamide, cisplatin, and carmustine conditioning regimen, compared to a 0.44% 4-yr risk found by Fisher et al. *(11)* in BC patients receiving standard adjuvant therapy. However, whether this dose–response effect continues with increasing cumulative doses, or plateaus at some level, is unclear. Furthermore, whether a high single dose of alkylators (as occurs in the transplant setting) further increases the risk, compared to a high cumulative-dose effect, is also unclear, although it appears that the cumulative dose is the more likely culprit. This latter point is exemplified by the data from Stone et al. *(8)* at the Dana-Farber Cancer Institute (DFCI), who found, in univariate analysis, that there was a significant correlation between the number of months of alkylator therapy pretransplant and the subsequent development of sMDS/sAML. This point is also borne out by the fact that, in the lymphoma transplant setting, the timing of the cases of sMDS/sAML (approx 6 yr from initial therapy to sMDS/sAML) corresponds closely to the typical alkylator-induced sMDS/sAML incubation period *(9)*. It should also be noted that all alkylators do not appear to be equal regarding leukemogenic risk: Melphalan and carmustine appear to be more leukemogenic than cyclophosphamide *(26)*. Last, the combination of multiple alkylating agents may be additive, or even synergystic, in terms of their leukemogenic potential.

Data regarding a dose–response effect for epipodophyllotoxins is less clear. In the solid tumor setting, Bokemeyer et al. *(14)* found, in their series of more than 1800 patients, that low doses of etoposide (i.e., less than 2 g/m^2) had only a 0.6% risk at 5 yr of causing sMDS/sAML. Some have found evidence of a dose–response effect with epipodophyllotoxins *(1,27)*. However, a recent report from the Cancer Therapy Evaluation Group of the National Cancer Institute, involving 2291 solid tumor patients, did not find any evidence of a direct correlation between cumulative dose of etoposide and incidence of sMDS/sAML. Data from this report, regarding dose of etoposide and risk of sMDS/sAML, are set forth in Table 3: This report did not find any evidence of a cumulative dose–response effect for etoposide; rather, there was an increased risk of sMDS/sAML at lower cumulative doses. In contrast to the solid tumor setting, data from the lymphoma and lymphoid leukemia area indicate a substantially increased risk of sMDS/sAML with the use of epipodophyllotoxins. Regimens without epipodophyllotoxins report cumulative risks of less than 1% *(28)*, regimens involving epipodophyllotoxins report cumulative risks in excess of 5% *(29–31)*. The rationale for this difference

Table 3
Cumulative Risk of sMDS/sAML with Etoposide

Cumulative dose of etoposide	No. of patients	4-yr risk	6-yr risk
Less than 1.5 g/m^2	451	2.1% (upper 95% CI, 3.7%)	3.3% (upper 95% CI, 5.9%)
1.5–3.9 g/m^2	1270	0.4% (upper 95% CI, 1.0%)	0.7% (upper 95% CI, 1.6%)
4.0 g/m^2 or more	570	1.4% (upper 95% CI, 2.9%)	2.2% (upper 95% CI, 4.6%)

CI, confidence interval.

is unclear, but it may be because higher cumulative doses are used in the leukemia setting, and/or because of a difference in schedule of administration (18).

Agents that target topoisomerase II (e.g., anthracyclines, etoposide) have also been implicated in the development of sMDS/sAML (1,31–33). The City of Hope found that, in their transplant series involving lymphoma patients, both pretransplant and transplant exposure, in the form of stem cell priming with 2 g/m^2 of etoposide, were associated with the development of sMDS/sAML (7,31). In contrast to classic sMDS/sAML arising from CT, sMDS/sAML associated with topoisomerase II agents has a shorter latency period between treatment with CT and subsequent development of sMDS/sAML. As described below, in Subheading 5, sMDS/sAML arising from topoisomerase II agents generally results in different cytogenetic abnormalities than seen with other agents (1).

Platinum agents were recently found to increase the risk of sMDS/sAML in a dose-dependent fashion, in a standard therapy review of patients with ovarian cancer (34). This may prove to be significant in the transplant setting, because cisplatin is frequently used in the conditioning regimen for BC patients. However, the low incidence of sMDS/sAML reported by Duke University (10) in their series of BC patients conditioned with cisplatin (among other agents), weighs against this agent being significantly leukemogenic, when used only as part of the conditioning regimen.

4.2. Genetics

Two recent reports indicate that there may be a genetic predisposition to the development of sMDS/sAML. Chen et al. (35) found a significantly increased frequency of the glutathione S-transferase theta-1 null genotype in sMDS/sAML patients, compared to controls. More recently, Felix et al. (36) analyzed a polymorphism in the *CYP3A4* gene, which is part of the cytochrome P-450 system involved with metabolizing epipodophyllotoxins. They found a significant difference in a particular *CYP3A4* genotype in sMDS/sAML patients, compared with patients who developed *de novo* acute myeloid leukemia. They postulate that the variant may increase production of potentially DNA-damaging metabolites. In a retrospective study at the DFCI (37), involving 104 female patients undergoing HDCT with ASCT for NHL, and the subsequent development of six cases of sMDS/sAML, clonal hematopoesis detected pretransplant, using X-inactivation clonality assay at the human androgen receptor locus, was found to be predictive of the development of sMDS/sAML (four of 10 patients with clonal hematopoesis pretransplant developed sMDS/sAML; $p = 0.004$). If these or other data prove to be predictive of an increased risk for development of sMDS/sAML, this may prove useful in tailoring therapy for particular patients at increased risk of sMDS/sAML by avoidance of more leukemogenic agents, or utilizing allogeneic rather than autologous stem cells (20).

4.3. Radiation Therapy

Several groups have found that radiation (particularly total body irradiation [TBI]) in the transplant setting increases the risk for the development of sMDS/sAML. Darrington et al. (6), at the University of Nebraska, found all of their cases of sMDS/sAML in NHL patients who received TBI as a part of their conditioning regimen. They also noted that four of the five patients, in Miller's series of NHL patients from the University of Minnesota, received TBI as part of their induction regimen (6,38). This increased risk for TBI was also found by the EBMT Lymphoma and Late Effects Working Parties in their report on 4998 lymphoma patients (relative risk 3.22; $p < 0.001$) (2). Although Stone et al. (9), at the DFCI, found that prior RT increased the risk of sMDS/sAML (univariate analysis), Stone does note that five of their nine patients with sMDS/sAML received CT alone, and thus questions whether TBI plays a significant role in leukemogenesis. In their series of lymphoma patients, the City of Hope did not find that TBI or prior RT contributed significantly to the risk of sMDS/sAML (7,31).

4.4. Source of Stem Cells

Some groups have noted a possible link between the use of PBSCs vs BM-derived stem cells as a potential risk factor for the development of sMDS/sAML. In a univariate analysis, Miller et al. (3), at the University of Minnesota, found, in their series of NHL autotransplant patients, a higher actuarial incidence of sMDS/sAML if PBSCs were used ($31 \pm 33\%$ vs $10 \pm 12\%$; $p = 0.0035$). Traweek et al. (7), at the City of Hope, found a trend of decreased risk for sMDS/sAML, if BM was used, with or without the addition of PBSCs (relative risk = 0.28; $p = 0.07$), in lymphoma patients undergoing ASCT. In an apparent update of this series of lymphoma patients from the City of Hope (31), this risk for PBSCs vs BM reached statistical significance, with peripheral stem cells having a relative risk of 1.5 ($p = 0.05$). Resolution of this issue will likely require a randomized study, but is of significant importance, given the increasing use of PBSCs in ASCT.

4.5. Age

Given the overall trend of an increased incidence of myelodyplasia with increasing age, coupled with the trend of lower posttransplant survival with increasing age, several groups have noted increasing age as a risk factor for the development of sMDS/sAML. Most recently, the EBMT, in their series of 4998 lymphoma patients, noted a relative risk of 3.2 ($p < 0.001$) for older patients, and the development of sMDS/sAML (2). Similar conclusions were reached by other studies of sMDS/sAML in lymphoma patients, with two groups (4,6) finding an increased risk for patients over age 40. However, the City of Hope data did not find any correlation between risk of sMDS/sAML and age (7,31).

4.6. Other Factors

Numerous other risk factors have been found to be significant in various series, including an increasing interval between standard therapy and ASCT *(2)*, HD vs NHL *(2)*, splenectomy (in HD) *(1,39,40)*, and increased duration of exposure to alkylating agents or standard CT *(8)*.

5. CYTOGENETIC FINDINGS

The most common cytogenetic findings in patients with sMDS/sAML are abnormalities of chromosome 5 and/or 7: Some series report this finding in up to 90% of the patients *(1,41–43)*. These abnormalities are most typical of patients treated with alkylating agents; patients treated with topoisomerase II inhibitors more typically display abnormalities involving t11q23 and/or t21q22 *(1,32,33)*. These same abnormalities are seen in patients with *de novo* MDS/AML, but their frequency, as is the frequency of all chromosomal abnormalities, is much higher in sMDS/sAML. In their review on this topic, Thirman and Larson *(1)* note that, in data from 240 sMDS/sAML patients from the University of Chicago, 69% had abnormalities involving chromosome 5 and/ or 7, 3% had t11q23, and 13% of patients had random chromosomal abnormalities. As noted in this and other series, not all patients with sMDS/sAML have chromosomal abnormalities: 9% of patients in this series had no clonal abnormalities *(1,41–43)*.

Although chromosomal abnormalities are typical of sMDS/sAML, they are probably not diagnostic thereof. Stone *(9)* reports that the DFCI group has found that 50% of sporadically tested, posttransplant, hematologically normal patients have clonal karyotypic abnormalities, including monosomy 7. Furthermore, some of these patients have remained hematologically normal for years despite these abnormal chromosomal findings *(9)*. Also, in the City of Hope series *(7)* involving 10 patients with post-HDCT sMDS/sAML, three of the 10 patients showed no evidence of myelodysplasia in their peripheral blood counts, although the number of karyotypically abnormal cells is increasing.

To try to decrease the risk of posttransplant sMDS/sAML, many transplant centers routinely perform pretransplant cytogenetic analysis, to screen out patients with detectable cytogenetic abnormalities *(20)*. However, as indicated by the City of Hope series of 10 lymphoma patients with sMDS/sAML *(7)*, and the Duke series of five BC patients with sMDS/sAML *(10)*, all of whom had normal pretransplant cytogenetics, the presence of normal chromosomes at the time of stem cell collection does not completely eliminate the risk of subsequently developing sMDS/sAML. Furthermore, as demonstrated by Abruzzese et al. *(19)*, normal cytogenetic screening may well not be sensitive enough to detect the abnormal clone.

6. DIAGNOSIS

The diagnosis of sMDS/sAML is rather straightforward in those patients who exhibit classic cytogenetic changes, as well as significant cytopenias and/or evidence of evolving leukemia *(44)*. In the classic form of sMDS/sAML, the blood and BM findings are similar to those found in primary MDS/AML. Anemia and thrombocytopenia are common, and leukopenia is not uncommon. Significant dysplastic changes are often observed in all three cell lines. The BM is usually hypercellular, and some reticulin fibrosis may be present. At times, there is some difficulty classifying either sMDS or

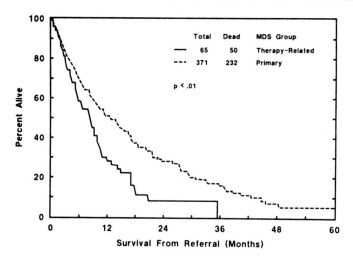

Fig. 1. Survival of patients at MD Anderson Cancer Center with therapy-related versus primary myelodysplastic syndrome. (With permission.)

sAML according to standard French-American-British Cooperative Group criteria used for MDS or AML (1).

Additionally, some series of sMDS/sAML patients include those patients who exhibit karyotypes typical of sMDS/sAML, regardless of whether there is other evidence of sMDS/sAML (3). Furthermore, methods more sensitive than standard cytogenetics are being developed that can detect less obvious chromosomal abnormalities. New methods being adopted include the use of panels of FISH probes for the more common cytogenetic abnormalities (19), and clonal analysis of X-linked polymorphisms (useful only in females) (37,45). Thus, more cases of sMDS/sAML may be diagnosed, although, as noted by Stone (9), the significance of such abnormalities in the absence of other manifestations of sMDS/sAML is somewhat unclear.

7. PROGNOSIS

In general, the prognosis for sMDS/sAML is worse than for *de novo* MDS or AML. For sMDS, this is well illustrated by Fig. 1, which reflects data from MD Anderson Cancer Center (MDACC) (46). This poorer outcome may result from the higher incidence of unfavorable (e.g., chromosome 5 and 7) cytogenetic abnormalities in these patients. In one of the largest series of sMDS/sAML patients published (46), the MDACC group found a median survival of 10 mo for their sMDS patients ($n = 50$), and 3.5 mo for their sAML patients ($n = 155$). Recently, a group of prognostic factors was developed at an International MDS Risk Analysis Workshop for patients with primary MDS (47). After analyzing a number of variables, a prognostic model was developed, based on percentage of BM blasts, number of cytopenias, and cytogenetic subgroup (good cytogenetics were normal, del[5q], del[20q], and −Y; poor-risk cytogenetics included those with three or more anomalies, or chromosome 7 anomalies; intermediate risk include all other cytogenetic categories). The applicability of this system to sMDS is unclear. It may well be that it will apply to create prognostic groups for purposes of evolution to AML and survival, but that, for patients with sMDS,

Table 4
CR Rates in sAML

Ref.	No. patients	CR rate (%)
49	121	16
50	28	18
51	23	52
52	36	47
46	148	34

these will portend faster evolution and shorter survival than their counterparts with primary MDS.

Regardless of the applicability of this prognostic index to patients with sMDS, it is clear that there are at least two distinct clinical subsets of patients with sMDS/sAML. The first group is those with abnormalities of chromosome 5 and/or 7, which are usually secondary to treatment with alkylating agents. Most of these patients have evidence of sMDS prior to transforming to sAML, and they generally respond poorly to induction CT, as well as having a poor long-term survival. The second group consists of those patients with balanced translocations involving 11q23 or 21q22, which is often secondary to prior treatment with topoisomerase II agents. As described in Subheading 3, this group has a much shorter latency period between treatment and development of sMDS/sAML. This group responds better to induction CT, but ultimately has poor long-term survival (1,48).

8. TREATMENT

8.1. CT for sAML

There is very little data regarding treatment of sAML induced by HDCT with ASCT: Accordingly, the following discussion is based primarily on data derived from series reporting patients with sAML induced by standard-dose CT. It is possible that posttransplant-sAML patients may fare worse, given the more cytotoxic therapy to which their marrow has been subjected. Generally, the results of studies reporting on the results of CT in sAML have been disappointing. Complete remission (CR) rates of 20 to >50% are reported, but average 35–40%, and the long-term disease-free survival (DFS) rates are low (46) (see Table 4 for CR rates reported in selected studies in sAML). In one of the largest series of sAML patients described (n = 148), MDACC reported (46) a 34% CR rate and 36% death rate during induction CT. Various regimens were used, with the highest CR rate occurring with high-dose cytarabine alone (45%). However, in a recent series of 16 sMDS patients reported by MDACC (53), 11 (69%) achieved a CR with topotecan and high-dose cytarabine. Others (51,54) have also tended to find higher CR rates with high-dose cytarabine. Treatment with low-dose cytarabine appears to yield lower CR rates than with conventional or HDCT. In reviews (55,56) on the use of low-dose cytarabine, CR rates of 16% were found in patients with sMDS/sAML.

In trying to ascertain prognostic factors for response and survival of sAML patients, it appears that the leukemic cell karyotype may be the most significant factor in predicting response. Patients with abnormalities of chromosome 5 and/or 7 have the lowest response rates; those with a normal karyotype t(8;21), t(15:17), or inversion 16,

Table 5
CR Rates in sAML with Favorable Cytogenetics
[t(18;21), t(15;17), and inv(16)]

Ref.	No. patients	CR rate (%)
46	13	69
57	5	100
58	35	80

have higher response rates. This is seen in data reported by MDACC *(46)*, in a series of 148 patients with sAML, which noted a 66–75% CR rate in those with favorable karyotypes, 43% CR rate for patients with normal karyotypes, and 17% CR rate for patients with chromosome 5 and/or 7 abnormalities (*see* Table 5 for CR rates in patients with favorable cytogenetics). Futhermore, they note that the more unfavorable cytogenetics found in sAML patients may explain much of the difference in response and survival of sAML patients versus *de novo* AML patients. The presence of prior hematologic disorder may also indidate a worse prognosis *(46,49)*.

Recently, the Southwest Oncology Group has reported data that indicates that sAML patients may fare worse with their response to induction CT than cytogenetically similar patients with *de novo* AML. Additionally, they note that the multidrug resistance gene *MDR1* appears to be highly expressed in sAML, and this may account for their poor response to standard CT, as well as explain the better response of these patients to high-dose cytarabine *(59,60)*.

CRs obtained in patients with sAML do not appear to be very durable, given the median survival of 3.5 mo noted by MDACC *(46)*, and the less than 10% 3-yr survival.

8.2. Allogeneic Stem Cell Transplantation for sAML

Given the poor outcome associated with standard-dose CT in sAML, a number of groups have explored the use of allogeneic stem cell transplantation (allo-SCT) in these patients. These results are set forth in Table 6. The numbers in these studies are relatively small, but they do seem to indicate that a minority of patients may survive this procedure with long-term DFS. It does appear from these series that patients transplanted in first remission do better than those transplanted with CT-resistant disease *(62,64)*. Concerning prognostic factors, one series *(60)* found that, in a univariate analysis, a shorter time from diagnosis of sAML to transplant was associated with a significantly lower risk of nonrelapse mortality and higher DFS. It should be noted that the above allotransplant series almost exclusively involve patients with sAML arising from standard-dose CT. Thus, this data may not be applicable to those already transplanted as part of their initial disease therapy, because this group may well not be able to tolerate second transplantation.

This point is borne out by a recent series of 50 patients undergoing allotransplantation for sMDS/sAML or recurrent disease after initially undergoing auto- (five patients) or allotransplant (45 patients), a median of 14 mo after their initial transplant *(66)*. At a median follow-up of 33 mo, only 10% (3/31) of patients over 18 were alive, and only 6% (2/31) were disease-free. Univariate predictors of DFS included age less than 18, and interval between transplants of greater than 1 yr (0% survival for those transplanted

Table 6
Allo-transplantation for sAML

Ref.	No. patients	TRM (%)	DFS (%)
60	46	44	24 (5 yr)
61	4	50	50 (~2 yr)
62	13	38	18 (2 yr)
63	5 sAML 6sMDS	36	27 (5 yr)
64	17	~40	18 (30 mo)
65	77	47	24 OS (5 yr)

DFS, disease-free survival; TRM, transplant-related mortality.

within 1 yr vs 16% for those more than 1 yr; $p = 0.004$) (66). However, with the advent of nonmyeloablative conditioning regimens for allo-SCT, second transplant to treat sAML may be more realistic. In a series of 10 patients with hematologic malignancy (two with sAML) after undergoing initial auto- or allotransplant, one group (65) reported 10% transplant-related mortality, 20% relapse rate, and 70% DFS at a median follow-up of 7 mo postsecond transplant, using a nonmyeloablative conditioning regimen for allo-transplantation (both matched sibling and unrelated donors being used).

8.3. Therapy for sMDS

The above discussion regarding CT and allo-SCT for sAML applies, to some degree, to sMDS, because some of the above series included patients with sMDS, and many of the patients in these series had their sAML evolve from sMDS. There is some data pertaining directly to the treatment of sMDS; however, much of it must be gleaned from treatment of primary MDS, because there are no large series reporting on treatment of sMDS. Patients with sMDS appear to have a shorter survival than patients with primary MDS. MDACC (46) reported a median survival of 10 mo in these patients, and less than 20% 2-yr survival. A variety of therapies have been tried in MDS, including biologic therapies (including interferons, growth factors, vitamin D, and retinoids), CT, and BM transplantation.

Interferon-α and/or -γ alone, or in combination with other agents, including low-dose cytarabine, have shown little effectiveness, with interferon alone being particularly ineffective (46,67,68). Vitamin D trials have also been disappointing, with Vitamin D being used as an agent to inhibit proliferation and induce differentiation. Similarly, retinoids have been ineffective, with one trial noting no survival difference vs placebo (46,69). Growth factors have likewise been relatively ineffective, although some patients have achieved increases in hemoglobin with the use of erythropoietin (70).

Concerning CTs, 5-azacytidine, an antimetabolite that produces in vitro cellular differentiation, has shown some promise with overall response rates being reported of 48 and 62% in studies by the Cancer and Leukemia Group B (71,72). Amifostine has been shown to have some efficacy in MDS (73,74). However, intensive CT regimens have produced the highest CR rates of any form of conventional therapy for MDS, with CR rates ranging from 40 to 70%. Response to therapy is, in many series, better for younger patients and those with more favorable karyotypes. These remissions are only moderately durable, with MDACC *(46)* reporting a median CR duration in 38 patients with priamry MDS of 10 mo, and 2-yr DFS of 25%. CR rates in sMDS appear to be lower, probably because of the more unfavorable karyotypes. This is reflected in MDACC data *(43)* comparing 50 patients with primary MDS with 13 patients with sMDS. Those patients with primary MDS achieved a CR rate of 68%; those with sMDS only achieved a 31% CR rate ($p = 0.03$).

9. CONCLUSION

Although no firm conclusion regarding treatment for sMDS/sAML is possible, a reasonable approach with these patients would be to consider their age, availability of an allogeneic donor, and likelihood of achieving CR with standard CT (based on karyotype). For younger patients with an available donor and poor cytogenetics, immediate transplantation using a nonmyeloablative regimen should be considered.

REFERENCES

1. Thirman M and Larson R. Therapy-related myeloid leukemia, *Hematol. Oncol. Clin. North Am.,* **10** (1996) 293–320.
2. Milligan D, Ruiz de Elvira M, Goldstone A, et al. Secondary leukemia and myelodysplasia after autografting for lymphoma; results from the EBMT, *Blood,* **92(Suppl)** (1998) 493a.
3. Miller J, Arthur D, Litz C, et al. Myelodysplastic syndrome after autologous bone marrow transplantation: an additional late complication of curative cancer therapy, *Blood,* **83** (1994) 3780–3786.
4. Andre M, Henry-Amar M, Blaise D, et al. Treatment-related deaths and second cancer risk after autologous stem-cell transplantation for Hodgkin's disease, *Blood,* **92** (1998) 1933–1940.
5. Taylor P, Jackson G, Lennard A, et al. Low incidence of myelodysplastic syndrome following transplantation using autologous non-cryopreserved bone marrow, *Leukemia,* **11** (1997) 1650–1653.
6. Darrington D, Vose J, Anderson J, et al. Incidence and characterization of secondary myelodysplastic syndrome and acute myelogenous leukemia following high-dose chemoradiotherapy and autologous stem-cell transplantation for lymphoid malignancies, *J. Clin. Oncol.,* **12** (1994) 2527–2534.
7. Traweek S, Slovak M, Nademanee At, et al. Clonal karyotopic hematopoetic cell abnormalities occurring after autologous bone marrow transplantation for Hodgkin's disease and non-Hodgkin's lymphoma, *Blood,* **84** (1994) 957–963.
8. Stone R, Neuberg D, Soiffer R, et al. Myelodysplastic syndrome as a late complication following autologous bone marrow transplantation for non-Hodgkin's lymphoma, *J. Clin. Oncol.,* **12** (1994) 2535–2542.
9. Stone R. Myelodysplastic syndrome after autologous transplantation for lymphoma: the price of progress, *Blood,* **83** (1994) 3437–3440.
10. Laughlin M, McGaughey D, Crews J, et al. Secondary myelodysplasia and acute leukemia in breast cancer patients after autologous bone marrow transplant, *J. Clin. Oncol.,* **16** (1998) 1008–1012.
11. Fisher B, Rockette H, Fisher E, et al. Leukemia in breast cancer patients following adjuvant chemotherapy or postoperative radiation: the NSABP experience, *J. Clin. Oncol.,* **12** (1985) 1640–1658.
12. Saso R, Kulkarni S, Powles R, et al. Secondary mds/aml in patients treated for myeloma, *Blood,* **92(Suppl)** (1998) 455a.
13. Govindarajan R, Jagannath S, Flick J, et al. Preceding standard therapy is the likely cause of MDS after autotransplants for multiple myeloma, *Br. J. Haemotol.,* **95** (1996) 349–353.
14. Bokemeyer C and Schmoll H. Secondary neoplasms following treatment of malignant germ cell tumors, *J. Clin. Oncol.,* **11** (1993) 1703–1709.
15. Boshoff C, Begent R, Oliver R, et al. Secondary tumours following etoposide containing therapy for germ cell cancer, *Ann. Oncol.,* **6** (1993) 5–40.

16. Nichols C, Breeden E, Loehrer P, et al. Secondary leukemia associated with a conventional dose of etoposide: review of serial germ cell tumor protocols. *J. Natl. Cancer Inst.*, **85** (1993) 36–40.

17. Kollmannsberger C, Beyer J, Droz J, et al. Secondary leukemia following high cumulative doses of etoposide in patients treated for advanced germ cell tumors, *J. Clin. Oncol.*, **16** (1998) 3386–3391.

18. Smith M, Rubinstein L, Anderson J, et al. Secondary leukemia or myelodysplastic syndrome after treatment with epipodophyllotoxins, *J. Clin. Oncol.*, **17** (1999) 569–577.

19. Abruzzese E, Radford J, Miller J, et al. Detection of abnormal clones in progenitor cells of patients who developed myelodysplasia after autologous stem cell transplantation, (1999), submitted.

20. Chao N, Nademanee A, Long G, et al. Importance of bone marrow cytogenetic evaluation before autologous bone marrow transplantation for Hodgkin's disease, *J. Clin. Oncol.*, **9** (1991) 1575.

21. Pedersen-Bjergaard J and Rowley J. Risk of therapy-related leukemia and preleukemia after Hodgkin's disease. Relation to age, cumulative dose of alkylating agents, and time from chemotherapy, *Lancet*, **2** (1987) 82.

22. Greene M, Boice J, Greer B, et al. Acute non-lymphocytic leukemia after therapy with alkylating agents for ovarian cancer, *N. Engl. J. Med.*, **307** (1982) 1416–1421.

23. Greene M, Young R, Merrill J, et al. Evidence of a treatment dose response in acute nonlymphocytic leukemias which occur after therapy for non-Hodgkin's lymphoma, *Cancer Res.*, **43**(1983) 1891–1909.

24. Pedersen-Bjergaard J, Sprecht L, Larsen S, et al. Risk of therapy-related leukemia and preleukemia after Hodgkin's disease. Relation to age, cumulative dose of alkylating agents, and time from chemotherapy, *Lancet*, **2** (1987) 83.

25. Curtis R, Boice J, Stovall M, et al. Risk of leukemia after chemotherapy and radiation treatment for breast cancer, *N. Engl. J. Med.*, **326** (1992) 1745–1751.

26. Levine E and Bloomfield C. Leukemias and myelodysplastic syndromes secondary to drug, radiation and environmental exposure, *Semin. Oncol.*, **19** (1992) 47–84.

27. Ratain M, Kaminer L, Bitran J, et al. Acute nonlymphocytic leukemia following etoposide and cisplatin combination chemotherapy for advanced non-small cell carcinoma of the lung, *Blood*, **70** (1987) 1412.

28. Kreissman S, Gelber R, Cohen H, et al. Incidence of secondary acute myelogenous leukemia after treatment of childhood acute lymphocytic leukemia, *Cancer*, **70** (1992) 2208–2213.

29. Katz J, Shuster J, Ravindranaath Y, et al. Secondary acute myelogenous leukemia (AML) following intensive treatment of childhood T-cell acute lymphoblastic leukemia (T-ALL) and advanced-stage lymphoblastic lymphoma (LL) treated with teniposide (VM-26): a Pediatric Oncology Group (POG) study, *Proc. Am. Soc. Clin. Oncol.*, **14** (1995) 344 (Abstract).

30. Pui C, Ribeiro R, Hancock M, et al. Acute myelogenous leukemia in children treated with epipodophyl-lotoxins for acute lymphoblastic leukemia, *N. Engl. J. Med.*, **325** (1991) 1682–1687.

31. Krishman A, Bhatia S, Bhatia R, et al. Risk factors for development of therapy-related leukemia (t-MDS/t-AML) following autologous transplantation (ABMT) for lymphoma, *Blood*, **92(Suppl)** (1998) 493a.

32. Larson R, Le Beau M, Ratain M, et al. Balanced translocations involving chromosome bands 11q23 and 21q22 in therapy-related leukemia, *Blood*, **79** (1992) 1892–1893.

33. Ratain M and Rowley J. Therapy-related acute myelogenous leukemia secondary to inhibitors of topoisomerase II: from bedside to the target genes, *Ann. Oncol.*, **3** (1992) 107–111.

34. Travis L, Holowaty E, Bergfeldt K, et al. Risk of leukemia after platinum-based chemotherapy for ovarian cancer, *N. Engl. J. Med.*, **340** (1999) 351–357.

35. Chen H, Sandler D, Taylor J, et al. Increased risk for myelodysplasic syndromes in individuals with glutathione transferase theta-1 (GSTT1) gene defect, *Lancet*, **347** 295–297.

36. Felix C, Walker A, Lange B, et al. Genetic predisposition to treatment-related leukemia: association of CYP3A4 genotype with epipodophyllotoxin-induced cases, *Blood*, **92(Suppl)** (1998) 311a.

37. Mach-Pascual S, Legare R, Lu D, et al. Predictive value of clonality analysis in patients with non-Hodgkin's lymphoma (NHL) undergoing autologous bone marrow transplant (ABMT), *Blood*, **90(Suppl)** (1997) 591a.

38. Anderson J, Vose J, and Kessinger A. Letter to the editor, *Blood*, **84** (1994) 3988.

39. Van Leeuwen F, Somers R, Taal B, et al. Increased risk of lung cancer, non-Hodgkin's lymphoma, and leukemia following Hodgkin's disease, *J. Clin. Oncol.*, **7** (1989) 1046–1058.

40. Kaldor J, Day N, Clarke E, et al. Leukemia following Hodgkin's disease, *N. Engl. J. Med.*, **322** (1990) 7.

41. Rowley J, Golomb H, Vardiman J, et al. Nonrandom chromosome abnormalities in acute leukemia and dysmyelopoetic syndromes in patients with previously treated malignant disease, *Blood*, **58** (1981) 759–767.

42. Heim S. Cytogenetic findings in primary and secondary MDS, *Leukemia Res.*, **16** (1992) 43–46.

43. Pedersen-Bjergaard J, Phillip P, Pedersen P, et al. Therapy-related myelodysplasia and acute myeloid luekemia: cytogenetic characteristics of 115 consecutive cases and risk in seven cohorts of patients intensively treated for malignant diseases in the Copenhagen series, *Leukemia*, **7** (1993) 1975–1986.

44. Bennett J, Catovsky D, Daniel M, et al. Proposals for the classification of the myelodysplastic syndromes, *Br. J. Haematol.*, **51** (1982) 189.

45. Gale R, Bunch C, Moir D, et al. Demonstration of developing myelodysplasia/acute myeloid leukemia in haemotologically normal patients after high-dose chemotherapy and autologous bone marrow transplantation using X-chromosome inactivation patterns, *Br. J. Haemotol.*, **93** (1996) 53–58.

46. Kantarjian H, Estey E, and Keating M. Treatment of therapy-related leukemia and myelodysplastic syndrome, *Hematol. Oncol. Clin. North Am.*, **7** (1993) 81–107.

47. Greenberg P, Cox C, LeBeau M, et al. International scoring system for evaluating prognosis in myelodysplastic syndromes, *Blood*, **89** (1997) 2079–2088.

48. Pedersen-Bjergaard J and Rowley J. The balanced and unbalanced chromosome abberations of acute myeloid leukemia may develop in different ways and may contribute to malignant transformation, *Blood*, **83** (1994) 2780.

49. Grunwald H and Rosner F. Acute myeloid leukemia following treatment of Hodgkin's disease, *Cancer*, **50** (1982) 676–683.

50. Lebeau M, Albain K, Larson R, et al. Clinical and cytogenetic correlations in 63 patients with therapy-related myelodysplastic syndromes and acute nonlymphocytic leukemia: further evidence for characteristic abnormalities of chromosome no. 5 and 7, *J. Clin. Oncol.*, **4** (1986) 325–345.

51. Preisler H, Raza A, Barcos M, et al. High-dose cytosine arabinoside as the initial treatment of poor-risk patients with acute non-lymphocytic leukemia. A Leukemia Intergroup study, *J. Clin. Oncol.*, **5** (1987) 75–82.

52. Perdersen-Bjergaard J, Phillip P, Larsen S, et al. Chromosome abberations and prognostic factors in therapy-related myelodysplasia and acute nonlymphocytic leukemia, *Blood*, **76** (1990) 1083–1091.

53. Beran M, Kantarjian H, and Estey E. Topotecan and high-dose cytarabine is an active combination regimen in myelodysplastic syndromes and chronic myelomonocytic leukemia, *Blood*, **92(Suppl)** (1998) 714a.

54. Larson R, Wernli M, LeBeau M, et al. Short remission durations in therapy-related leukemia despite cytogenetic complete responses to high-dose cytarabine, *Blood*, **72** (1988) 1333–1339.

55. Bolwell B, Cassileth P, and Gale P. Low dose cytosine arabinoside in myelodysplasioa and acute myelogenous leukemia: a review, *Leukemia*, **1** (1987) 575–579.

56. Cheson B, Jasperse D, Simon R, et al. Critical appraisal of low-dose cytosine arabinoside in patient with acute non-lymphocytic leukemia and myelodysplastic syndromes, *J. Clin. Oncol.*, **4** (1986) 1857–1864.

57. Fenaux P, Lucidarme D, Ilai J, et al. Favorable cytogenetic abnormalities in secondary leukemia, *Cancer*, **63** (1989) 2505–2508.

58. Quesnel B, Kantarjian H, Bjeergaard J, et al. Therapy related acute myeloid leukemia with t(8;21), inv(16), and t(8;16): a report on 25 cases and review of the literature, *J. Clin. Oncol.*, **11** (1993) 2370–2379.

59. List A. Role of multidrug resistance and its pharmacologic modulation in acute myeloid leukemia, *Leukemia*, **10** (1996) 946–951.

60. Appelbaum F, Le Beau M, and Willman C. "Secondary leukemia" in *Hematology 1996 Education Program*, American Society of Hematology, pp. 33–47.

61. Geller G, Vogelsang G, Wingard J, et al. Successful marrow transplantation for acute myelogenous leukemia following therapy for Hodgkin's disease, *J. Clin. Oncol.*, **6** (1988) 1558–1561.

62. Dewitte T, Zwaan F, Hermans J, et al. Allogeneic bone marrow transplantation for secondary leukaemia and myelodysplastic syndrome: a survey by the Leukaemia Working Party of the European Bone Marrow Transplantation Group (EBMTG), *Br. J. Haemotol.*, **74** (1990) 151–155.

63. Longmore G, Guinan E, Weinstein H, et al. Bone marrow transplantation for myelodysplasia and secondary acute nonlymphocytic leukemia, *J. Clin. Oncol.*, **8** (1990) 1707–1714.

64. Sutton L, Leblong V, LeMaignan C, et al. Bone marrow transplantation for myelodysplastic syndrome and secondary leukemia: outcome of 86 patients, *Bone Marrow Transplant.*, **7(Suppl 2)** (1991) 39.

65. Nagler A, Or R, Naparstek E, et al. Secondary allogeneic stem cell transplantation (allosct) using a non-myeloablative conditioning regimen for patients with hematological malignancies, *Blood*, **92(Suppl)** (1998) 137a.

66. Childs B, Boulad F, Castro-Malspina H, et al. Second allogeneic bone marrow transplant for relapsed or secondary malignancies, *Blood*, **90(Suppl)** (1997) 551a.

67. Elias L, Hoffman R, Boswell S, et al. A trial of recombinant alpha-interferon in the myelodysplastic syndromes, *Leukemia*, **1** (1987) 105–107.

68. Robert K, Hellstrom E, Einhorn S, et al. Acute myelogenous leukemia of unfavorable prognosis treated with retinoic acid, vitamin D, alpha-interferon and low doses of cytosine arabinoside, *Scand. J. Haemotol.*, **34(Suppl 44)** (1986) 61–74.

69. Koeffler H, Heitjan D, Mertelsmann R, et al. Randomized study of 13-cis retinoic acid vs placebo in the myelodysplastic disorders, *Blood*, **74** (1987) 703–708.

70. Geisslert R, Schulte P, and Ganser A. Clinical use of haematopoetic growth factors in patients with myelodysplastic syndromes, *Int. J. Haemotol.*, **65** (1997) 339–354.

71. Silverman L, Davis R, Holland J, et al. 5-azacytidine as a low-dose continuous infusion is an effective therapy for patients with myelodysplastic syndromes, *Proc. Am. Soc. Clin. Oncol.*, **8** (1989) 198.

72. Silverman L, Holland J, Nelson D, et al. Trilineage response of myelodysplastic syndromes to subcutaneous azacytidine, *Proc. Am. Soc. Clin. Oncol.*, **10** (1991) 222.

73. DeCastro C, Gockerman J, Moore J, et al. Treatment of myelodysplastic syndrome (MDS) with amifostine, *Blood*, **92** (1998) 251b.

74. List A, Brasfield F, Heaton R, et al. Stimulation of hematopoesis by amifostine in patients with myelodysplasia, *Blood*, **90** (1997) 3364–3369.

20   Can *Aspergillus* Infections Be Prevented in Allogeneic Bone Marrow Transplant Recipients?

Sherif B. Mossad, MD, and David L. Longworth, MD

CONTENTS

1. INTRODUCTION

Members of the genus *Aspergillus* are ubiquitous saprophytic fungi that reproduce asexually, more so during the summer months, producing thousands of conidia. The relatively small size of these conidia (1.5–6 µm) allows their suspension in air currents for long periods of time, and permits them to reach terminal bronchioles of the human lung, where they may grow and replicate. The clinical spectrum of human aspergillosis includes asymptomatic colonization, tissue invasion, and widespread visceral dissemination. Patients with prolonged granulocytopenia are at particular risk of developing serious infections with these organisms. Diagnostic techniques for early detection are limited, and accurate diagnosis often requires invasive procedures, such as transbronchial biopsy or open lung biopsy. Therapeutic options, including antifungal chemotherapeutic agents and surgical resection, are also far from perfect. The rapidly progressive course of the disease often precludes antemortem diagnosis.

Aspergillosis is the second most common fungal infection in bone marrow transplant (BMT) recipients. Diagnostic measures to detect early disease are currently insensitive, and, unfortunately, despite aggressive therapy, the outcome is frequently fatal. The utility of several prophylactic measures to prevent invasive aspergillosis has been debated in the literature. None seem to be perfect. This chapter reviews the available data and offers the authors' opinions regarding the best options available to prevent *Aspergillus* infections in BMT recipients.

2. EPIDEMIOLOGY

Aspergillus species are the second most common cause of opportunistic fungal infections, after *Candida* species, in granulocytopenic patients and transplant recipients *(1)*. Most infections are caused by *A. fumigatus* or *A. flavus*.

The incidence of *Aspergillus* infections in allogeneic BMT (allo-BMT) recipients is higher than in autologous BMT (ABMT) recipients, because of the much higher degree of immunosuppression in allogeneic recipients. A review of the early infectious complications in 219 ABMT recipients revealed only one case (0.5%) of *Aspergillus* pneumonia *(2)*. Another review of 66 patients undergoing peripheral blood stem cell transplantation revealed no invasive fungal infections *(3)*. The incidence of *Aspergillus* infections in allo-BMT recipients in various studies has ranged between 3.6 and 10.5%, depending on the duration of follow-up *(4–8)*. One autopsy study, involving 40 allo-BMT and 16 ABMT recipients, found *Aspergillus* infection in 11% of patients, two-thirds of which were only identified postmortem *(9)*.

Most *Aspergillus* infections occur in the pre-engraftment period during hospitalization, but patients who develop chronic graft-vs-host disease (GVHD) remain at risk for years after BMT. The median survival from the time of diagnosis is 28 d, and the attributable mortality ranges from 68 to 85% *(4,7,8)*. The most commonly involved organ is the lung *(4,6,8)*, followed by the sinuses *(10,11)*. Cutaneous involvement from direct inoculation at the site of central catheters may also occur *(12)*. Dissemination occurs in up to 60% of patients with fatal invasive aspergillosis *(1)*, particularly to the central nervous system *(13)*.

Risk factors for early-onset *Aspergillus* infection (within 3 mo of BMT) include prolonged neutropenia *(5,7)*, BMT for myelodysplastic syndrome *(8)*, hematologic malignancy in other than first remission *(6)*, human leukocyte antigen donor-recipient mismatch *(6)*, BMT from an unrelated donor *(8)*, receiving T-cell-depleted marrow *(7)*, positive-recipient cytomegalovirus (CMV) serostatus *(7)*, acute GVHD *(5,7,8)*, and use of high-dose (0.5–1 mg/kg/d) corticosteroids as a component of GVHD prophylaxis *(5)*.

Risk factors for late-onset *Aspergillus* infection (beyond 3 mo of BMT) include recipient age >40 yr *(6)*, BMT from an unrelated donor *(6)*, delayed engraftment *(6)*, chronic GVHD *(6)*, use of high-dose steroids (>1 mg/kg/d for more than 1 wk) *(6)*, and graft rejection *(4)*. Two other important epidemiologic risk factors for the development of invasive aspergillosis are exposure to construction work at the hospital site *(14,15)* and smoking contaminated marijuana *(16)*.

Up to one-third of patients with invasive *Aspergillus* infection prior to BMT are at particular risk for recurrence after transplant *(17)*; however, several reports have documented successful BMT after effective treatment for invasive aspergillosis *(4,18,19)*.

3. PROPHYLACTIC MEASURES AGAINST *ASPERGILLUS* INFECTIONS

Given the imperfect therapy of aspergillosis, significant attention has been devoted to the development of preventive strategies. Several studies and reviews have addressed this issue *(20–23)*. Prophylactic measures include preventing acquisition of the organism by reducing environmental exposure, specific antifungal chemoprophylactic agents, and the use of agents that boost the host's defense mechanisms. Many studies examining these issues must be interpreted with caution, given that *Aspergillus* infections may be seasonal, and may occur in clusters.

3.1. Reduction in Environmental Exposure

Recent guidelines for the management of ABMT and allo-BMT recipients *(24,25)* have recommended the use of high-efficiency particulate air (HEPA) filters, air-controlled units, laminar airflow (LAF) rooms, and avoidance of plants in patients' rooms to help prevent acquisition of *Aspergillus* species. Using whole-wall HEPA filtration units with horizontal LAF in patients' rooms significantly reduces the number of *Aspergillus* organisms in the air, and has been associated with a reduction in the number of nosocomial *Aspergillus* infections *(26)*. Strict protective isolation, sterile diets, and intestinal microbial decontamination with oral nonabsorbable antibiotics are not effective strategies for the prevention of *Aspergillus* infections *(27,28)*. Limited data suggest that, in institutions with low rates of *Aspergillus* infections, BMT may be done safely without the use of HEPA filters or any protective isolation *(29)*.

Barrier measures that have been successfully used to interrupt nosocomial outbreaks of aspergillosis associated with hospital construction include building airtight plastic and dry wall barriers around the construction sites, use of negative pressure ventilation in the work area, decontamination of the air-handling systems in special care units with copper-8-quinolinolate, and restricting traffic between construction areas and adjoining patient care areas *(30)*.

Commentary. Given the difficulties in the diagnosis and treatment of *Aspergillus* infections in BMT recipients, the authors favor the use of preventive strategies to minimize exposure for which data suggest potential efficacy. These include the use of whole-wall HEPA filtration with horizontal LAF in patients undergoing allo-BMT, and the strategies outlined above during hospital construction-associated outbreaks. Though data are lacking to support efficacy, the authors also favor the use of HEPA filters, either portable or whole-wall, in patients undergoing ABMT, and the use of protective respiratory masks while allo-BMT and ABMT recipients are outside their rooms on the BMT unit, and during transportation to other areas of the hospital.

3.2. Antifungal Chemoprophylaxis

Two strategies have been employed in the use of antifungal agents to prevent the development of invasive *Aspergillus* infections in BMT recipients: prophylactic use (i.e., administering antifungal agents to high-risk patients before the appearance of any suggestive symptoms or signs), and preemptive or empiric use (i.e., administering antifungal agents to patients with suspicious findings, but not definitive for invasive fungal infections). Most authorities agree that patients with persistent neutropenic fever for 3–5 d, despite receiving broad-spectrum antibacterial agents, should be started on antifungal agents *(20–23)*. Amphotericin B and itraconazole are the two available agents with activity against *Aspergillus* species. Side effects profile and in vitro susceptibility studies favor itraconazole *(31)*; however, animal studies have shown a poor correlation between minimum inhibitory concentration (MIC) in vitro and treatment outcome in vivo *(32)*.

3.2.1. AMPHOTERICIN B

Low-dose amphotericin B (0.15–0.25 mg/kg/d), started on the first day of the pretransplant conditioning regimen, and continued until the absolute neutrophil count is ≥1000/mm^3, resulted in a significant reduction in the incidence and mortality of invasive aspergillosis, and was well tolerated in one nonrandomized study (33). However, the historical controls in this study were not all nursed in rooms with LAF or HEPA filters. Effective treatment for CMV disease was also not available for the historical controls, which might have been associated with less protection against aspergillosis, given the immunosuppressive properties of CMV infection.

Subsequent studies using a slightly lower dose of amphotericin B (0.1 mg/kg/d) showed a reduction in oropharyngeal yeast colonization, a reduction in the overall incidence of fungal infections, and a delay in switching to high-dose amphotericin B (5,34,35). However, in these studies, the observed improvement in survival was not attributable to the prevention of fungal infections, and a specific reduction in *Aspergillus* infections was not observed. Moreover, an unexplained reduction in cyclosporine levels was found in patients receiving low-dose amphotericin B, leading to an increased rate of GVHD in one study (5). In addition, the infusion-related toxicities of amphotericin B were significantly greater than placebo in the study in ABMT recipients (34).

A fundamental problem with amphotericin B, despite its activity against *Aspergillus* species, is that only a small proportion of the administered dose is diffusible and bioactive. One autopsy study showed that only 3.2% of the total dose of amphotericin B given to cancer patients was recovered from the lungs and that tissue titers were seldom fungicidal (36).

Commentary. Given that measures to reduce environmental exposure to *Aspergillus* are not always successful, administering amphotericin B at a low dose of 0.1–0.25 mg/kg/d, started on the first day of the pretransplant conditioning regimen, is an acceptable prophylactic measure, particularly in patients with risk factors for early-onset infection, as outlined above. Close attention to the possible deterioration of renal function, particularly when using other nephrotoxic agents, is essential. Slower infusions, saline hydration, and symptomatic treatment of infusion-related sides effects are usually effective in minimizing amphotericin-associated toxicities.

Beyond engraftment, and following hospital discharge, the authors favor the continued use of amphotericin B in allogeneic recipients at higher risk for late-onset infection (*see* Subheading 2.), although data to support this recommendation are lacking. The optimal dose and duration of prophylactic amphotericin B in such individuals is unknown. At this center, the authors routinely administer 0.5–1 mg/kg amphotericin B 2–3 ×/wk in allogeneic recipients who are receiving more than 0.5 mg/kg/d prednisone. More frequent dosing is sometimes utilized in those with prior proven aspergillosis.

3.2.2. INHALED AMPHOTERICIN B

Inhaled antimicrobial agents have been used successfully in several patient populations, such as in patients with cystic fibrosis receiving inhaled tobramycin for the prevention of recurrent pneumonia caused by *Pseudomonas aeruginosa*, and in patients with the acquired immune deficiency syndrome receiving inhaled pentamidine for the prevention of *Pneumocystis carinii* pneumonia.

Several studies in BMT recipients have examined the utility of inhaled amphotericin

B in the prevention of aspergillosis. Unfortunately, almost all of these studies have been nonrandomized, and have used historical controls for comparison *(37–43)*. The usual dose ranged from 5 to 20 mg/d administered via a nebulizer or a face mask, at a flow rate of 6–8 mL/min over 10–20 min, in 2–4 divided doses, from the onset of granulocytopenia until the total granulocyte count returned to ≥1000/mm^3. A reduction in the number of cases of invasive aspergillosis, and in the use of intravenous (iv) amphotericin B, was reported in some of these studies. However, these results were confounded by several factors, including the introduction of HEPA filters *(37,40,43)*, nursing patients in new buildings with better airflow *(38)*, elimination of hospital equipment contaminated with *Aspergillus* spores *(38)*, variable pretransplant conditioning regimens and GVHD prophylactic regimens *(40)*, introduction of CMV prophylactic regimens *(40)*, and concomitant use of prophylactic biweekly iv amphotericin B *(42)*, or oral amphotericin B lozenges *(38,41)*, or suspension *(40)*. Another important variable in these studies was the lack of standardization in the inhalation techniques, and in the compliance of individual patients, resulting in different amounts of retained amphotericin B in thc ncbulizer *(41)*.

All studies of inhaled amphotericin B have reported minimal side effects, except for nasal irritation, unpleasant taste, and mild nausea. Treatments were easily administered, even to pediatric patients *(42)*, despite the high prevalence of mucositis. The only prospective randomized multicenter trial *(44)*, comparing inhaled amphotericin B to no inhaled therapy, was conducted in Germany on patients not housed in LAF units, and it found no significant reduction in the incidence of invasive pulmonary aspergillosis. In this study, 23% of patients stopped taking inhaled amphotericin B because of side effects. Concerns were also raised in this study regarding the potential increased risk for bacterial pneumonia in patients receiving inhaled amphotericin B.

Minimal systemic absorption was found in studies that measured amphotericin B serum concentrations following inhaled therapy *(39,41,42)*. A large proportion of amphotericin B in aerosols is trapped in the nasopharynx and in large airways *(39,41,42)*, because of the large size of the particles and their lipophilic properties. This might be viewed as an advantage, given that the upper airways are the main portal of entry of *Aspergillus* spores.

Commentary. Administering amphotericin B by aerosol makes intuitive sense. The drug is delivered to the site where the organism is most likely to colonize, and from which invasion and dissemination subsequently occurs. Despite the lack of compelling data to support efficacy, the authors recommend this strategy in patients at high risk for late-onset infection (Subheading 2.), particularly during hospital readmissions for treatment of GVHD. In the hospital setting, the authors administer 10 mg aerosolized amphotericin B bid if tolerated.

3.2.3. LIPID FORMULATIONS OF AMPHOTERICIN B

Three new formulations of amphotericin B have been introduced during the past few years, with the aim of better efficacy and fewer side effects. These include amphotericin B lipid complex (ABLC), liposomal amphotericin B (LAB) and amphotericin B colloidal dispersion (ABCD).

Studies in BMT recipients have suggested that ABCD is effective in preemptive (empiric) treatment of febrile neutropenia *(45)*, as well as in documented invasive aspergillosis *(46)*. Studies have shown that ABCD (up to 7.5 mg/kg/d) has a renal-sparing effect compared to conventional amphotericin B *(45–47)*, but produces more infusion-related toxicities *(45)*. Studies using ABLC (5 mg/kg/d) for suspected or documented invasive aspergillosis had a response rate of approx 40%, even after the failure of conventional amphotericin B *(48,49)*. Three studies, using LAB prophylactically or preemptively, showed a reduction in fungal colonization and in invasive fungal infections, but not in deaths caused by *Aspergillus* infections *(50–52)*. Two of these studies, however, reported results on the same group of patients in two different journals *(50,51)*, and the third study *(52)* also included patients reported in the former two studies. Two other nonrandomized studies *(53,54)* using LAB for documented or suspected mycosis suggested that it was well-tolerated and somewhat effective. In fact, all patients with invasive aspergillosis died in one of these studies *(54)*, despite LAB. Again, there was a great deal of overlap in the data reported in these two studies from the same institution. Another caveat is that other antifungal agents with activity against *Aspergillus* species were used concomitantly in some patients in these studies, including itraconazole *(53,54)*, aerosolized amphotericin B *(54)*, iv conventional amphotericin B *(52,54)*, and oral amphotericin B *(53)*. Changes in GVHD and CMV prophylactic regimens were also implemented at the same time that LAB was introduced *(52)*, making it hard to assess the relative impact of these variables on the incidence of aspergillosis.

The effect of the various lipid formulations of amphotericin B on renal and hepatic functions is difficult to ascertain in some of these studies, because of other confounding variables affecting these functions, such as GVHD, veno-occlusive disease of the liver, and the use of other medications with similar side effects.

Commentary. Despite the renal-sparing effect of these lipid formulations of amphotericin B, none has proven to be superior to conventional amphotericin B in preventing *Aspergillus* infections in BMT recipients. Moreover, given their much higher cost (15–40-× that of conventional amphotericin B), the authors do not recommend using these agents upfront for prophylaxis in this setting. It may be appropriate to use these formulations in the treatment of patients with invasive aspergillosis refractory to conventional amphotericin B, or if renal insufficiency progresses despite saline hydration.

3.2.4. IMIDAZOLES

In one large study, fluconazole has been shown to be effective and safe in preventing systemic fungal infections after BMT *(55)*, with the caveat that the incidence of *Candida krusei* infections was increased *(56)*. Miconazole has also been effective in preventing fungal sepsis in neutropenic patients *(57)*, but is now off the market in the United States. Ketoconazole is much less effective than itraconazole in preventing fatal fungal infections in patients with severe granulocytopenia *(58)*, and is associated with more significant drug interactions. Fluconazole, miconazole, and ketoconazole all have negligible activity against *Aspergillus* species.

Itraconzole, on the other hand, is a highly lipophilic triazole, which has been shown to be effective in reducing proven and probable aspergillosis, as well as in reducing fungal colonization and the need for iv amphotericin B use, in one nonrandomized trial *(59)* in patients with hematological malignancies. However, patients in this study also received nasal amphotericin B, and the effects of LAF or HEPA filters were not addressed. The optimum prophylactic dose has not been determined, but one small pharmacokinetic study in ABMT recipients suggested that 5 mg/kg/d, given in 1–2 divided doses, achieves steady state within 15 d *(60)*. The MIC_{50} of *A. fumigatus* for itraconazole is 250 ng/mL *(61)*, and in vitro-acquired resistance is rare (<4%). The occurrence of fungal infections, particularly caused by *Aspergillus* species, correlated with itraconzaole plasma levels of less than 250 ng/mL, which lasted more than 2 wk in one prospective study *(62)*. Oral absorption of itraconazole in BMT recipients is highly variable, because of poor oral intake, vomiting, chemotherapy-induced damage to the intestinal epithelium (mucositis), and the concomitant use of H_2-receptor blockers. An oral solution appears to be more bioavailable than the tablet form. The effect of itraconazole on liver function in BMT recipients is difficult to assess, because of multiple confounding factors.

Voriconazole *(63)* and SCH-56592 *(64)* are two new triazoles with even more potent anti-*Aspergillus* activity than itraconazole, and are currently being evaluated in clinical trials.

Commentary. Itraconazole at a dose of 5 mg/kg/d appears to be a safe agent for preventing *Aspergillus* infections after BMT in patients who can tolerate oral medications. The oral suspension form is better absorbed, and serum drug levels should be monitored and, ideally, maintained at or above 250 ng/mL. The authors recommend prophylactic itraconazole to all allo-BMT recipients following engraftment, to be continued after discharge from the hospital, as long as they receive significant immunosuppression with steroids or other agents used for treatment of GVHD. Because of the low incidence of invasive aspergillosis in ABMT recipients, the authors do not advocate routine antifungal prophylaxis following engraftment.

3.2.5. OTHER COMBINATIONS AND NEW ANTIFUNGAL AGENTS

Several agents that act synergistically with amphotericin B against *Aspergillus* species are being investigated in in vitro and animal studies, including rifabutin *(65)* and azithromycin *(66)*. These agents do not have intrinsic anti-*Aspergillus* activity by themselves, but the data clearly show that their use in combination with amphotericin B reduces MICs of the latter drug against *Aspergillus* species, probably as the result of inhibition of fungal protein synthesis. The use of these agents may allow lower doses of amphotericin B to be used effectively, thus reducing its toxicity. There are no good clinical data to support the incorporation of these agents into antifungal prophylactic regimens.

Echinocandins and pneumocandins are new antifungal agents currently still in the preliminary phases of investigation. In vitro studies and animal data show enhanced activity against *Aspergillus* species *(67,68)*, with MICs significantly lower than itraconazole and amphotericin B.

3.3. Immunomodulatory Agents

Given the limitations of strategies to reduce exposure and prevent colonization, several agents have been used to either passively support the immune system, such as iv immunoglobulin (IVIg), or to assist in a more rapid recovery of cellular immune function, such as granulocyte colony-stimulating factor (G-CSF) and granulocyte-macrophage colony-stimulating factor (GM-CSF).

3.3.1. IV Immunoglobulin

A recent study in ABMT recipients showed that IVIg had no value in preventing infections *(69)*. In allo-BMT recipients, however, IVIg decreased the risk of acute GVHD, and of infections in general, but had no effect on the overall occurrence of fungal infections *(70)*.

3.3.2. Granulocyte Transfusions

Debate concerning the utility of granulocyte transfusions, in neutropenic patients with suspected or confirmed infections has been ongoing for several decades *(71)*. A study published 20 yr ago *(72)* suggested that granulocyte transfusions, given prophylactically during the first 3 wk after BMT, prevented the occurrence of septicemia. However, there was no effect on survival, and no comment on the incidence of fungal infections in general, or *Aspergillus* infections in particular. A few reports *(73,74)* have suggested that granulocyte transfusions can be given as an adjunctive measure in treating invasive aspergillosis in BMT recipients. Data on the dose and quality of transfused granulocytes are variable, and concerns regarding alloimmunization persist.

3.3.3. Colony-stimulating Factors

G-CSF and GM-CSF are widely used in BMT to facilitate peripheral blood stem cell collection pretransplant, and to promote neutrophil recovery posttransplant. Studies with both of these agents in ABMT *(2)* and allo-BMT *(75)* recipients have shown a reduction in the duration of neutropenia, in the length of hospital stay, and in the incidence of infections in general, but these drugs have had no specific effect on the incidence of infections caused by *Aspergillus* species, or on the use of amphotericin B.

Studies utilizing macrophage colony-stimulating factor have shown an improvement in survival in allo-BMT recipients with invasive fungal infections *(76)*. However, the beneficial effect was much more pronounced for infections caused by *Candida* species than *Aspergillus* species, and thrombocytopenia was a common dose-related side effect.

In vitro studies have shown that the oxidative response, and damage caused by human neutrophils and macrophages to *Aspergillus* hyphae, were enhanced by both G-CSF and interferon-γ *(77,78)*. This observation has been applied successfully to the clinical care of patients with chronic granulomatous disease *(79)*.

Commentary. Immunomodulatory agents appear to have no direct benefit when administered prophylactically on the incidence of aspergillosis in BMT recipients. Nevertheless, these agents may shorten the duration of neutropenia and reduce the overall incidence of infectious complications following both ABMT and allo-BMT; their use has become standard of care in the early posttransplant period following BMT. Granulocyte transfusions appear to have no role in preventing *Aspergillus* infections.

4. MEASURES FOR EARLY DETECTION

4.1. Clinical Suspicion

Specific attention to subtle early symptoms and clinical signs of invasive aspergillosis remains the most important measure for early detection. These may include sinus headache, dry cough, and nonspecific skin rash or redness at the site of iv catheters. Such findings should prompt closer follow-up and a more detailed evaluation with imaging studies or biopsies of involved organs. Regrettably, these findings are insensitive and nonspecific.

4.2. Surveillance Cultures

Surveillance cultures in BMT recipients have had limited value in predicting infections in general *(80,81)*. Sensitivity and negative predictive value of orointestinal surveillance cultures for infections with *Candida albicans*, however, may approach 100%; thus, a negative fungal surveillance culture may be useful in excluding infections with the organism *(80)*. One German study *(81)* found that 62% of BMT recipients were colonized with *Candida* species during the course of their hospitalization, and suggested that most patients harbored the organism before BMT.

A study done in leukemic patients two decades ago *(82)* showed that a positive nasal culture for *Aspergillus* species was highly predictive for the subsequent development of aspergillosis. A sterile nasal culture was also somewhat predictive of aspergillosis, suggesting that a sterilized nose by antibacterial agents can then be invaded by *Aspergillus* species, in the appropriate environmental setting. A more recent study in neutropenic patients found that 20% were colonized by *Aspergillus* species, in the absence of clinically significant infection *(38)*. One large study in BMT recipients *(6)* showed that 25% of patients who had *Aspergillus* organisms identified were either colonized or had contaminated cultures.

4.3. Serologic and Polymerase Chain Reaction-based Tests

Several European studies *(14,83,84)* have assessed the value of detecting circulating galactomannan antigen, a cell wall component of *Aspergillus* that appears to be a specific indicator of invasive disease. Antigenemia preceded clinical and radiological manifestations of invasive aspergillosis by approx 2 wk, with a sensitivity of 40% and a specificity of 80%. It is thus clear that antigenemia is not a specific sign of invasive aspergillosis, but may indicate colonization or latent infection, and the predictive value of a transiently positive test is as yet unclear. Enzyme immunoassay is a more accurate test than latex agglutination, with a lower limit of detection of galactomannan as low as 1 ng/mL. Levels of antigenemia are higher in disseminated than in localized disease, and correlate with the outcome of antifungal therapy *(85)*. Some investigators *(86,87)* have compared the detection of galactomannan antigenemia with antigenuria, and have demonstrated poor correlation between these tests in individual patients. Applying these tests to bronchoalveolar lavage (BAL) fluid for the detection of galactomannan antigen in patients with suspected *Aspergillus* pneumonia was of limited value in one study *(88)*. *Aspergillus* antibody detection is not useful in detecting invasive aspergillosis *(89)*.

Detection of *Aspergillus* DNA by using an oligonucleotide probe hybridization assay, and amplification of the polymerase chain reaction (PCR) products in blood, is a promising new measure for early diagnosis of aspergillosis. In one study *(90)*, this assay was 88% sensitive (100%, if repeated twice), and 98% specific in patients with invasive disease. Antigenemia preceded radiographic evidence of disease by a median of 4 d. In patients who responded well to antifungal therapy, PCR assays became persistently negative; those who did not respond remained PCR-positive *(90)*.

The major drawback of PCR-based detection methods is the risk of contamination, given the ubiquitous distribution of *Aspergillus* organisms in the environment. In patients at risk for aspergillosis, the predictive value of PCR-positive results on BAL fluid is low, because of the high rate of false-positive results *(91)*. PCR may be used to establish the diagnosis when performed on lung biopsy specimens in patients with negative cultures because of previous antifungal therapy. Molecular typing methods of fungal pathogens, such as DNA fingerprinting, may be helpful in defining the epidemiology of aspergillosis, but their role in early diagnosis remains to be determined *(92)*.

Commentary. A high index of suspicion has to be maintained throughout the period of transplantation, and for a variable duration thereafter, to detect symptoms or signs suggestive of early *Aspergillus* infection. Performing surveillance nasal cultures for *Aspergillus* would be most useful in the setting of an apparent outbreak. Serologic and PCR-based tests may be used to assess the response to antifungal therapy in documented cases of invasive aspergillosis, but they presently have no role as surveillance measures.

5. SUMMARY, CONCLUSIONS, AND RECOMMENDATIONS

Aspergillosis is a serious and rapidly fatal illness in allo-BMT recipients. Prevention of exposure and of invasive disease is clearly desirable, given the lack of uniformly effective therapy. Currently, reduction of environmental exposure to *Aspergillus* spores seems to be the most effective prophylactic strategy. Amphotericin B is fungicidal, and using it prophylactically at a low dose, around the time of BMT, seems partially effective, but renal and systemic toxicities remain major concerns. Lipid formulations of amphotericin B appear to have less toxicity, but are considerably more expensive than the conventional formulation, and their efficacy is probably comparable. Inhaled amphotericin B makes theoretical sense, because the respiratory tract is the main portal of entry of *Aspergillus* spores, but data supporting its efficacy are limited. Itraconazole is a fungistatic agent that has a good safety profile, but it must be administered orally, which can be a problem in patients with mucositis or nausea. Immunomodulatory agents are promising, but none have been proven effective as prophylactic agents against aspergillosis at this time. The authors recommend the following prophylactic strategies against aspergillosis in allo-BMT recipients.

1. Resection of residual *Aspergillus* pulmonary nodules should be attempted before BMT, whenever possible, to avoid reactivation during periods of maximum immunosuppression.
2. Reducing environmental exposure by using HEPA filters, avoiding flowers in patients' rooms, avoiding travel outside the BMT unit unless absolutely necessary (and the use of repository masks during such travel), and implementing strict barrier precautions during periods of construction work in or close to the BMT ward.
3. Amphotericin B at a dose of 0.1–0.25 mg/kg/d, started on the first day of the pretransplant conditioning regimen, and continued throughout the period of transplantation until engraftment, or until the dose is increased to 0.5–1 mg/kg/d with persistent neutropenic fever. Close attention should be paid to renal function and electrolyte balance. The authors do not recommend lipid formulations of amphotericin B to be used as prophylactic agents, unless patients are intolerant to conventional amphotericin B, or have a serum creatinine above 3 mg/dL.
4. Itraconazole, at a dose of 200 mg/d, should be started after engraftment, when the patient can tolerate oral medications. The optimum duration of therapy with this drug is unclear, but it should be continued as long as patients receive significant immunosuppression. Monitoring serum itraconazole levels is desirable, particularly in patients with gastrointestinal GVHD, but assays for serum itraconazole levels are not available in many

laboratories, and the optimal monitoring schedule is not currently known. Patients taking antacids or H_2-receptor blockers should be advised to take itraconazole at least 2 h before or after these medications, because an acidic stomach pH is essential for absorption of itraconazole.

5. Inhaled amphotericin B, at a dose of 10 mg bid, is recommended, if tolerated, for patients readmitted to the hospital for management of GVHD, in addition to some other systemic form of antifungal prophylaxis, such as oral itraconazole or iv low-dose amphotericin B. Patients should be monitored for proper administration of the aerosols.

6. Patients with documented gastrointestinal GVHD are less likely to absorb oral itraconazole. Individuals receiving >0.5 mg/kg/d of prednisone are perhaps best served by continuing iv low-dose daily amphotericin B, or 0.5–1 mg/kg 2–3×/wk, as long as tolerated. There is no literature to support this approach, but the authors believe that it is reasonable in this high-risk patient population, until further data become available.

Early detection of invasive aspergillosis, based upon clinical suspicion, is very important, given that surveillance cultures are expensive and insensitive, except in an outbreak setting. The detection of *Aspergillus* galactomannan antigen in serum, urine, or BAL fluid does not differentiate colonization from infection, although the level of antigenemia correlates with the likelihood of disseminated disease, and with the response to antifungal therapy. PCR-based tests performed on blood are very specific and sensitive, when repeated more than once, but more studies are needed before implementing these tests in clinical practice. The authors therefore do not recommend using serologic or PCR-based tests routinely, at the present time, in the care of allo-BMT recipients. The authors do believe, however, that such tests may be useful in specific clinical settings, such as in patients with clinical and radiological findings suggestive of aspergillosis, but with negative cultures because of prior antifungal therapy.

Because *Aspergillus* infection is closely related to the occurrence of GVHD and CMV infection, better prevention and safer treatment for both of these conditions may have a favorable impact on the incidence of aspergillosis in BMT recipients.

Despite advances in the past two decades in the prevention, diagnosis, and therapy of aspergillosis, this infection remains a major threat to patients undergoing allo-BMT and a major challenge to physicians caring for them. Although this threat can be minimized through the judicious application of the principles outlined above, it cannot presently be entirely eliminated. Invasive aspergillosis remains the foremost infectious disease challenge in allo-BMT. Further research studies are desperately needed to define better techniques for early diagnosis, better antifungal chemotherapeutic agents, and optimal strategies to prevent late-onset disease, especially in patients with chronic GVHD.

REFERENCES

1. Wheat J. Fungal infections in the immunocompromised host. In Rubin RH, Young LS (eds.), *Clinical Approach to Infection in the Compromised Host*, 3rd ed., Plenum, New York, 1994, pp. 211–237.
2. Mossad SB, Longworth DL, Goormastic M, Serky JM, Keys TF, and Bolwell BJ. Early infectious complications in autologous bone marrow transplantation: a review of 219 patients, *Bone Marrow Tranplant.*, **18** (1996) 265–271.
3. Kolbe K, Domkin D, Derigs HG, Bhakdi S, Huber C, and Aulitzky WE. Infectious complications during neutropenia subsequent to peripheral blood stem transplantation, *Bone Marrow Transplant.*, **19** (1997) 143–147.
4. McWhinney PHM, Kibbler CC, Hamon MD, Smith OP, Gandhi L, Berger LA, et al. Progress in the

diagnosis and management of aspergillosis in bone marrow transplantation: 13 years experience, *Clin. Infect. Dis.*, **17** (1993) 397–404.

5. O Donnell MR, Schmidt GM, Tegtmeier BR, Faucett C, Fahey JL, Ito J, et al. Prediction of systemic fungal infection in allogeneic marrow recipients: impact of amphotericin prophylaxis in high-risk patients, *J. Clin. Oncol.*, **12** (1994) 827–834.

6. Wald A, Leisering W, van Burik J, and Bowden RA. Epidemiology of *Aspergillus* infections in a large cohort of patients undergoing bone marrow transplantation, *J. Infect. Dis.*, **175** (1997) 1459–1466.

7. Morrison VA, Haake RJ, and Weisdorf DJ. Non-*Candida* fungal infections after bone marrow transplantations: risk factors and outcome, *Am. J. Med.*, **96** (1994) 497–503.

8. Jantunen E, Ruutu P, Niskanen L, Volin L, Parkkali T, Koukila-Kähkölä P, et al. Incidence and risk factors for invasive fungal infections in allogeneic MBT recipients, *Bone Marrow Transplant.*, **19** (1997) 801–808.

9. Chandrasekar PH, Weinmann A, Shearer C and Bone Marrow Transplantation Team. Autopsy-identified infections among bone marrow transplant recipients: a clinico-pathologic study of 56 patients, *Bone Marrow Transplant.*, **16** (1995) 678–681.

10. Drakos PE, Nagler A, Or R, Naparstek E, Kapelushnik J, Engelhard D, et al. Invasive fungal sinusitis in patients undergoing bone marrow transplantation, *Bone Marrow Transplant.*, **12** (1993) 203–208.

11. Choi SS, Milmoe GJ, Dinndrof PA, and Quinones RR. Invasive *Aspergillus* sinusitis in pediatric bone marrow transplant patients, *Arch. Otolaryngol. Head Neck Surg.*, **121** (1995) 1188–1192.

12. Allo MD, Miller J, Townsend T, and Tan C. Primary cutaneous aspergillosis associated with Hickman intravenous catheters, *N. Engl. J. Med.*, **317** (1987) 1105–1108.

13. Ribaud YM, Williams M, Guermazi A, Gluckman E, Brocheriou C, and Laval-Jeantet M. MR of cerebral aspergillosis in patients who have had bone marrow transplantation, *Am. J. Neuroradiol.*, **16** (1995) 555–562.

14. Ansorg R, van den Boom R, von Heinegg EH, and Rath PM. Association between incidence of *Aspergillus* antigenemia and exposure to construction work at a hospital site, *Zbl. Bakt.*, **284** (1996) 146–152.

15. Loo VG, Bertrand C, Dixon C, Vityé D, Eng B, DeSalis B, et al. Control of construction-associated nosocomial aspergillosis in an antiquated hematology unit, *Infect. Control Hosp. Epidemiol.*, **17** (1996) 360–364.

16. Hamadeh R, Ardehali A, Locksley RM, and York MK. Fatal aspergillosis with smoking contaminated marijuana in a marrow transplant recipient, *Chest*, **94** (1998) 432–433.

17. Offner F, Cordonnier C, Ljungman P, Prentice HG, Engelhard D, De Bacquer D, et al. Impact of previous aspergillosis on the outcome of bone marrow transplantation, *Clin. Infect. Dis.*, **26** (1998) 1098–1103.

18. Michailov G, Laporte JP, Lesage S, Fouillard L, Isnard F, Noel-Walter MP, et al. Autologous bone marrow transplantation is feasible in patients with a prior history of invasive pulmonary aspergillosis, *Bone Marrow Transplant.*, **17** (1996) 569–572.

19. Martino R, Lopez R, Sureda A, Brunet S, and Domingo-Albós A. Risk of reactivation of a recent invasive fungal infection in patients with hematologic malignancies undergoing further intensive chemo-radiotherapy. A single-center experience and review of the literature, *Haematologica*, **82** (1997) 297–304.

20. Gubbins PO, Bowman JL, and Penzak SR. Antifungal prophylaxis to prevent invasive mycoses among bone marrow transplantation recipients, *Pharmacotherapy*, **18** (1998) 549–564.

21. Uzun O and Anaissie EJ. Antifungal prophylaxis in patients with hematologic malignancies: a reappraisal, *Blood*, **86** (1995) 2063–2072.

22. Richardson MD and Kokki MH. Antifungal therapy in 'bone marrow failure', *Br. J. Hematol.*, **100** (1998) 619–628.

23. Castagnola E, Bucci B, Montinaro E, and Viscoli C. Fungal infections in patients undergoing bone marrow transplantation: an approach to a rational management protocol, *Bone Marrow Transplant.*, **18S** (1996) 97–106.

24. Rowe JM, Ciobanu N, Ascensao J, Stadtmauer EA, Weiner RS, Schenkein DP, et al. Recommended guidelines for the management of autologous and allogeneic bone marrow transplantation. A report of the Eastern Cooperative Oncology Group (ECOG), *Ann. Intern. Med.*, **120** (1994) 143–158.

25. Momin F and Chandrasekar PH. Antimicrobial prophylaxis in bone marrow transplantation, *Ann. Intern. Med.*, **123** (1995) 205–215.

26. Sherertz RJ, Belani A, Kramer BS, Elfenbein GJ, Weiner RS, Sullivan ML, et al. Impact of air filtration on nosocomial *Aspergillus* infections. Unique risk of bone marrow transplant recipients, *Am. J. Med.*, **83** (1987) 709–718.

27. Petersen FB, Buckner CD, Clift RA, Lee S, Nelson N, Counts GW, et al. Laminar air flow isolation and decontamination: a prospective randomized study of the effects of prophylactic systemic antibiotics in bone marrow transplant patients, *Infection*, **14** (1986) 115–121.

28. Skinhøj P, Jacobsen N, Hølby N, Faber V, and the Copenhagen Bone Marrow Transplant Group. Strict protective isolation in allogeneic bone marrow transplantation: effect on infectious complications, fever and graft versus host disease, *Scand. J. Infect. Dis.*, **19** (1987) 91–96.

29. Russell J, Poon MC, Jones AR, Woodman RC, and Ruether BA. Allogeneic bone-marrow transplantation without protective isolation in adults with malignant disease, *Lancet*, **339** (1992) 38–40.

30. Opal SM, Asp AA, Cannady PB Jr, Morse PL, Burton LJ, et al. Efficacy of infection control measures during a nosocomial outbreak of disseminated aspergillosis associated with hospital construction, *J. Infect. Dis.*, **153** (1986) 634–637.

31. Hennequin C, Benailly N, Silly C, Sorin M, Scheinman P, Lenoir G, et al. In vitro susceptibilities to amphotericin B, itraconazole, and miconazole of filamentous fungi isolated from patients with cystic fibrosis, *Antimicrob. Agents Chemother.*, **41** (1997) 2064–2066.

32. Odds FC, Van Gervan F, Espinel-Ingroff A, Bartlett MS, Ghannoum MA, Lancaster MV, et al. Evaluation of possible correlations between antifungal susceptibilities of filamentous fungi in vitro and antifungal treatment outcomes in animal infection models, *Antimicrob. Agents Chemother.*, **42** (1998) 282–288.

33. Rousey SR, Rusler S, Gottlieb M, and Ash RC. Low-dose amphotericin B prophylaxis against invasive *Aspergillus* infections in allogeneic marrow transplantation, *Am. J. Med.*, **91** (1991) 484–491.

34. Perfect JR, Klotman ME, Gilbert CC, Crawford DD, Rosner GL, Wright KA, et al. Prophylactic intravenous amphotericin B in neutropenic autologous bone marrow transplant recipients, *J. Infect. Dis.*, **165** (1992) 891–897.

35. Riley DK, Pavia AT, Beatty PG, Petersen FB, Spruance JL, Stokes R, et al. The prophylactic use of low-dose amphotericin B in bone marrow transplant patients, *Am. J. Med.*, **97** (1994) 509–514.

36. Collette N, Van Der Auwera P, Lopez AP, Heymans C, and Meunier F. Tissue concentrations and bioactivity of amphotericin B in cancer patients treated with amphotericin B-deoxycholate, *Antimicrob. Agents Chemother.*, **33** (1989) 362–368.

37. Conneally E, Cafferkey MT, Daly PA, Keane CT, and McCann SR. Nebulized amphotericin B as prophylaxis against invasive aspergillosis in granulocytopenic patients, *Bone Marrow Transplant.*, **5** (1990) 403–406.

38. Jeffery GM, Beard MEJ, Ikram RB, Chua J, Allen JR, and Heaton DC. Intranasal amphotericin B reduces the frequency of invasive aspergillosis in neutropenic patients, *Am. J. Med.*, **90** (1991) 685–692.

39. Myers SE, Devine SM, Topper RL, Ondrey M, Chandler C, O'Toole K, et al. A pilot study of prophylactic aerosolized amphotericin B in patients at risk for prolonged neutropenia, *Leukemia and Lymphoma*, **8** (1992) 229–233.

40. Hertenstein B, Kern WV, Schmeiser T, Stefanic M, Bunjes D, Wiesneth M, et al. Low incidence of invasive fungal infections after bone marrow transplantation in patients receiving amphotericin B inhalations during neutropenia, *Ann. Hematol.*, **68** (1994) 21–26.

41. Beyer J, Schwartz S, Barzen G, Risse G, Dullenkopff K, Weyer C, et al. Use of amphotericin B aerosols for the prevention of pulmonary aspergillosis, *Infection*, **22** (1994) 143–148.

42. Trigg ME, Morgan D, Burns TL, Kook H, Rumelhart SL, Holida MD, et al. Successful program to prevent aspergillus infections in children undergoing marrow transplantation: use of nasal amphotericin, *Bone Marrow Transplant.*, **19** (1997) 43–47.

43. Withington S, Chambers ST, Beard ME, Inder A, Allen JR, Ikram RB, et al. Invasive aspergillosis in severely neutropenic patients over 18 years: impact of intranasal amphotericin B and HEPA filtration, *J. Hosp. Infect.*, **38** (1998) 11–18.

44. Behre GF, Schwartz S, Lenz K, Ludwig WD, Wandt H, Schilling E, et al. Aerosol amphotericin B inhalations for prevention of invasive pulmonary aspergillosis in neutropenic cancer patients, *Ann. Hematol.*, **71** (1995) 287–291.

45. White MH, Bowden RA, Sandler ES, Graham ML, Noskin GA, Wingard JR, et al. Randomized, double-blind clinical trial of amphotericin B colloidal dispersion vs. amphotericin B in the empirical treatment of fever and neutropenia, *Clin. Infect. Dis.*, **27** (1998) 296–302.

46. Bowden RA, Cays M, Gooley T, Mamelok RD, and van Burik J. Phase I study of amphotericin B colloidal dispersion for the treatment of invasive fungal infections after marrow transplant, *Clin. Infect. Dis.*, **173** (1996) 1208–1215.

47. Amanda MA, Bowden RA, Forest A, Working PK, Newman MS, and Mamelok RD. Population pharmacokinetics and renal function-sparing effects of amphotericin B colloidal dispersion in patients receiving bone marrow transplants, *Antimicrob. Agents Chemother.*, **39** (1995) 2042–2047.

48. Wingard JR. Efficacy of amphotericin B lipid complex injection (ABLC) in bone marrow transplant recipients with life-threatening systemic mycoses, *Bone Marrow Transplant.*, **19** (1997) 343–347.

49. Mehta J, Kelsey S, Chu P, Powles R, Hazel D, Riley U, et al. Amphotericin B lipid complex (ABLC) for the treatment of confirmed or presumed fungal infections in immunocompromised patients with hematologic malignancies, *Bone Marrow Transplant.*, **20** (1997) 39–43.

50. Tollemar J, Ringdén O, Andersson S, Sundberg B, Ljungman P, and Tydén G. Randomized double-blind study of liposomal amphotericin B (Ambisome) prophylaxis of invasive fungal infections in bone marrow transplant rcipients, *Bone Marrow Transplant.*, **12** (1993) 577–582.

51. Tollemar J, Ringdén O, Andersson S, Sundberg B, Ljungman P, Sparrelid E, et al. Prophylactic use of liposomal amphotericin B (Ambisome) against fungal infections: a randomized trial in bone marrow transplant recipients, *Transplant. Proc.*, **25** (1993) 1495–1497.

52. Andström EE, Ringdón O, Remberger M, Svahn BM, and Tollemar J. Safety and efficacy of liposomal amphotericin B in allogeneic bone marrow transplant recipients, *Mycoses*, **39** (1996) 185–193.

53. Krüger W, Stockschläder M, Rüssmann B, Berger C, Hoffknecht M, Sobottka I, et al. Experience with liposomal amphotericin-B in 60 patients undergoing high-dose therapy and bone marrow or peripheral blood stem cell transplantation, *Br. J. Haematol.*, **91** (1995) 684–690.

54. Krüger W, Stockschläder M, Sobottka I, Betker R, De Wit M, Kröger N. Antimycotic therapy with liposomal amphotericin-B for patients undergoing bone marrow or peripheral blood stem cell transplantation, *Leukemia and Lymphoma*, **24** (1997) 491–499.

55. Slavin MA, Osborne B, Adams R, et al. Efficacy and safety of fluconazole prophylaxis for fungal infections after marrow transplantation: a prospective, randomized, double-blind study, *J. Infect. Dis.*, **171** (1995) 1545–1552.

56. Wingard JR, Merz WG, Rinaldi MG, Johnson TR, Karp JE, Saral R. Increase in *Candida krusei* infection among patients with bone marrow transplantation and neutropenia treated prophylactically with fluconazole, *N. Engl. J. Med.*, **325** (1991) 1274–1277.

57. Wingard JR, Vaughan WP, Braine HG, Merz WG, and Saral R. Prevention of fungal sepsis in patients with prolonged neutropenia: a randomized, double-blind, placebo-controlled trial of intravenous miconazole, *Am. J. Med.*, **83** (1987) 1103–1110.

58. Tricot G, Joosten E, Boogaerts MA, Vande Pitte J, and Cauwenbergh G. Ketoconazole vs. itraconazole for antifungal prophylaxis in patients with severe granulocytopenia: preliminary results of two nonrandomized studies, *Rev. Infect. Dis.*, **9** (1987) S94–S99.

59. Todeschini G, Murari C, Bonesi R, et al. Oral itraconazole plus nasal amphotericin B for prophylaxis of invasive aspergillosis in patients with hematological malignancies, *Eur. J. Clin. Microbiol. Infect. Dis.*, **12** (1993) 614–619.

60. Prentice AG, Warnock DW, Johnson SAN, Phillips MJ, and Oliver DA. Multiple dose pharmacokinetics of an oral solution of itraconazole in autologous bone marrow transplant recipients, *J. Antimicrob. Chemother.*, **34** (1994) 247–252.

61. Chryssanthou E. In vitro susceptiblity of respiratory isolates of aspergillus species to itraconazole and amphotericin B. Acquired resistance to itraconazole, *Scand. J. Infect. Dis.*, **29** (1997) 509–512.

62. Boogaerts MA, Verhoef GE, Zachee P, Demuynck H, Verbist L, and De Beule K. Antifungal prophyaxis with itraconazole in prolonged neutropenia: correlation with plasma levels, *Mycoses*, **32** (1989) S103–S108.

63. Murphy M, Bernard E, Ishimaru T, and Armstrong D. Activity of voriconazole (UK-109,496) against clinical isolates of *Aspergillus* species and its effectiveness in an experimental model of invasive pulmonary aspergillosis, *Antimicrob. Agents Chemother.*, **41** (1997) 696–698.

64. Oakley K, Moore CB, and Denning DW. In vitro activity of SCH-56592 and comparison with activities of amphotericin B and itraconazole against *Aspergillus* spp., *Antimicrob. Agents Chemother.*, **41** (1997) 1124–1126.

65. Clancy CJ, Yu YC, Lewin A, and Nguyen MH. Inhibition of RNA synthesis as a therapeutic strategy against *Aspergillus* and *Fusarium*: demonstration of in vitro synergy between rifabutin and amphotericin B, *Antimicrob. Agents Chemother.*, **42** (1998) 509–513.

66. Nguyen MH, Clancy CJ, Yu YC, and Lewin AS. Potentiation of antifungal activity of amphotericin B by azithromycin against *Aspergillus* species, *Eur. J. Clin. Microb. Infect. Dis.*, **16** (1997) 846–848.

67. Pfaller MA, Marco F, Messer SA, and Jones RN. In vitro activity of two echinocandin derivatives, LY303366 and MK-0991 (L-743,792), against clinical isolates of *Aspergillus, Fusarium, Rhizopus*, and other filamentous fungi, *Diagn. Microbiol. Infect. Dis.*, **30** (1998) 251–255.

68. Kurtz MB, Bernard EM, Edwards FF, et al. Aerosol and parenteral pneumocandins are effective in a rat model of pulmonary aspergillosis, *Antimicrob. Agents Chemother.*, **39** (1995) 1784–1789.

69. Wolff SN, Fay JW, Herzig RH, Greer JP, Dummer S, Brown RA, et al. High-dose weekly intravenous immunoglobulin to prevent infections in patients undergoing autologous bone marrow transplantation or severe myelosuppressive therapy. A study of the American Bone Marrow Transplant Group., *Ann. Intern. Med.*, **118** (1993) 937–942.

70. Sullivan KM, Kopecky KJ, Jocom J, Fisher L, Buckner CD, Meyers JD, et al. Immunomodulatory and antimicrobial efficacy of intravenous immunoglobulin in bone marrow transplantation, *N. Engl. J. Med.*, **323** (1990) 705–712.

71. Strauss RG. Therapeutic granulocyte transfusions in 1993, *Blood*, **81** (1993) 1675–1678.

72. Clift RA, Sanders JE, Thomas ED, Williams B, Buckner CD. Granulocyte transfusions for the prevention of infection in patients receiving bone-marrow transplants, *N. Engl. J. Med.*, **298** (1978) 1052–1057.

73. Clarke K, Szer J, Shelton M, Coghlan D, and Grigg A. Multiple granulocyte transfusions facilitating successful unrelated bone marrow transplantation in a patient with very severe aplastic anemia complicated by suspected fungal infection, *Bone Marrow Transplant.*, **16** (1995) 723–726.

74. Catalano L, Fontana R, Scarpato N, Picardi M, Rocco S, and Rotoli B. Combined treatment with amphotericin-B and granulocyte transfusion from G-CSF-stimulated donors in an aplastic patient with invasive aspergillosis undergoing bone marrow transplantation, *Haematologica*, **82** (1997) 71–72.

75. Nemunaitis J, Rosenfeld CS, Ash R, et al. Phase III randomized, double-blind placebo-controlled trial of rhGM-CSF following allogeneic bone marrow transplantation, *Bone Marrow Transplant.*, **15** (1995) 949–954.

76. Nemunaitis J, Meyers JD, Buckner CD, et al. Phase I trail of recombinant human macrophage colony-stimulating factor in patients with invasive fungal infections, *Blood*, **78** (1991) 907–913.

77. Roilides E, Uhlig K, Venzon D, Pizzo PA, and Walsh TJ. Enhancement of oxidative response and damage caused by human neutrophils to *Aspergillus fumigatus* hyphae by granulocyte colony-stimulating factor and gamma interferon, *Infect. Immun.*, **61** (1993) 1185–1193.

78. Murray HW. Interferon-gamma and host antimicrobial defense: current and future clinical applications, *Am. J. Med.*, **97** (1994) 459–467.

79. Rex JH, Bennett JE, Gallin JI, Malech HL, DeCarlo ES, and Melnick DA. In vivo interferon-γ therapy augments the in vitro ability of chronic granulomatous disease neutrophils to damage *Aspergillus* hyphae, *J. Infect. Dis.*, **163** (1991) 849–852.

80. Riley DK, Pavia AT, Beatty PG, Denton D, and Carroll KC. Surveillance cultures in bone marrow transplant recipients: worthwhile or wasteful?, *Bone Marrow Transplant.*, **15** (1995) 469–473.

81. Hoppe JE, Klingebiel T, and Neithammer D. Orointestinal yeast colonization of paediatric bone marrow transplant recipients: surveillance by quantitative culture and serology, *Mycoses*, **30** (1995) 51–57.

82. Aisner J, Murillo J, Schimpff SC, and Steere AC. Invasive aspergillosis in acute leukemia: correlation with nose cultures and antibiotic use, *Ann. Intern. Med.*, **90** (1979) 4–9.

83. Rohrlich P, Sarfati J, Mariani P, Duval M, Carol A, Saint-Martin C, et al. Prospective sandwich enzyme-linked immunosorbent assay for serum galactomannan: early predictive value and clinical use in invasive aspergillosis, *Pediatr. Infect. Dis. J.*, **15** (1996) 32–37.

84. Sulahian A, Tabouret M, Ribaud P, Sarfati J, Gluckman E, Latgé JP, et al. Comparison of an enzyme immunoassay and latex agglutination test for detection of galactomannan in the diagnosis of invasive aspergillosis, *Eur. J. Clin. Microbial. Infect. Dis.*, **15** (1996) 139–145.

85. Patterson TF, Miniter P, Patterson JE, Rappeport JM, and Andriole VT. *Aspergillus* antigen in the diagnosis of invasive aspergillosis, *J. Infect. Dis.*, **171** (1995) 1553–1558.

86. Ansorg R, von Heinegg EH, and Rath PM. *Aspergillus* antigenuria compared to antigenemia in bone marrow transplant recipients, *Eur. J. Clin. Microbiol. Infect. Dis.*, **13** (1994) 582–589.

87. Stynen D, Goris A, Sarfati J, and Latgé JP. A new sensitive sandwich enzyme-linked immunosorbent assay to detect galactofuran in patients with invasive aspergillosis, *J. Clin. Microbiol.*, **33** (1995) 497–500.

88. Rath PM, Oeffleke R, Müller KD, and Ansorg R. Non-value of *Aspergillus* antigen detection in

bronchoalveolar lavage fluids of patients undergoing bone marrow transplantation, *Mycoses*, **39** (1996) 367–370.

89. Patterson JE, Zidouh A, Miniter P, Andriole VT, and Patterson TF. Hospital epidemiologic surveillance for invasive aspergillosis: patient demographics and the utility of antigen detection, *Infect. Control Hosp. Epidemiol.*, **18** (1997) 104–108.

90. Einsele H, Hebart H, Roller G, Löffler J, Rothenhofer I, Müller CA, et al. Detection and identification of fungal pathogens in blood by using molecular probes, *J. Clin. Microbiol.*, **35** (1997) 1353–1360.

91. Bretagne S, Costa J-M, Marmorat-Khuong A, Poron F, Cordonnier C, Vidaud M, et al. Detection of *Aspergillus* species DNA in bronchoalveolar lavage samples by competitive PCR, *J. Clin. Microbiol.*, **33** (1995) 1164–1168.

92. Pfaller MA. Epidemiology of fungal infections: the promise of molecular typing, *Clin. Infect. Dis.*, **20** (1995) 1535–1539.

21 Prevention of Cytomegalovirus Infection After Allogeneic Bone Marrow Transplantation

Karim A. Adal, MD,
and Robin K. Avery, MD

CONTENTS

1. BACKGROUND: CLINICAL SIGNIFICANCE OF CYTOMEGALOVIRUS AFTER BONE MARROW TRANSPLANTATION

Despite advances in prophylaxis, diagnostic methods, and antiviral therapy, cytomegalovirus (CMV) infection remains a pervasive problem after allogeneic bone marrow transplantation (allo-BMT). The mainstay of antiviral therapy has been ganciclovir *(1,2)*, but universal ganciclovir prophylaxis, while diminishing the risk of CMV infection and disease during the prophylaxis period, has been associated with a significantly higher incidence of neutropenia *(1–5)*, leading to early discontinuation in some patients, as well as to an incidence of late CMV infections *(6–12)*. Preemptive strategies, basing the use of antiviral therapy on an early detection test from blood, bronchoalveolar lavage (BAL) fluid, or other source, have been devised in attempt to identify a subset of patients most likely to benefit from ganciclovir *(13–15)*.

Whether or not such an approach is preferable to universal ganciclovir prophylaxis is the subject of considerable debate. This chapter presents the data on both prophylactic and preemptive strategies, and discusses newer diagnostic modalities for CMV, as well as the use of immunoglobulin (Ig) (either unselected or CMV hyperimmune globulin). Future directions may include the use of newer antivirals such as foscarnet and other agents *(16–24)*, combination antiviral therapy, adoptive T-cell immunotherapy *(25–32)*,

From: *Current Controversies in Bone Marrow Transplantation*
Edited by: B. Bolwell © Humana Press Inc., Totowa, NJ

donor leukocyte infusions *(33)*, or other immunomodulatory therapy, based on advances in understanding the biology of host response to CMV infection after BMT. Because CMV infection is much less frequent and severe in recipients of autologous or syngeneic BMTs and stem cell transplants, this chapter concentrates on the recipient of an allo-BMT or stem cell transplant.

An overview of the impact of CMV infection after BMT should encompass both classical clinical presentations and newer insights into CMV pathogenesis. In the era before antiviral therapy, 80% or more of CMV seropositive BMT recipients developed evidence of CMV reactivation (or superinfection from the donor) *(34)*. One-third of seronegative recipients developed CMV primary infection, particularly if the donor was seropositive, or if the patient received granulocyte transfusions *(35)*. This incidence was found to be considerably reduced in seronegative recipients with seronegative donors, with the administration of CMV-free blood products *(36–40)*. The most-feared complication of CMV infection after BMT has been CMV pneumonitis, with a case-fatality rate of 85% or more in the preganciclovir era. Even with the most effective therapy yet described, that of ganciclovir plus unselected immunoglobulin (IVIg) or CMV hyperimmune globulin (CMVIg), up to 50% (or more, in some series) of patients with CMV pneumonitis will not survive *(12,41–45)*. For this reason, efforts have been concentrated on prevention.

CMV pneumonitis *(46–49)* has been considered a subset of interstitial pneumonitis, and constitutes about one-half of interstitial pneumonitis cases in the classical literature. About one-third of interstitial pneumonitis has been considered idiopathic, with the remainder of cases being caused by *Pneumocystis carinii* and other viruses, such as herpes simplex virus (HSV) and adenovirus. Human herpesvirus-6 may account for a significant percentage of the cases previously considered idiopathic *(50,51)*. Interstitial pneumonitis and CMV pneumonitis are seen more frequently in patients with unrelated donors *(8,52–55)*, patients who have received total body irradiation as part of their conditioning regimen *(45,52,53,56–58)*, and in patients with acute graft-vs-host disease (GVHD) *(11,35,52,56,59–62)*, although fatal pneumonitis can occur without GVHD *(63)*. Recipients of T-cell-depleted (TCD) grafts also appear to be at higher risk *(4,33,52,61,64–67)*. The use of antilymphocyte therapy, such as OKT3 or antithymocyte globulin (ATG), may also predispose to development of symptomatic CMV *(11,35,52,56)*, and the use of tacrolimus (FK506) for GVHD prophylaxis also may increase CMV risk *(67)*. Pretransplant pulmonary function may play a role *(68)*. CMV pneumonitis is most common in the period 30–90 d after transplantation, and, in the early years of BMT, occurred in up to 60% of patients, although, in more recent years, this has fallen to 30% or less *(34)*.

It has long been suggested that CMV pneumonitis is an immunopathologic process *(26,48,69–72)*. This idea is supported by the fact that antiviral therapy alone is often ineffective, but the combination of antiviral therapy with IVIg or CMVIg significantly increases survival *(41–45,73)*. The importance of anti-CMV cytotoxic activity by BAL cells has been stressed *(74)*. Patients who recover a detectable systemic cytotoxic T-cell response against CMV appear to be at less risk for developing severe CMV disease *(6,7,59,75)*, and the lack of helper cell response appears to correlate with the severity of CMV disease *(53)*. Indeed, CMV seropositive recipients with a seronegative donor (D–/R+) may be at particular risk, given the lack of preexisting donor T-cell immunity to CMV, in a recipient whose immune system is being reconstituted by donor cells

(76–80); such recipients tend to manifest a higher viral load in quantitative CMV studies *(76)*. The immunopathologic process may reflect not only deficiencies in cellular immune function, but also a skew in the Th2 vs Th1 cellular response, with a disproportionate production of Th2-type cytokines *(72)*.

Because patients with acute GVHD often have delayed return of more complex immune functions, either because of GVHD itself, or its treatment, it is not surprising that such patients are also at higher risk *(35,42,52,56,59–62)*. Patients with unrelated donors are also at higher risk, presumably because of their greater overall incidence and severity of GVHD *(8,52–55)*. Patients who received TCD grafts are at higher risk of CMV, and possibly other viral infections, probably because of the early absence of virus-specific cytotoxic T-cell responses *(4,33,52,61,64–67)*. For these reasons, the possibility of restoring healthy anti-CMV T-cell responses by adoptive immunotherapy, including genetically modified T-cell clones, has become an active area of research *(25–32)*.

In addition, as in solid organ transplantation *(58)*, CMV after BMT appears to have an impact well beyond direct infectious syndromes caused by the virus. The association of CMV infection with leukopenia, thrombocytopenia, pancytopenia, and graft loss has been well described *(81,82)*. A potential mechanism for this phenomenon has recently been elucidated, with the finding that CMV infection leads to downregulation of hematopoietic factors in the stromal cell microenvironment *(83,84)*. CMV may also delay immune reconstitution short of pancytopenia, or may alter the pattern of immune reconstitution with a relative weight toward CD8[+] T-cells, and relatively fewer CD4[+] T-cells and CD20[+] B-cells *(85)*. Recent work *(86,87)* has suggested that CMV antigens can induce expansion of clonal CD8[+] T-cells after BMT. A possible association between CMV infection and chronic GVHD has been described *(11,60,88–91)*, and an association with bronchiolitis obliterans, which may be a form of chronic GVHD, has also been suggested *(69)*. CMV infection has been linked with CD13-bearing mononuclear cells, which appear to trigger autoimmunity, and which may play a role in chronic GVHD *(85,88,90–94)*. CMV disease has been associated with increased immune activation with soluble interleukin-2 receptor as a marker *(95)*, and has been found to exert a proinflammatory effect with upregulation of lymphocyte function-associated antigen 2 (LFA-2) and intercellular adhesion molecule 1 (ICAM-1) *(89)*. In addition, CMV infection has been associated with an increased risk for fungal and other opportunistic infections in solid organ transplantation *(58,96)*, and this appears to be the case in allo-BMT recipients as well, although the immunosuppression conferred by GVHD and its treatment may partially account for this in the BMT population.

Gastrointestinal CMV infection can occur in any area of the gastrointestinal tract, and may be characterized clinically by diarrhea, abdominal pain and cramping, and/ or nausea and vomiting, with or without fever *(97)*. Because these are also symptoms characteristic of gastrointestinal GVHD, endoscopy or colonoscopy with mucosal biopsies are very helpful in differentiating these two entities (or their combination), which would considerably affect the course of treatment *(98)*. CMV hepatitis is also a well-described entity, and may be confused with liver GVHD or medication toxicity; in some cases, a liver biopsy may be helpful. CMV may occasionally present with reference to other organ systems, such as the central nervous system; direct viral detection studies, such as polymerase chain reaction (PCR) on cerebrospinal fluid may be helpful.

With the advent of newer methods of CMV detection, such as CMV antigenemia, CMV DNA by PCR, and CMV DNA by hybrid capture, which are more sensitive for detection of low levels of viremia than the shell vial centrifugation and tissue culture assays, there is potential for CMV detection in an early stage of reactivation. Because symptomatic CMV disease is frequently, though not always, preceded by CMV viremia, early therapy may prevent development of clinical disease (99). As detection of asymptomatic viremia increases, it is possible that new and expanded clinical categories of CMV may be seen. These may include more frequent detection of CMV during the neutropenic pre-engraftment phase of transplant (66,100–101), which traditionally has been uncommon, but has been associated with the presence of other opportunistic infections and a high fatality rate. Another clinical phenomenon recently noted, with the initiation of quantitative molecular diagnosis, has been low-level breakthrough viremia while on prophylaxis or therapy (102,103; R. Avery, personal communication). Although this offers the opportunity for intensification of antiviral therapy, the clinical significance of such breakthrough viremia has not yet been elucidated.

In the ganciclovir prophylaxis era, there may be an increased incidence of late-occurring CMV after the prophylaxis period (d +100 in programs following a protocol in common use) (6 12). Evaluation of proposed prophylaxis regimens should include information on CMV infection and disease occurring after termination of prophylaxis, as well as during the period in which antiviral therapy is administered. The question has been raised as to whether or not ganciclovir may delay the development of an effective anti-CMV immune response (6).

Although antiviral resistance has been far less common in transplant recipients than in patients with AIDS or severe combined immunodeficiency (104), the widespread use of ganciclovir has occasioned some concern about the potential for increasing resistance to develop. Such resistance may already be more common than generally thought (18,23,104–109). The use of foscarnet as an alternative anti-CMV agent, with relatively little marrow-suppressive effect in BMT patients, has been described (16–24,110,111). It may be the drug of choice for CMV occurring in the neutropenic pre-engraftment period. Foscarnet also has the advantage of activity against ganciclovir-resistant strains of CMV, but its nephrotoxicity may limit its usefulness, especially in patients receiving concomitant amphotericin B, cyclosporine, or tacrolimus. In addition to studies on antiviral resistance, a relatively new area of investigation is the possible biological differences between different strains or genotypes of CMV (35,112,113), which may also contribute to differing severity of disease.

A considerable amount of research into CMV pathogenesis, diagnostic methods, prophylaxis, and treatment has paralleled advances in understanding the reconstitution of the immune system after BMT. However, many questions still remain. The subheadings which follow examine the literature in these areas in more detail, as well as future directions for inquiry.

2. CMV DIAGNOSTIC MODALITIES

In the past, diagnosis of CMV viremia relied generally on the shell vial centrifugation culture or tissue culture performed on blood buffy coats. Shell vial is the only culture method with a rapid turnaround time (less than 48 h), but both shell vial and conventional tissue culture methods are qualitative, and of limited value for monitoring the therapeutic response, because they generally become rapidly negative on therapy, regardless of clinical outcome. In the past few years, several new rapid diagnostic tests for CMV have been developed, which can also provide quantitation of CMV DNA copies *(114,115)*. These newer, more sensitive assays also have made it possible to detect viremia earlier, and at a lower level, than previous assays. Therefore, in many centers, culture-based assays have been superseded by direct antigen or DNA detection methods, because culture methods are time-consuming and have a low sensitivity *(116)*, although their advantage is the availability of the virus in culture, if susceptibility testing is needed.

The CMV antigenemia assay is performed by staining polymorphonuclear leukocytes with monoclonal antibodies directed against protein pp65, present inside CMV-infected leukocytes *(117–119)*. It provides some information regarding viral load, but is considered less quantitative than the PCR or DNA hybrid capture. It is more sensitive than culture methods, and provides an assessment of the therapeutic response. Drawbacks include the limitations of the test in neutropenic patients, because peripheral blood leukocytes are the basis for the assay, and the fact that it is labor-intensive, and specimens must be processed immediately. Quantitative PCR assays require standardization *(120)*, and are time-consuming and more appropriate for batch testing, but the commercially available kits provide sensitive and reliable quantitation of CMV DNA *(121,122)*. Reverse transcription-PCR is a method that detects late viral mRNA (CMV pp67) in leukocytes, as opposed to viral DNA, and has been found to be less sensitive, but more predictive of the onset of CMV-related clinical symptoms *(123)*. The hybrid-capture CMV DNA assay is a rapid and simple procedure that can easily be done on a daily basis in a smaller laboratory, but requires controls for quantitative testing, and has the same limitations as antigenemia, regarding neutropenia. Another advantage of the hybrid-capture assay is that collected blood can be stored and processed at a later time. This is true for PCR assays as well.

In one of the best comparative studies of the various diagnostic methods to date, 402 immunosuppressed patients at risk for CMV (HIV-infected, solid organ transplant, and BMT recipients) were evaluated prospectively *(124)*. Results of the study showed that the hybrid-capture assay, the antigenemia assay, and the shell vial and tube culture methods were 95, 94, 43, and 46% sensitive, respectively. If shell vial and tube culture were assumed to be 100% specific, hybrid capture and antigenemia were found to be 95 and 94% specific, respectively. Similar results, showing that the DNA-based methods and antigenemia assay are comparable or far more sensitive than shell vial culture, are obtained when comparing PCR to antigenemia *(125)*, or hybrid-capture assay and PCR to shell vial *(126)*. Similarly, studies in BMT recipients have shown the superiority of PCR and/or antigenemia to culture assays *(100,102,103,127–130)*.

Other methods are in the process of being developed, but, from a clinical point of view, culture is no longer the gold standard for CMV diagnosis, and it is clear that, at this point in time, antigenemia or DNA detection methods have become the preferred methods for diagnosis.

3. CMV PROPHYLAXIS IN ALLO-BMT RECIPIENTS

CMV was recognized as a serious problem in allo-BMT recipients well before the development of early, sensitive tests for CMV diagnosis, which allow for preemptive therapy. Thus, considerable research has addressed the question of CMV prophylaxis, i.e., antiviral or adjunctive medical strategies, not based on CMV detection tests, administered to entire groups of BMT recipients. The mainstay of such prophylactic protocols has been the antiviral ganciclovir (1,2,47), but acyclovir (131–133), foscarnet (19–20,22,110), and other antivirals have been studied. In addition, there is considerable literature on the value of IVIg and CMVIg, both for CMV prevention and for other benefits after BMT. Many centers incorporate both antivirals (either prophylactic or preemptive) and Ig administration in their early posttransplant protocols. In general, ganciclovir-based protocols have been successful in reducing the symptomatic manifestations of CMV disease during the prophylaxis period, but neutropenia during ganciclovir therapy has led to early discontinuation or attenuation of prophylaxis in some patients (1–3). It also has been more difficult to show a difference in mortality because of ganciclovir prophylaxis, and some late CMV infections after the prophylaxis period have occurred (1,2,6–12).

The role of CMV-free blood products, particularly in protecting the seronegative BMT recipient from CMV infection, has been well established (36–39). A randomized trial of filtered vs seronegative blood products showed, in a secondary analysis, that the probability of CMV disease was greater with filtered products (2.4 vs 0%), but was within acceptable limits, according to the authors' definition (37).

Before discussing prophylaxis with antiviral agents, the use of IVIg and CMVIg in CMV prophylaxis is now reviewed. It is generally agreed that Ig therapy, in some form in the early post-BMT period probably has preventive activity against bacterial infection, CMV, interstitial pneumonia, and acute GVHD (134,135). In addition, it is well established that the most effective therapy for CMV pneumonitis after BMT is a combination of ganciclovir and IVIg or CMVIg (41–45,73), which significantly increases survival, compared to antiviral therapy alone or globulin therapy alone.

Early studies suggested that prophylactic, intermittent administration of CMVIg (136–138) and IVIg (134,139) significantly reduced the risk of CMV. However, more recent studies (39,140,141) have brought this into question, and subsequent meta-analyses and compilations of published trials have concluded that CMVIg and IVIg probably have a protective effect, but do not abolish the risk of CMV after allo-BMT (142–146). One review (147) concluded that the evidence for a role for IVIg in prevention of GVHD was more solid than for prevention of CMV, but another meta-analysis (144) suggested that the reduction in fatal CMV infection, CMV pneumonitis, interstitial pneumonitis, and total mortality was more significant than the reduction in acute GVHD. The risk for acute GVHD may correlate with IgG trough levels (148). There is little to suggest that IVIg and CMVIg are different in efficacy.

Acyclovir was the principal antiviral utilized in transplantation prior to the introduction of ganciclovir (56), and is still used frequently for prophylaxis and treatment of HSV and varicella-zoster virus (VZV) infections after transplantation. Acyclovir lacks a virus-specific thymidine kinase, and thus has relatively little in vitro activity against CMV, far less than ganciclovir. However, acyclovir has been shown in some studies to have a protective effect. Meyers et al. (131) randomized allo-BMT recipients to receive iv acyclovir, vs no antiviral therapy, from d −5 to d +30 after transplantation. Isolation of CMV from any site occurred in 59% of acyclovir patients, compared to 75% of controls, though viremia was not significantly different (39 vs 48%). CMV pneumonitis was significantly reduced (19 vs 31%) within the first 100 d after transplantation. Mortality at 100 d was also significantly reduced (71% survival in the acyclovir group, compared to 46% among controls). These results were confirmed and extended in a European multicenter study (132), which found that 1 mo of iv acyclovir followed by 6 mo of oral acyclovir at high dose (800 mg qid) significantly improved survival at 7 mo (79/105 patients vs 60/102 patients in the control groups), and decreased CMV viremia in the first 210 d after BMT (24 vs 36%), although the incidence of CMV disease was similar between the groups.

Many programs now incorporate acyclovir into the early posttransplant prophylactic protocol, based on these and other results. However, few centers currently rely on acyclovir alone for prevention of CMV, since significant residual CMV infection appears to occur on such regimens *(149)*. As of 1993, 42/70 European BMT centers used the strategy of high-dose acyclovir, and used preemptive strategies of various kinds for early CMV detection and treatment *(56)*; however, much of the published literature on ganciclovir prophylaxis in BMT is from 1993 on, and predominant practices may have changed after that point. Valacyclovir, the acyclovir prodrug that achieves higher levels than acyclovir, has been tested in solid organ recipients, as a potential form of CMV prophylaxis *(150)*, but has yet to be evaluated in BMT recipients.

Many centers base their current prophylaxis on two randomized controlled trials of ganciclovir prophylaxis published in 1993 *(1,2)*. Prior to this, nonrandomized data has suggested a benefit to ganciclovir prophylaxis *(151)*. Winston et al. *(1)* performed a randomized, placebo-controlled, double-blind trial of 85 CMV-seropositive allo-BMT recipients who were treated with iv ganciclovir (2.5 mg/kg/8 h) for 1 wk before transplant, then 6 mg/kg ganciclovir iv Monday through Friday from engraftment to d +120 after transplant. This study showed a reduction in CMV infection from 56 to 20%, and in CMV disease from 24 to 10%, in the ganciclovir-treated group. However, reversible neutropenia requiring interruption of prophylaxis occurred in 58% of ganciclovir-treated patients vs 28% of the placebo group. Overall survival was not significantly different *(1)*.

Goodrich et al. *(2)* randomized seropositive recipients to 5 mg/kg ganciclovir, for 5 d, followed by 5 mg/kg QD until d +100 after transplant. Although 45% of the placebo group developed CMV infection during the first 100 d, only 3% of the ganciclovir group did, and CMV disease developed in 29% of placebo recipients vs 0% of ganciclovir recipients. However, neutropenia occurred in 30% of ganciclovir recipients vs none of the placebo recipients, and those patients who became neutropenic were at greater risk of bacterial infection. Mortality at 100 and 180 d did not differ significantly between the groups *(2)*, although an earlier trial by the same group, which used ganciclovir as preemptive therapy in patients with positive surveillance cultures from any site, did in fact show a survival benefit *(152)*.

Additional studies of prophylactic ganciclovir have confirmed these results. One study *(153)* demonstrated a dramatic decrease in CMV-related interstitial pneumonitis with the introduction of ganciclovir prophylaxis, but no reduction in idiopathic interstitial pneumonitis. Another *(154)* reported a reduction in symptomatic CMV and pneumonitis, but no difference in mortality.

A further study by Salzberger et al. *(3)* assessed risk factors and patterns of ganciclovir-related neutropenia. In this study, 58% of patients receiving universal ganciclovir prophylaxis, to d +100, developed an absolute neutrophil count (ANC) less than 1500/μL; 41% had an ANC less than 1000/μL. This study identified low marrow cellularity from d +21 to +28, hyperbilirubinemia during the first 20 d (possibly from veno-occlusive disease-related tubular dysfunction), and elevated serum creatinine after d 21 as risk factors for ganciclovir-induced neutropenia. Ganciclovir dose adjustments for renal dysfunction were made when the creatinine clearance fell below 50 mL/min. Neutropenia negatively predicted overall and event-free survival *(3)*. Those authors concluded that high-risk patients (with two or more of the above risk factors) might be candidates for alternative strategies of prophylaxis, intensive drug monitoring and early dose adjustments, and/or targeted ganciclovir dosing *(3)*. They also suggested that ganciclovir should be discontinued when the ANC falls to 1000 (not 750), because neutropenia at that level is predictive of further neutropenia and mortality *(3)*.

Attempts to reduce toxicity caused by ganciclovir-related neutropenia have included thrice-weekly ganciclovir prophylaxis regimens. Although apparently effective in some patient groups *(155)*, concerns have been raised about breakthrough CMV infection in patients with unrelated donors and/or TCD grafts *(4,8,64)*. In one study of TCD graft recipients, neutropenia occurred in a significant fraction of patients, despite the lower dose *(4)*, bacteremia was common in the neutropenic patients, and CMV prevention was incomplete *(4)*. In another study, which compared thrice-weekly with 5× per wk ganciclovir prophylaxis *(67)*, it was found that active CMV disease, CMV pneumonia, and CMV-attributable mortality were significantly less frequent in recipients with TCD grafts who were prophylaxed with the 5×/wk regimen. It should be noted that, in evaluating the efficacy of ganciclovir-based prophylaxis regimens, nonculture methods, such as antigenemia *(102)* or CMV-DNA by PCR or hybrid capture, are more likely to detect breakthrough viremia than are shell culture *(102)*; this may be particularly important in centers that use less frequent ganciclovir prophylaxis dosing intervals, such as thrice weekly regimens, in which breakthrough viremia may be more likely.

Because of its poor bioavailability, and lack of certainty of absorption in patients with active gastrointestinal GVHD, oral ganciclovir has not yet received much attention as a potential prophylactic agent in allo-BMT recipients, although it has become useful in some groups of solid organ transplant recipients *(156,157)*. Valganciclovir, a much more orally absorbable form of the drug, will be available in the future, and may make oral ganciclovir-based regimens a more realistic option for BMT patients.

Other potential problems with universal ganciclovir prophylaxis have been raised. Li et al. *(6)* noted that late CMV infections occurred more frequently in patients who had received early ganciclovir prophylaxis. They found that fewer ganciclovir-treated BMT recipients showed recovery of CMV-specific cytotoxic T-cell responses between d +40 and +90, and the recovery of such a response appeared to be protective vis-a-vis late CMV *(6)*. Those authors suggested that assessment of CMV-specific T-cell responses at various times might identify subgroups of patients who had reconstituted immunity enough not to need further ganciclovir prophylaxis, thereby decreasing overall toxicity *(6)*. In addition, this group has developed and strongly advocated the use of adoptive transfer of CMV-specific cytotoxic lymphocyte clones *(25,27–32)*. Other groups *(7–12)* have also noted the late incidence of CMV beyond the prophylaxis period, and have suggested the need for ongoing prophylaxis in selected groups, especially those with ongoing chronic GVHD *(8)*. One study of late CMV (after d +100) identified the significant risk factors to be the use of ATG, a peripheral blood stem cell transplant, severe acute or chronic GVHD, CMV disease within the first 100 d posttransplant, and CMV excretion after d +100 *(11)*. It is clear that late CMV disease is an increasing problem, and identification of subgroups at higher risk may lead to extension of prophylaxis or modification of prophylactic protocols for these subgroups.

Because of these difficulties with neutropenia and other issues in ganciclovir-based regimens, despite their striking reduction in CMV infection during the prophylaxis period, ongoing research is addressing novel strategies for CMV prevention (5). Preemptive strategies, described in subheading 4 below, have been studied as a means of potentially preserving the efficacy, but reducing the toxicity, of universally administered antiviral prophylaxis. There are, as yet, few direct comparisons of prophylactic and preemptive strategies (13). Boeckh et al. (13) randomized patients to universal ganciclovir prophylaxis vs preemptive ganciclovir therapy, based on CMV antigenemia. More CMV disease before d +100 was seen in the antigenemia group (14 vs 2.7%), but there was no significant difference in CMV disease by d +180, and neutropenia and survival were also not significantly different. The similarity in survival rates was attributed to more late CMV disease and more early invasive fungal infections in the universal prophylaxis group (13). This study also demonstrated that the risk of progression of asymptomatic antigenemia to symptomatic CMV disease was greater in patients with significant-grade GVHD.

Foscarnet is an antiviral agent with efficacy against many members of the herpesvirus family, including ganciclovir-resistant CMV. Because of its nephrotoxicity, its use in transplantation has been limited until recently, but its lack of myelotoxicity is a potential advantage in BMT. One prophylaxis study (19) utilized foscarnet in patients temporarily unable to receive ganciclovir, because of delayed engraftment or ganciclovir-induced neutropenia. Foscarnet was well-tolerated at a (relatively low) dose of 60 mg/kg/d for a median of 22 d. CMV was not entirely prevented, with a detection rate of 15% and CMV-related mortality of 5% (19). In another study of patients with TCD grafts, foscarnet prophylaxis significantly reduced CMV antigenemia and mortality, compared to historical controls who received acyclovir (20). Foscarnet has also been used for CMV treatment in patients who are anticipated to have difficulties with ganciclovir-induced neutropenia (21), or who have CMV viremia prior to engraftment. Its nephrotoxicity appears to be increased in patients receiving concomitant amphotericin B (22), and probably also in patients receiving cyclosporine or tacrolimus.

Studies with agents such as foscarnet, which do not display crossresistance with ganciclovir, will assume increasing importance if the small number of ganciclovir-resistant isolates from BMT patients increases (18,23,104–109). Although relatively common in patients with advanced HIV and CMV retinitis, especially in the era prior to combination antiretroviral therapy, CMV resistance to ganciclovir has not been a widespread problem in transplant patients, to date. Whether that will change, with the increasing use of ganciclovir over time, is a concern. Unfortunately, foscarnet resistance has also been described (105).

Other research is ongoing to identify potential protective mechanisms against CMV that do not depend solely on antiviral therapy. Studies in murine CMV have shown that IL-2 activated bone marrow cells vigorously lyse murine CMV-infected cells, and prolong survival of immunocompromised mice (158); this strategy has yet to be shown effective in humans.

Recently, increasing interest has focused on posttransplant immunomodulation using additional donor cells. Donor leukocyte or lymphocyte infusions have been advocated to prevent relapse (159), but there may be additional benefit in infection prevention as well. Infusion of donor leukocytes, containing Epstein-Barr virus (EBV)-specific cytotoxic lymphocyte activity, has been shown to be effective in the treatment of EBV-related posttransplant lymphoproliferative disease in allo-BMT recipients (160). Recent work has highlighted the potential role of adoptive immunotherapy for CMV, using donor CMV-specific cytotoxic lymphocyte clones *(25,27–32)*. This exciting field of research provides a potential means of accelerating the reconstitution of the immune response to a specific infectious stimulus, namely CMV, and may alter the approach to CMV prophylaxis in the future, depending on the results of ongoing studies.

4. CMV PREEMPTIVE STRATEGIES

In 1991, a landmark article by Schmidt et al. *(161)*, and an accompanying editorial by Rubin *(162)*, officially introduced the era of preemptive therapy for CMV disease in allo-BMT recipients. Schmidt et al. *(161)* screened patients on d +35 with cultures of BAL fluid by the shell vial culture method, and treated patients with positive cultures with ganciclovir. That same year, Goodrich et al. *(152)* published their experience with preemptive therapy based on monitoring patients with weekly cultures of throat swabs, blood, urine, or BAL on d +35. Both studies demonstrated the profound efficacy of ganciclovir in reducing the incidence of CMV pneumonia and death.

The concept of preemptive therapy tries to balance a variety of issues. On the one hand, prophylaxis of an entire group of patients includes those who may be at less risk for developing disease, thus leading to excess morbidity from drug toxicity and significantly increased costs *(14)*, as well as delay in the reconstitution of protective CMV-specific T-cells *(6)*. On the other hand, the concern is that waiting for screening tests to turn positive prior to instituting therapy may result in a higher risk of more severe disease in some patients. The ideal screening test for preemptive therapy should have the following characteristics: use of easily available body fluids (e.g., blood or urine, as opposed to BAL fluid); a quick turnaround time, while maintaining a high degree of reproducibility; a sensitivity approaching 100%; a high negative predictive value for invasive disease; and a potential for quantitative results, which would allow monitoring response to therapy in a more precise fashion.

In the case of CMV, there is a spectrum of illness ranging from asymptomatic viremia, to CMV syndrome, to invasive end-organ disease *(5,9,34,47–49,58)*. The assumption and hope of preemptive therapy is that asymptomatic viremia always precedes development of disease, so that rapid institution of therapy would abort progression to more advanced stages of clinical illness. In BMT recipients, viremia has been recognized as the major virologic risk factor for the progression to clinical disease, with a negative predictive value of 86% for conventional blood cultures *(99)*, and approaching 100% for antigen or DNA detection methods.

One of the most informative studies on preemptive therapy was published in 1996 by Boeckh et al. *(13)*, in which 226 BMT recipients were randomized at engraftment to receive placebo or ganciclovir until d +100 in a double-blind protocol. In patients who developed high-grade antigenemia (three or more positive cells in two slides) or viremia, the study drug was discontinued, and ganciclovir was started for at least 3 wk, or until the antigenemia resolved. Despite the fact that more patients in the placebo group developed CMV disease, there was no significant difference by d +180, because of more late CMV disease in the ganciclovir group, no difference in CMV-related death, transplant survival, and neutropenia. In addition, the ganciclovir group had a significantly higher incidence of early invasive fungal infections. The antigenemia detection method used in this study led to a lower incidence of early CMV disease than preemptive trials in which the shell vial culture method was used *(152,161)*.

Even lower rates of CMV disease could potentially have been achieved if patients with low-grade antigenemia had been treated immediately, or if therapy had not been discontinued after 3 wk or resolution of the antigenemia. Patients with low-grade antigenemia developed CMV disease rapidly, if they had severe GVHD (grades III–IV), and not, if they had milder GVHD. In another study *(10)* of 117 recipients of allo-BMT treated with preemptive ganciclovir, late CMV infections (pneumonitis or gastroenteritis) developed in seven patients after d +150, and this occurrence was associated with a high CMV load at some point during the monitoring period, as determined by quantitative PCR. Thus, preemptive therapy does not eliminate totally the risk for late CMV disease, and it may be that patients lacking CMV-specific Th-cell response may benefit from continued screening for CMV infection after d +100 *(7)*. As more is learned about the pathogenesis of CMV and the diagnostic armamentarium is refined for better predictive power, more sophisticated algorithms may be developed using more than one preemptive trigger.

Other uncontrolled studies have shown that the preemptive approach is a successful option. In one report *(62)*, preemptive therapy, based on antigenemia, was used successfully in a pediatric population. That same group later demonstrated that CMV DNA by PCR was a somewhat more sensitive test than antigenemia or shell vial culture *(163)*. A study by Einsele et al. *(164)* compared preemptive therapy in two groups of patients monitored with PCR or culture, and concluded that the group monitored with PCR had earlier detection of virus and institution of therapy, lower incidence of CMV disease and CMV-associated mortality, and a shorter duration of ganciclovir therapy with a lower duration and incidence of neutropenia and nonviral infections. Other studies with encouraging results include studies by Zaia et al. *(15)* and Mandanas et al. *(14)*, as in the studies by Schmidt et al. *(161)* and Goodrich et al. *(152)* respectively, and two studies by Ljungman et al. *(17,165)*, in which patients were monitored by PCR, and successfully treated with ganciclovir or foscarnet. Ljungman et al. retrospectively analyzed patients treated with PCR-based preemptive therapy vs culture-based preemptive therapy vs no therapy, and were able to show a decreased incidence in CMV disease (2.2 vs 6.2 vs 11.7%) and death caused by CMV (0 vs 2.9 vs 10.1%) during the first 100 d after BMT *(111)*. Various other uncontrolled studies have assessed the feasibility of the preemptive approach, mostly with good results *(128,166)*. There is no consensus regarding the duration of therapy in preemptive protocols. More data are needed, but for now many believe that, when a preemptive approach is used, a minimum of 3 wk of therapy, or until the diagnostic test becomes negative (whichever occurs later), is warranted *(167)*. Continuing ganciclovir longer than that should be decided on an individual basis in each case. Some studies have had success with a 2-wk course of therapy *(168)*

At this center, the authors et al. have been using universal prophylaxis with iv ganciclovir (5 mg/kg/d) from time of engraftment until d +100 *(1,2)*, including seronegative recipients who receive marrow from seronegative donors, because there have been occasional cases of CMV viremia in this population. Although the authors acknowledge the real problem with side effects such as neutropenia, and the concern for a potential increase in incidence of invasive fungal infections, this strategy has considerably reduced, though not eliminated, CMV disease in this population. Late CMV infections have occurred, mostly in patients with severe GVHD and significant immunosuppression. At this institution, the quantitative hybrid-capture CMV DNA assay is used for diagnosis, because of its sensitivity, especially for early or low-level viremia. Also, it does not remain positive for prolonged periods while on therapy, as can occur with PCR testing, in which it becomes more difficult to determine when to stop treatment. The authors are currently considering how to proceed with preemptive ganciclovir therapy in a low-risk group of patients who would be defined as seronegative patients with seronegative donors, and seropositive cases (donor or recipient) with grade I or no GVHD. Excluding seropositive recipients of seronegative donors may be warranted, because these patients may be at higher risk for CMV disease. Another consideration would be to restrict preemptive therapy to patients receiving a transplant from matched-sibling donors *(54)*. A similar approach was taken by Verdonck et al. *(168)* with good results: Their study enrolled CMV-seropositive recipients of BMTs from HLA-identical siblings who were given ganciclovir, either preemptively when CMV antigenemia was detected, or prophylactically when high-dose steroids were given for grade 2 or more GVHD. They elected to monitor patients with grade 2 GVHD who did not require high doses of steroids (only 4/20 patients with grade 1 GVHD), although the authors believe that prophylaxis should be extended to this group as well, because of the close association and interaction between GVHD and CMV reactivation. The results of Verdonck et al.'s study are encouraging, however, because none of the patients developed invasive CMV disease, and the authors feel that more studies with similar designs should be done. Further comparisons of preemptive vs universal prophylactic protocols, or hybrid strategies assigning patients to different protocols, based on such factors as serostatus, occurrence of GVHD, TCD, or poor reconstitution of anti-CMV cellular immune response, will be of interest.

5. CONCLUSION

Much research remains to be done in the challenging field of CMV prophylaxis. It is still unclear whether universal ganciclovir-based prophylaxis regimens or early detection-based preemptive therapy for CMV infection is more efficacious, or if a hybrid approach should be implemented. Given the lack of definitive data proving the superiority of one strategy over another, practice among centers continues to be varied and in accordance with the clinical experience at that center. In fact, in a recent questionnaire-based survey of the majority of BMT centers in the United States, the authors were struck by the lack of uniformity regarding individual protocols for CMV prophylaxis. Of a total of 81 centers responding to the survey, more than half are currently using preemptive therapy for CMV (R. Avery et al., manuscript in preparation). The other centers are divided between universal prophylaxis and hybrid strategies (using universal prophylaxis for higher-risk groups and preemptive therapy for other groups). Neutropenia is a problem for over half the centers regardless of the approach used, but several centers commented that the early use of granulocyte colony-stimulating factor can minimize this problem. The most common diagnostic method used is PCR, followed by antigenemia, shell vial, tissue culture, and hybrid capture assay. These results illustrate the lack of consensus among programs in the United States regarding the optimal method of CMV prevention, and the need for more standardization.

CMV prophylaxis in the past 5 yr has focused primarily on either universal ganciclovir-based prophylaxis regimens or early detection-based preemptive therapy for CMV infection. Ganciclovir universal prophylaxis is effective in reducing CMV infection and disease during the prophylaxis period, but potential problems include a significant incidence of neutropenia, and possible consequent increase in bacterial and fungal infections; an incidence of late CMV infections and delayed development of specific anti-CMV responses; and an inability to show, in many studies, an improvement in survival in ganciclovir-treated patients. Although preemptive strategies are becoming more popular, they have not totally replaced universal prophylaxis. The challenge is to identify the subgroup of patients, and the time of administration, which will maximize the benefits of ganciclovir *(5,9)*, or to develop a less toxic and equally effective antiviral strategy. Certain subgroups of patients, such as those with severe GVHD, TCD grafts, or who receive certain immunosuppressive agents such as FK506 (tacrolimus) or ATG, may be candidates for more aggressive prophylaxis strategies *(4,11,33,64,67)*.

Ig therapy, either IVIg or CMVIg, continues to be considered a useful adjunct to prophylaxis of CMV, interstitial pneumonitis, bacterial infection, and acute GVHD, but is not generally relied on as the sole modality for CMV prevention. Similarly, many centers utilize acyclovir for HSV and VZV prophylaxis, some in the early posttransplant period, and some for extended periods of time, but rarely rely on acyclovir as the principal modality of CMV prevention. Foscarnet has been successfully utilized in patients who are neutropenic, or who cannot tolerate ganciclovir, but its potential nephrotoxicity remains a concern. It has been used more extensively in European programs. Newer antivirals, such as valacyclovir, cidofovir, valganciclovir, and other agents, are yet to be shown effective in CMV prevention after BMT. The small but growing number of reports of ganciclovir-resistant CMV in this population may also alter prophylactic strategies in the future.

Finally, as newer immunosuppressive agents are developed for the prophylaxis and treatment of GVHD, their differential effects on CMV risk will be important to examine. Mycophenolate mofetil, for example, has been highly effective in reducing the risk for rejection in solid organ transplantation, but its possible augmentation of CMV risk in some subgroups of patients remains controversial *(169,170)*. The use of FK506 for GVHD prophylaxis has been associated in one study *(67)* with a higher risk for CMV. Newer monoclonal antibody treatments *(171–174)* for GVHD have yet to be fully studied in terms of CMV and overall infection risk. An intriguing new immunosuppressive agent, leflunomide, has been reported to have novel anti-CMV activity *(175)*. Given the changing landscape of GVHD and its treatment, and the availability of newer diagnostic modalities for CMV and newer antivirals, it is likely that CMV prevention strategies, too, will evolve over time in response to these developments.

ACKNOWLEDGMENTS

The authors would like to acknowledge and thank Belinda Yen-Lieberman, Ph.D., for her review and comments on the section on diagnosis of CMV infection.

REFERENCES

1. Winston DJ, Ho WG, Bartoni K, et al. Ganciclovir prophylaxis of cytomegalovirus infection and disease in allogeneic bone marrow transplant recipients. Results of a placebo-controlled, double-blind trial, *Ann. Intern. Med.*, **118** (1993) 179–184.

2. Goodrich JM, Bowden RA, Fisher L, Keller C, Schoch G, and Meyers JD. Ganciclovir prophylaxis to prevent cytomegalovirus disease after allogeneic marrow transplant, *Ann. Intern. Med.*, **118** (1993) 173–178.

3. Salzberger B, Bowden RA, Hackman RC, Davis C, and Boeckh M. Neutropenia in allogeneic marrow transplant recipients receiving ganciclovir for prevention of cytomegalovirus disease: risk factors and outcome, *Blood*, **90** (1997) 2502–2508.

4. Przepiorka D, Ippoliti C, Panina A, et al. Ganciclovir three times per week is not adequate to prevent cytomegalovirus reactivation after T cell-depleted marrow transplantation, *Bone Marrow Transplant.*, **13** (1994) 461–464.

5. Goodrich JM, Boeckh M, and Bowden R. Strategies for the prevention of cytomegalovirus disease after marrow transplantation, *Clin. Infect. Dis.*, **19** (1994) 287–298.

6. Li CR, Greenberg PD, Gilbert MJ, Goodrich JM, and Riddell SR. Recovery of HLA-restricted cytomegalovirus (CMV)-specific T-cell responses after allogeneic bone marrow transplant: correlation with CMV disease and effect of ganciclovir prophylaxis, *Blood*, **83** (1994) 1971–1979.

7. Krause H, Hebart H, Jahn G, Muller CA, and Einsele H. Screening for CMV-specific T-cell proliferation to identify patients at risk of developing late onset CMV disease, *Bone Marrow Transplant.*, **19** (1997) 1111–1116.

8. Atkinson K, Arthur C, Bradstock K, et al. Prophylactic ganciclovir is more effective in HLA-identical family member marrow transplant recipients than in more heavily immune-suppressed HLA-incidental unrelated donor marrow transplant recipients. Australasian Bone Marrow Transplant Study Group, *Bone Marrow Transplant.*, **16** (1995) 401–405.

9. Zaia JA and Forman SJ. Cytomegalovirus infection in the bone marrow transplant recipient, *Infect. Dis. Clin. North Am.*, **9** (1995) 879–900.

10. Zaia JA, Gallez-Hawkins GM, Tegtmeier BR, et al. Late cytomegalovirus disease in marrow transplantation is predicted by virus load in plasma, *J. Infect. Dis.*, **176** (1997) 782–785.

11. Maltezou HC, Whimbey E, Champlin RE, et al. Late CMV disease in adult allogeneic bone marrow transplant (BMT) and peripheral blood stem cell (PBSC) recipients, in *Program Abstr. Intersci. Conf. Antimicrob. Agents Chemother.*, 1996, Abstract, H1.

12. Nguyen Q, Champlin R, Giralt S, et al. Late cytomegalovirus pneumonia in adult allogeneic blood and marrow transplant recipients, *Clin. Infect. Dis.*, **28** (1999) 618–623.

13. Boeckh M, Gooley TA, Myerson D, Cunningham T, Schoch G, and Bowden RA. Cytomegalovirus pp65 antigenemia-guided early treatment with ganciclovir versus ganciclovir at engraftment after allogeneic marrow transplantation: a randomized double-blind study, *Blood*, **88** (1996) 4063–4071.

14. Mandanas RA, Saez RA, Selby GB, and Confer DL. Cytomegalovirus surveillance and prevention in allogeneic bone marrow transplantation: examination of a preemptive plan of ganciclovir therapy, *Am. J. Hematol.*, **51** (1996) 104–111.

15. Zaia JA, Schmidt GM, Chao NJ, et al. Preemptive ganciclovir administration based solely on asymptomatic pulmonary cytomegalovirus infection in allogeneic bone marrow transplant recipients: long-term follow-up, *Biol. Bone Marrow Transplant.*, **1** (1995) 88–93.

16. Chang J, Powles R, Singhal S, et al. Foscarnet therapy for cytomegalovirus infection after allogeneic bone marrow transplantation, *Clin. Infect. Dis.*, **22** (1996) 583–584.

17. Ljungman P, Oberg G, Aschan J, et al. Foscarnet for pre-emptive therapy of CMV infection detected by a leukocyte-based nested PCR in allogeneic bone marrow transplant patients, *Bone Marrow Transplant.*, **18** (1996) 565–568.

18. Reusser P, Cordonnier C, Einsele H, et al. European survey of herpesvirus resistance to antiviral drugs in bone marrow transplant recipients. Infectious Diseases Working Party of the European Group for Blood and Marrow Transplantation (EBMT), *Bone Marrow Transplant.*, **17** (1996) 813–817.

19. Ippoliti C, Morgan A, Warkentin D, et al. Foscarnet for prevention of cytomegalovirus infection in allogeneic marrow transplant recipients unable to receive ganciclovir, *Bone Marrow Transplant.*, **20** (1997) 491–495.

20. Bacigalupo A, Tedone E, Van Lint MT, et al. CMV prophylaxis with foscarnet in allogeneic bone marrow transplant recipients at high risk of developing CMV infections, *Bone Marrow Transplant.*, **13** (1994) 783–788.

21. Bacigalupo A, van Lint MT, Tedone E, et al. Early treatment of CMV infections in allogeneic bone marrow transplant recipients with foscarnet or ganciclovir, *Bone Marrow Transplant.*, **13** (1994) 753–758.

22. Reusser P, Gambertoglio JG, Lilleby K, and Meyers JD. Phase I–II trial of foscarnet for prevention of cytomegalovirus infection in autologous and allogeneic marrow transplant recipients, *J. Infect. Dis.*, **166** (1992) 473–479.

23. Razis E, Cook P, Mittelman A, and Ahmed T. Treatment of gancyclovir resistant cytomegalovirus with foscarnet: a report of two cases occurring after bone marrow transplant, *Leuk. Lymphoma*, **12** (1994) 477–480.

24. Aschan J, Ringden O, Ljungman P, Lonnqvist B, and Ohlman S. Foscarnet for treatment of cytomegalovirus infections in bone marrow transplant recipients, *Scand. J. Infect. Dis.*, **24** (1992) 143–150.

25. Greenberg PD, Finch RJ, Gavin MA, et al. Genetic modification of T-cell clones for therapy of human viral and malignant diseases, *Cancer J. Sci. Am.*, **4(Suppl 1)** (1998) S100–105.

26. Riddell SR. Pathogenesis of cytomegalovirus pneumonia in immunocompromised hosts, *Semin. Respir. Infect.*, **10** (1995) 199–208.

27. Riddell SR and Greenberg PD. Cellular adoptive immunotherapy after bone marrow transplantation, *Cancer Treat. Res.*, **76** (1995) 337–369.

28. Steffens HP, Kurz S, Holtappels R, and Reddehase MJ. Preemptive CD8 T-cell immunotherapy of acute cytomegalovirus infection prevents lethal disease, limits the burden of latent viral genomes, and reduces the risk of virus recurrence, *J. Virol.*, **72** (1998) 1797–1804.

29. Walter EA, Greenberg PD, Gilbert MJ, et al. Reconstitution of cellular immunity against cytomegalovirus in recipients of allogeneic bone marrow by transfer of T-cell clones from the donor, *N. Engl. J. Med.*, **333** (1995) 1038–1044.

30. Dazzi F and Goldman JM. Adoptive immunotherapy following allogeneic bone marrow transplantation, *Annu. Rev. Med.*, **49** (1998) 329–340.

31. Riddell SR, Watanabe KS, Goodrich JM, Li CR, Agha ME, and Greenberg PD. Restoration of viral immunity in immunodeficient humans by the adoptive transfer of T cell clones, *Science*, **257** (1992) 238–241.

32. Riddell SR, Walter BA, Gilbert MJ, and Greenberg PD. Selective reconstitution of CD8$^+$ cytotoxic T lymphocyte responses in immunodeficient bone marrow transplant recipients by the adoptive transfer of T cell clones, *Bone Marrow Transplant.*, **14(Suppl 4)** (1994) S78–84.

33. Couriel D, Canosa J, Engler H, Collins A, Dunbar C, and Barrett AJ. Early reactivation of cytomegalovirus and high risk of interstitial pneumonitis following T-depleted BMT for adults with hematological malignancies, *Bone Marrow Transplant.*, **18** (1996) 347–353.

34. Bowden RA and Meyers JD. Prophylaxis of cytomegalovirus infection, *Semin. Hematol.*, **27(Suppl 1)** (1990) 17–21, 28–29.

35. Meyers JD, Flournoy N, and Thomas ED. Risk factors for cytomegalovirus infection after human bone marrow transplantation, *J. Infect. Dis.*, **153** (1986) 478–488.

36. Bowden RA, Slichter SJ, Sayers MH, Mori M, Cays MJ, and Meyers JD. Use of leukocyte-depleted platelets and cytomegalovirus-seronegative red blood cells for prevention of primary cytomegalovirus infection after marrow transplant, *Blood*, **78** (1991) 246–250.

37. Bowden RA, Slichter SJ, Sayers M, et al. A comparison of filtered leukocyte-reduced and cytomegalovirus (CMV) seronegative blood products for the prevention of transfusion-associated CMV infection after marrow transplant, *Blood*, **86** (1995) 3598–3603.

38. Mackinnon S, Burnett AK, Crawford RJ, Cameron S, Leask BG, and Sommerville RG. Seronegative blood products prevent primary cytomegalovirus infection after bone marrow transplantation, *J. Pathol.*, **41** (1988) 948–950.

39. Bowden RA, Sayers M, Flournoy N, et al. Cytomegalovirus immune globulin and seronegative blood products to prevent primary cytomegalovirus infection after marrow transplantation, *N. Engl. J. Med.*, **314** (1986) 1006–1010.

40. Bowden RA, Sayers M, Gleaves CA, Banaji M, Newton B, and Meyers JD. Cytomegalovirus-seronegative blood components for the prevention of primary cytomegalovirus infection after marrow transplantation. Considerations for blood banks, *Transfusion*, **27** (1987) 478–481.

41. Ljungman P, Niederwieser D, Pepe MS, Longton G, Storb R, and Meyers JD. Cytomegalovirus infection after marrow transplantation for aplastic anemia, *Bone Marrow Transplant.*, **6** (1990) 295–300.

42. Schmidt GM, Kovacs A, Zaia JA, et al. Ganciclovir/immunoglobulin combination therapy for the treatment of human cytomegalovirus-associated interstitial pneumonia in bone marrow allograft recipients, *Transplantation*, **46** (1998) 905–907.

43. Reed EC, Bowden RA, Dandliker PS, Lilleby KE, and Meyers JD. Treatment of cytomegalovirus pneumonia with ganciclovir and intravenous cytomegalovirus immunoglobulin in patients with bone marrow transplants, *Ann. Intern. Med.*, **109** (1988) 783–788.

44. Emanuel D, Cunningham I, Jules-Elysee K, et al. Cytomegalovirus pneumonia after bone marrow transplantation successfully treated with the combination of ganciclovir and high-dose intravenous immune globulin, *Ann. Intern. Med.*, **109** (1988) 777–782.

45. Ljungman P, Engelhard D, Link H, et al. Treatment of interstitial pneumonitis due to cytomegalovirus with ganciclovir and intravenous immune globulin: experience of European Bone Marrow Transplant Group, *Clin. Infect. Dis.*, **14** (1992) 831–835.

46. Neiman P, Wasserman PB, Wentworth BB, et al. Interstitial pneumonia and cytomegalovirus infection as complications of human marrow transplantation, *Transplantation*, **15** (1973) 478–485.

47. Meyers JD. Prevention of cytomegalovirus infection after marrow transplantation, *Rev. Infect. Dis.*, **11(Suppl 7)** (1989) S1691–1705.

48. Ljungman P. Cytomegalovirus pneumonia: presentation, diagnosis, and treatment, *Semin. Respir. Infect.*, **10** (1995) 209–215.

49. Holland HK, Saral R. Cytomegaloviral virus infection in bone marrow transplantation recipients: strategies for prevention and treatment, *Support Care Cancer*, **1** (1993) 245–249.

50. Carrigan DR, Drobyski WR, Russler SK, Tapper MA, Knox KK, and Ash RC. Interstitial pneumonitis associated with human herpesvirus 6 infection after marrow transplantation, *Lancet*, **338** (1991) 147–149.

51. Cone RW, Hackman RC, Huang ML, et al. Human herpesvirus 6 in lung tissue from patients with pneumonitis after bone marrow transplantation, *N. Engl. J. Med.*, **329** (1993) 156–161.

52. Okada M and Takemoto Y. [Monitoring of CMV infection after bone marrow transplantation], *Nippon Rinsho.*, **56** (1998) 189–192.

53. Ljungman P, Aschan J, Azinge JN, et al. Cytomegalovirus viraemia and specific T-helper cell responses as predictors of disease after allogeneic marrow transplantation, *Br. J. Haematol.*, **83** (1993) 118–124.

54. Takenaka K, Gondo H, Tanimoto K, et al. Increased incidence of cytomegalovirus (CMV) infection and CMV-associated disease after allogeneic bone marrow transplantation from unrelated donors. The Fukuoka Bone Marrow Transplantation Group, *Bone Marrow Transplant.*, **19** (1997) 241–248.

55. Ringden O, Pihlstedt P, Volin L, et al. Failure to prevent cytomegalovirus infection by cytomegalovirus hyperimmune plasma: a randomized trial by the Nordic Bone Marrow Transplantation Group, *Bone Marrow Transplant.*, **2** (1987) 299–305.

56. Ljungman P, De Bock R, Cordonnier C, et al. Practices for cytomegalovirus diagnosis, prophylaxis and treatment in allogeneic bone marrow transplant recipients: a report from the Working Party for Infectious Diseases of the EBMT, *Bone Marrow Transplant.*, **12** (1993) 399–403.

57. Bowden RA and Meyers JD. Infection complicating bone marrow transplantation. In Rubin RH and Young LS (eds.), *Clinical Approach to Infection in the Compromised Host*, 3rd ed., Plenum, New York, 1994, pp. 601–628.

58. Rubin RH. Infection in the organ transplant recipient. In Rubin RH, Young LS (eds.), *Clinical Approach to Infection in the Compromised Host*, 3rd ed., Plenum, New York, 1994, pp. 629–705.

59. Einsele H, Ehninger G, Steidle M, et al. Lymphocytopenia as an unfavorable prognostic factor in patients with cytomegalovirus infection after bone marrow transplantation, *Blood*, **82** (1993) 1672–1678.

60. Matthes-Martin S, Aberle SW, Peters C, et al. CMV-viraemia during allogeneic bone marrow transplantation in paediatric patients: association with survival and graft-versus-host disease, *Bone Marrow Transplant.*, **21(Suppl 2)** (1998) S53–56.

61. Bacigalupo A, Tedone E, Isaza A, et al. CMV-antigenemia after allogeneic bone marrow transplantation: correlation of CMV-antigen positive cell numbers with transplant-related mortality, *Bone Marrow Transplant.*, **16** (1995) 155–161.

62. Locatelli F, Percivalle E, Comoli P, et al. Human cytomegalovirus (HCMV) infection in paediatric patients given allogeneic bone marrow transplantation: role of early antiviral treatment for HCMV antigenaemia on patients' outcome, *Br. J. Haematol.*, **88** (1994) 64–71.

63. Breuer R, Or R, Lijovetzky G, et al. Interstitial pneumonitis in T-cell-depleted bone marrow transplantation, *Bone Marrow Transplant.*, **3** (1988) 625–630.

64. Canpolat C, Culbert S, Gardner M, Whimbey E, Tarrand J, and Chan KW. Ganciclovir prophylaxis

for cytomegalovirus infection in pediatric allogeneic bone marrow transplant recipients, *Bone Marrow Transplant.*, **17** (1996) 589–593.

65. Hertenstein B, Hampl W, Bunjes D, et al. In vivo/ex vivo T cell depletion for GVHD prophylaxis influences onset and course of active cytomegalovirus infection and disease after BMT, *Bone Marrow Transplant.*, **15** (1995) 387–393.

66. Nagler A, Elishoov H, Kapelushnik Y, Breuer R, Or R, and Engelhard D. Cytomegalovirus pneumonia prior to engraftment following T-cell depleted bone marrow transplantation, *Med. Oncol.*, **11** (1994) 127–32.

67. Maltezou HC, Whimbey E, Champlin RE, et al. Comparison of two ganciclovir regimens for the prevention of CMV disease in adult allogeneic bone marrow transplant (BMT) recipients, In: *Program Abstr. Intersci. Conf. Antimicrob. Agents Chemother.*, (1996) 168 (Abstract).

68. Horak DA, Schmidt GM, Zaia JA, Niland JC, Ahn C, and Forman SJ. Pretransplant pulmonary function predicts cytomegalovirus-associated interstitial pneumonia following bone marrow transplantation, *Chest.*, **102** (1992) 1484–1490.

69. Chien J, Chan CK, Chamberlain D, et al. Cytomegalovirus pneumonia in allogeneic bone marrow transplantation. An immunopathologic process? *Chest.*, **98** (1990) 1034–1037.

70. Muller CA, Hebart H, Roos A, Roos H, Steidle M, and Einsele H. Correlation of interstitial pneumonia with human cytomegalovirus-induced lung infection and graft-versus-host disease after bone marrow transplantation, *Med. Microbiol. Immunol. (Berlin).*, **184** (1995) 115–121.

71. Tsinontides AC and Bechtel TP. Cytomegalovirus prophylaxis and treatment following bone marrow transplantation, *Ann. Pharmacother.*, **30** (1996) 1277–1290.

72. Sparrelid E, Emanuel D, Fehniger T, Andersson U, and Andersson J. Interstitial pneumonitis in bone marrow transplant recipients is associated with local production of TH2-type cytokines and lack of T cell-mediated cytotoxicity, *Transplantation*, **63** (1997) 1782–1789.

73. Schmidt GM, Kovacs A, Zaia JA, et al. Ganciclovir/immunoglobulin combination therapy for the treatment of human cytomegalovirus-associated interstitial pneumonia in bone marrow allograft recipients, *Transplantation*, **46** (1988) 905–907.

74. Bowden RA, Dobbs S, Kopecky KJ, Crawford S, and Meyers JD. Increased cytotoxicity against cytomegalovirus-infected target cells by bronchoalveolar lavage cells from bone marrow transplant recipients with cytomegalovirus pneumonia, *J. Infect.Dis.*, **158** (1988) 773–779.

75. Reusser P, Riddell SR, Meyers JD, and Greenberg PD. Cytotoxic T-lymphocyte response to cytomegalovirus after human allogeneic bone marrow transplantation: pattern of recovery and correlation with cytomegalovirus infection and disease, *Blood*, **78** (1991) 1373–1380.

76. Gor D, Sabin C, Prentice HG, et al. Longitudinal fluctuations in cytomegalovirus load in bone marrow transplant patients: relationship between peak virus load, donor/recipient serostatus, acute GVHD and CMV disease, *Bone Marrow Transplant.*, **21** (1998) 597–605.

77. Webster A, Blizzard B, Pillay D, Prentice HG, Pothecary K, and Griffiths PD. Value of routine surveillance cultures for detection of CMV pneumonitis following bone marrow transplantation, *Bone Marrow Transplant.*, **12** (1993) 477–481.

78. Foot AB, Caul EO, Roome AP, Darville JM, and Oakhill A. Cytomegalovirus pneumonitis and bone marrow transplantation: identification of a specific high risk group, *J. Clin. Pathol.*, **46** (1993) 415–419.

79. Lutz E, Ward KN, Szydlo R, and Goldman JM. Cytomegalovirus antibody avidity in allogeneic bone marrow recipients: evidence for primary or secondary humoral responses depending on donor immune status, *J. Med. Virol.*, **49** (1996) 61–65.

80. Grob JP, Grundy JE, Prentice HG, et al. Immune donors can protect marrow-transplant recipients from severe cytomegalovirus infections, *Lancet.*, **1** (1987) 774–776.

81. Verdonck LF, de Gast GC, van Heugten HG, Nieuwenhuis HK, and Dekker AW. Cytomegalovirus infection causes delayed platelet recovery after bone marrow transplantation, *Blood*, **78** (1991) 844–848.

82. Bilgrami S, Almeida GD, Quinn JJ, et al. Pancytopenia in allogeneic marrow transplant recipients: role of cytomegalovirus, *Br. J. Haematol.*, **87** (1994) 357–362.

83. Dobonici M, Podlech J, Steffens HP, Maiberger S, and Reddehase MJ. Evidence against a key role for transforming growth factor-beta 1 in cytomegalovirus-induced bone marrow aplasia, *J. Gen. Virol.*, **179** (1998) 867–876.

84. Steffens HP, Podlech J, Kurz S, Angele P, Dreis D, and Reddehase MJ. Cytomegalovirus inhibits

the engraftment of donor bone marrow cells by downregulation of hemopoietin gene expression in recipient stroma, *J. Virol.*, **72** (1998) 5006–5015.

85. Kook H, Goldman F, Padley D, et al. Reconstruction of the immune system after unrelated or partially matched T-cell-depleted bone marrow transplantation in children: immunophenotypic analysis and factors affecting the speed of recovery, *Blood*, **88** (1996) 1089–1097.

86. Dolstra H, Van de Wiel-van Kemenade E, De Witte T, and Preijers F. Clonal predominance of cytomegalovirus-specific CD8+ cytotoxic T lymphocytes in bone marrow recipients, *Bone Marrow Transplant.*, **18** (1996) 339–345.

87. Dolstra H, Preijers F, Van de Wiel-van Kemenade E, Schattenberg A, Galama J, and de Witte T. Expansion of CD8+CD57+ T-cells after allogeneic BMT is related with a low incidence of relapse and with cytomegalovirus infection, *Br. J. Haematol.*, **90** (1995) 300–307.

88. Muller CA and Einsele H. Influence of human cytomegalovirus on immune reconstitution after bone marrow transplantation, *Ann. Hematol.*, **64(Suppl)** (1992) A140–142.

89. Craigen JL and Grundy JE. Cytomegalovirus induced up-regulation of LFA-3 (CD58) and ICAM-1 (CD54) is a direct viral effect that is not prevented by ganciclovir or foscarnet treatment, *Transplantation*, **62** (1996) 1102–1108.

90. Soderberg C, Larsson S, Rozell BL, Sumitran-Karuppan S, Ljungman P, and Moller E. Cytomegalovirus-induced CD13-specific autoimmunity: a possible cause of chronic graft-vs-host disease, *Transplantation*, **61** (1996) 600–609.

91. Soderberg C, Sumitran-Karuppan S, Ljungman P, and Moller E. CD13-specific autoimmunity in cytomegalovirus-infected immunocompromised patients, *Transplantation*, **61** (1996) 594–600.

92. Larsson S, Soderberg-Naucler C, and Moller E. Productive cytomegalovirus (CMV) infection exclusively in CD13-positive peripheral blood mononuclear cells from CMV-infected individuals: implications for prevention of CMV transmission, *Transplantation*, **65** (1998) 411–415.

93. Torok-Storb B, Simmons P, Khaira D, Stachel D, and Myerson D. Cytomegalovirus and marrow function, *Ann. Hematol.*, **64(Suppl)** (1992) A128–131.

94. von Laer D, Meyer-Koenig U, Serr A, et al. Detection of cytomegalovirus DNA in CD34+ cells from blood and bone marrow, *Blood*, **86** (1995) 4086–4090.

95. Engelhard D, Nagler A, Singer R, and Barak V. Soluble interleukin-2 receptor levels in cytomegalovirus disease and graft versus host disease after T-lymphocyte depleted bone marrow transplantation for hematological neoplasias, *Leuk. Lymphoma.*, **12** (1994) 273–280.

96. George MJ, Snydman DR, Werner BG, et al. Independent role of cytomegalovirus as a risk factor for invasive fungal disease in orthotopic liver transplant recipients, *Am. J. Med.*, **103** (1997) 106–113.

97. Einsele H, Ehninger G, Hebart H, et al. Incidence of local CMV infection and acute intestinal GVHD in marrow transplant recipients with severe diarrhoea, *Bone Marrow Transplant.*, **14** (1994) 955–963.

98. Kraus MD, Feran-Doza M, Garcia-Moliner ML, Antin J, and Odze RD. Cytomegalovirus infection in the colon of bone marrow transplantation patients, *Mol. Pathol.*, **11** (1998) 29–36.

99. Meyers JD, Ljungman P, and Fisher LD. Cytomegalovirus excretion as a predictor of cytomegalovirus disease after marrow transplantation: importance of cytomegalovirus viremia, *J. Infect. Dis.*, **162** (1990) 373–380.

100. Yuen KY, Lo SK, Chiu EK, et al. Monitoring of leukocyte cytomegalovirus DNA in bone marrow transplant recipients by nested PCR, *J. Clin. Microbiol.*, **33** (1995) 2530–2534.

101. Limaye AP, Bowden RA, Myerson D, and Boeckh M. Cytomegalovirus disease occurring before engraftment in marrow transplant recipients, *Clin. Infect. Dis.*, **24** (1997) 830–835.

102. Nicholson VA, Whimbey E, Champlin R, et al. Comparison of cytomegalovirus antigenemia and shell vial culture in allogeneic marrow transplantation recipients receiving ganciclovir prophylaxis, *Bone Marrow Transplant.*, **19** (1997) 37–41.

103. Boeckh M, Gallez-Hawkins GM, Myerson D, Zaia JA, and Bowden RA. Plasma polymerase chain reaction for cytomegalovirus DNA after allogeneic marrow transplantation: comparison with polymerase chain reaction using peripheral blood leukocytes, pp65 antigenemia, and viral culture, *Transplantation*, **64** (1997) 108–113.

104. Wolf DG, Yaniv I, Honigman A, Kassis I, Schonfeld T, and Ashkenazi S. Early emergence of ganciclovir-resistant human cytomegalovirus strains in children with primary combined immunodeficiency, *J. Infect. Dis.*, **178** (1998) 535–538.

105. Knox KK, Drobyski WR, and Carrigan DR. Cytomegalovirus isolate resistant to ganciclovir and foscarnet from a marrow transplant patient, *Lancet*, **337** (1991) 1292–1293.

106. Boivin G, Erice A, Crane DD, Dunn DL, and Balfour HH, Jr. Ganciclovir susceptibilities of cytomegalovirus (CMV) isolates from solid organ transplant recipients with CMV viremia after antiviral prophylaxis, *J. Infect. Dis.*, **168** (1993) 332–335.

107. Drew WL, Miner RC, Busch DF, et al. Prevalence of resistance in patients receiving ganciclovir for serious cytomegalovirus infection, *J. Infect. Dis.*, **163** (1991) 716–719.

108. Slavin MA, Bindra RR, Gleaves CA, Pettinger MB, and Bowden RA. Ganciclovir sensitivity of cytomegalovirus at diagnosis and during treatment of cytomegalovirus pneumonia in marrow transplant recipients, *Antimicrob. Agents Chemother.*, **37** (1993) 1360–1363.

109. Erice A, Borrell N, Li W, Miller WJ, and Balfour HH Jr. Ganciclovir susceptibilities and analysis of UL97 region in cytomegalovirus (CMV) isolates from bone marrow recipients with CMV disease after antiviral prophylaxis, *J. Infect. Dis.*, **178** (1998) 531–534.

110. Lonnqvist B, Aschan J, and Ringden O. Foscarnet as inpatient prophylaxis only is insufficient to prevent cytomegalovirus infection after marrow transplantation, *J. Infect. Dis.*, **168** (1993) 1073.

111. Ljungman P. Cytomegalovirus infections in transplant patients, *Scand. J. Infect. Dis.*, **100(Suppl)** (1996) 59–63.

112. Woo PC, Lo CY, Lo SK, et al. Distinct genotypic distributions of cytomegalovirus (CMV) envelope glycoprotein in bone marrow and renal transplant recipients with CMV disease, *Clin. Diagn. Lab. Immunol.*, **4** (1997) 515–518.

113. Souza IE, Nicholson D, Matthey S, et al. Rapid epidemiologic characterization of cytomegalovirus strains from pediatric bone marrow transplant patients, *Infect. Control Hosp. Epidemiol.*, **16** (1995) 399–404.

114. Tong CYW. Diagnosis of cytomegalovirus infection and disease, *J. Med. Microbiol.*, **46** (1997) 717–719.

115. Boeckh M and Boivin G. Quantitation of cytomegalovirus: methodologic aspects and clinical applications, *Clin. Microbiol. Rev.*, **11** (1998) 533–554.

116. Mazzulli T, Rubin RH, Ferraro MJ, et al. Cytomegalovirus antigenemia: clinical correlations in transplant recipients and in persons with AIDS, *J. Clin. Microbiol.*, **31** (1993) 2824–2827.

117. The TH, van der Bij W, van den Berg AP, et al. Cytomegalovirus antigenemia, *Rev. Infect. Dis.*, **12(Suppl 7)** (1990) S737–744.

118. Hauw The T, van den Berg AP, Harmsen MC, van der Bij W, and van Son WJ. Cytomegalovirus antigenemia assay: a plea for standardization, *Scand. J. Infect. Dis.*, **99 (Suppl)** (1995) 25–29.

119. St George K and Rinaldo CR Jr. Comparison of commercially available antibody reagents for the cytomegalovirus pp65 antigenemia assay, *Clin. Diagn. Virol.*, **7** (1997) 147–152.

120. Grundy JE, Ehrnst A, Einsele H, et al. Three-center European external quality control study of PCR for detection of cytomegalovirus DNA in blood, *J. Clin. Microbiol.*, **34** (1996) 1166–1170.

121. Hiyoshi M, Tagawa S, Takubo T, et al. Evaluation of Amplicor CMV test for direct detection of cytomegalovirus in plasma specimens, *J. Clin. Microbiol.*, **35** (1997) 2692–2694.

122. Krajden M, Shankaran P, Bourke C, and Lau W. Detection of cytomegalovirus in blood donors by PCR using the Digene SHARP signal system assay: effects of sample preparation and detection methodology, *J. Clin. Microbiol.*, **34** (1996) 29–33.

123. Gozlan J, Laporte JP, Lesage S, et al. Monitoring of cytomegalovirus infection and disease in bone marrow recipients by reverse transcription-PCR and comparison with PCR and blood and urine cultures, *J. Clin. Microbiol.*, **34** (1996) 2085–2088.

124. Mazzulli T, Drew LW, Yen-Lieberman B, et al. Multicenter comparison of the digene hybrid capture CMV DNA assay (version 2.0), the pp 65 antigenemia assay, and cell culture for detection of cytomegalovirus viremia, *J. Clin. Microbiol.*, **37** (1999) 958–963.

125. Freymuth F, Gennetay E, Petitjean J, et al. Comparison of nested PCR for detection of DNA in plasma with pp65 leukocytic antigenemia procedure for diagnosis of human cytomegalovirus infection, *J. Clin. Microbiol.*, **32** (1994) 1614–1618.

126. Barrett-Muir WY, Aitken C, Templeton K, Raftery M, Kelsey SM, and Breuer J. Evaluation of the Murex hybrid capture cytomegalovirus DNA assay versus plasma PCR and shell vial assay for diagnosis of human cytomegalovirus viremia in immunocompromised patients, *J. Clin. Microbiol.*, **36** (1998) 2554–2556.

127. Vlieger AM, Boland GJ, Jiwa NM, et al. Cytomegalovirus antigenemia assay or PCR can be used to monitor ganciclovir treatment in bone marrow transplant recipients, *Bone Marrow Transplant.*, **9** (1992) 247–253.

128. Hebart H, Muller C, Loffler J, Jahn G, and Einsele H. Monitoring of CMV infection: a comparison of PCR from whole blood, plasma-PCR, pp65-antigenemia and virus culture in patients after bone marrow transplantation, *Bone Marrow Transplant.*, **17** (1996) 861–868.

129. Boeckh M, Bowden RA, Goodrich JM, Pettinger M, and Meyers JD. Cytomegalovirus antigen detection in peripheral blood leukocytes after allogeneic marrow transplantation, *Blood*, **80** (1992) 1358–1364.

130. Imbert-Marcille BM, Milpied N, Coste-Burel M, et al. Clinical and practical value of human cytomegalovirus DNAemia detection by semi-nested PCR for follow-up of BMT recipients, *Bone Marrow Transplant.*, **15** (1995) 611–617.

131. Meyers JD, Reed EC, Shepp DH, et al. Acyclovir for prevention of cytomegalovirus infection and disease after allogeneic marrow transplantation, *N. Engl. J. Med.*, **318** (1988) 70–75.

132. Prentice HG, Gluckman E, Powles RL, et al. Impact of long-term acyclovir on cytomegalovirus infection and survival after allogeneic bone marrow transplantation. European Acyclovir for CMV Prophylaxis Study Group, *Lancet*, **343** (1994) 749–753.

133. Prentice HG, Gluckman E, Powles RL, et al. Long-term survival in allogeneic bone marrow transplant recipients following acyclovir prophylaxis for CMV infection. The European Acyclovir for CMV Prophylaxis Study Group, *Bone Marrow Transplant.*, **19** (1997) 129–133.

134. Winston DJ, Ho WG, Lin CH, et al. Intravenous immunoglobulin for prevention of cytomegalovirus infection and interstitial pneumonia after bone marrow transplantation, *Ann. Intern. Med.*, **106** (1987) 12–18.

135. Sullivan KM, Kopecky KJ, Jocom J, et al. Immunomodulatory and antimicrobial efficacy of intravenous immunoglobulin in bone marrow transplantation, *N. Engl. J. Med.*, **323** (1990) 705–712.

136. Meyers JD, Leszczynski J, Zaia JA, et al. Prevention of cytomegalovirus infection by cytomegalovirus immune globulin after marrow transplantation, *Ann. Intern. Med.*, **98** (1983) 442–446.

137. Condie RM and O'Reilly RJ. Prevention of cytomegalovirus infection by prophylaxis with an intravenous, hyperimmune, native, unmodified cytomegalovirus globulin. Randomized trial in bone marrow transplant recipients, *Am. J. Med.*, **76** (1984) 134–141.

138. Einsele H, Vallbracht A, Schmidt H, et al. Prevention of CMV infection after BMT in high-risk patients using CMV hyperimmune globulin, *Cancer Detect. Prev.*, **12** (1988) 637–641.

139. Winston DJ, Ho WG, Lin CH, Budinger MD, Champlin RE, and Gale RP. Intravenous immunoglobulin for modification of cytomegalovirus infections associated with bone marrow transplantation. Preliminary results of a controlled trial, *Am. J. Med.*, **76** (1984) 128–133.

140. Ruutu T, Ljungman P, Brinch L, et al. No prevention of cytomegalovirus infection by anticytomegalovirus hyperimmune globulin in seronegative bone marrow transplant recipients. The Nordic BMT Group, *Bone Marrow Transplant.*, **19** (1997) 233–236.

141. Bowden RA, Fisher LD, Rogers K, Cays M, and Meyers JD. Cytomegalovirus (CMV)-specific intravenous immunoglobulin for the prevention of primary CMV infection and disease after marrow transplant, *J. Infect. Dis.*, **164** (1991) 483–487.

142. Sullivan KM. Immunoglobulin therapy in bone marrow transplantation, *Am. J. Med.*, **83** (1987) 34–45.

143. Messori A, Rampazzo R, Scroccaro G, and Martini N. Efficacy of hyperimmune anticytomegalovirus immunoglobulins for the prevention of cytomegalovirus infection in recipients of allogeneic bone marrow transplantation: a meta-analysis. *Bone Marrow Transplant.*, **13** (1994) 163–167.

144. Bass EB, Powe NR, Goodman SN, et al. Efficacy of immune globulin in preventing complications of bone marrow transplantation: a meta-analysis, *Bone Marrow Transplant.*, **12** (1993) 273–282.

145. Gale RP and Winston D. Intravenous immunoglobulin in bone marrow transplantation, *Cancer*, **68(Suppl)** (1991) 1451–1453.

146. Siadak MF, Kopecky K, and Sullivan KM. Reduction in transplant-related complications in patients given intravenous immuno globulin after allogeneic marrow transplantation, *Clin. Exp. Immunol.*, **97(Suppl 1)** (1994) 53–57.

147. Guglielmo BJ, Wong-Beringer A, and Linker CA. Immune globulin therapy in allogeneic bone marrow transplant: a critical review, *Bone Marrow Transplant.*, **13** (1994) 499–510.

148. Cottler-Fox M, Lynch M, Pickle LW, Cahill R, Spitzer TR, and Deeg HJ. Some but not all benefits of intravenous immunoglobulin therapy after marrow transplantation appear to correlate with IgG trough levels, *Bone Marrow Transplant.*, **8** (1991) 27–33.

149. Selby PJ, Powles RL, Easton D, et al. Prophylactic role of intravenous and long-term oral acyclovir after allogeneic bone marrow transplantation, *Br. J. Cancer*, **59** (1989) 434–438.

150. Lowance D, Legendre C, Neumayer H-H, et al. Valaciclovir reduces the incidence of cytomegalovirus

disease and acute graft rejection in CMV-seronegative recipients of a seropositive cadaveric renal allograft, In: *Program Abstr. Am. Soc. Transpl. Phys.* Chicago; (1998) 94 (Abstract).

151. Atkinson K, Downs K, Golenia M, et al. Prophylactic use of ganciclovir in allogeneic bone marrow transplantation: absence of clinical cytomegalovirus infection, *Br. J. Haematol.*, **79** (1991) 57–62.

152. Goodrich JM, Mori M, Gleaves CA, et al. Early treatment with ganciclovir to prevent cytomegalovirus disease after allogeneic bone marrow transplantation, *N. Engl. J. Med.*, **325** (1991) 1601–1607.

153. Atkinson K, Nivison-Smith I, Dodds A, Concannon A, Milliken S, and Downs K. Comparison of the pattern of interstitial pneumonitis following allogeneic bone marrow transplantation before and after the introduction of prophylactic ganciclovir therapy in 1989, *Bone Marrow Transplant.*, **21** (1998) 691–695.

154. von Bueltzingsloewen A, Bordigoni P, Witz F, et al. Prophylactic use of ganciclovir for allogeneic bone marrow transplant recipients [published erratum appears in *Bone Marrow Transplant*, **13** (1994) 232], *Bone Marrow Transplant.*, **12** (1993) 197–202.

155. Yau JC, Dimopoulos MA, Huan SD, et al. Prophylaxis of cytomegalovirus infection with ganciclovir in allogeneic marrow transplantation, *Eur. J. Haematol.*, **47** (1991) 371–376.

156. Gane E, Saliba F, Valdecasas GJ, et al. Randomised trial of efficacy and safety of oral ganciclovir in the prevention of cytomegalovirus disease in liver-transplant recipients. The Oral Ganciclovir International Transplantation Study Group, *Lancet*, **350** (1997) 1729–1733.

157. Brennan DC, Garlock KA, Singer GG, et al. Prophylactic oral ganciclovir compared with deferred therapy for control of cytomegalovirus in renal transplant recipients, *Transplantation*, **64** (1997) 1843–1846.

158. Agah R, Charak BS, Chen V, and Mazumder A. Adoptive transfer of anti-cytomegalovirus effect of interleukin-2- activated bone marrow: potential application in transplantation, *Blood*, **78** (1991) 720–727.

159. Barrett AJ, Mavroudis D, Tisdale J, et al. T cell-depleted bone marrow transplantation and delayed T cell add-back to control acute GVHD and conserve a graft-versus-leukemia effect, *Bone Marrow Transplant.*, **21** (1998) 543–551.

160. Papadopoulos EB, Ladanyi M, Emanuel D, et al. Infusions of donor leukocytes to treat Epstein-Barr virus-associated lymphoproliferative disorders after allogeneic bone marrow transplantation, *N. Engl. J. Med.*, **330** (1994) 1185–1191.

161. Schmidt GM, Horak DA, Niland JC, Duncan SR, Forman SJ, and Zaia JA. Randomized controlled trial of prophylactic ganciclovir for cytomegalovirus pulmonary infection in recipients of allogeneic bone marrow transplants. The City of Hope-Stanford-Syntex CMV Study Group, *N. Engl. J. Med.*, **324** (1991) 1005–1011.

162. Rubin RH. Preemptive therapy in immunocompromised hosts, *N. Engl. J. Med.*, **324** (1991) 1057–1059.

163. Gerna G, Furione M, Baldanti F, Percivalle E, Comoli P, and Locatelli F. Quantitation of human cytomegalovirus DNA in bone marrow transplant recipients, *Br. J. Haematol.*, **91** (1995) 674–683.

164. Einsele H, Ehninger G, Hebart H, et al. Polymerase chain reaction monitoring reduces the incidence of cytomegalovirus disease and the duration and side effects of antiviral therapy after bone marrow transplantation, *Blood*, **86** (1995) 2815–2820.

165. Ljungman P, Lore K, Aschan J, et al. Use of a semi-quantitative PCR for cytomegalovirus DNA as a basis for pre-emptive antiviral therapy in allogeneic bone marrow transplant patients, *Bone Marrow Transplant.*, **17** (1996) 583–587.

166. Koehler M, St. George K, Ehrlich GD, Mirro J Jr, Neudorf SM, and Rinaldo C. Prevention of CMV disease in allogeneic BMT recipients by cytomegalovirus antigenemia-guided preemptive ganciclovir therapy, *J. Pediatr. Hematol. Oncol.*, **19** (1997) 43–47.

167. Singhal S, Mehta J, and Powles R. Prevention of cytomegalovirus disease by a short course of preemptive ganciclovir or foscarnet, *Blood*, **84** (1994) 2055.

168. Verdonck LF, Dekker AW, Rozenberg-Arska M, and van den Hoek MR. A risk-adapted approach with a short course of ganciclovir to prevent cytomegalovirus (CMV) pneumonia in CMV-seropositive recipients of allogeneic bone marrow transplants, *Clin. Infect. Dis.*, **24** (1997) 901–907.

169. Sarmiento JM, Dockrell DH, Schwab TR, and Paya CV. The impact of mycophenolate mofetil (MMF) on cytomegalovirus (CMV) disease [Abstract #597], In: *ASTP 17th Annual Meeting.* Chicago; 1998.

170. First MR. Clinical application of immunosuppressive agents in renal transplantation, *Surg. Clin. North Am.*, **78** (1998) 61–76.

171. Vallera DA, Carroll SF, Snover DC, Carlson GJ, and Blazar BR. Toxicity and efficacy of anti-T-

cell ricin toxin A chain immunotoxins in a murine model of established graft-versus-host disease induced across the major histocompatibility barrier, *Blood*, **77** (1991) 182–194.

172. Herbelin C, Stephan J-L, Donadieu J, et al. Treatment of steroid-resistant acute graft-versus-host disease with an anti-IL-2-receptor monoclonal antibody (BT 563) in children who received T cell-depleted, partially matched, related bone marrow transplants, *Bone Marrow Transplant.*, **13** (1994) 563–569.

173. Racadot E, Milpied N, Bordigoni P, et al. Sequential use of three monoclonal antibodies in corticosteroid-resistant acute GVHD: a multicentric pilot study including 15 patients, *Bone Marrow Transplant.*, **15** (1995) 669–677.

174. Hale G, Zhang M-J, Bunjes D, et al. Improving the outcome of bone marrow transplantation by using CD52 monoclonal antibodies to prevent graft-versus-host disease and graft rejection, *Blood*, **92** (1998) 4581–4590.

175. Waldman WJ, Knight DA, Lurain N, et al. Novel mechanism of cytomegalovirus inhibition by leflunomide: equivalent activity against ganciclovir/foscarnet-sensitive and resistant isolates [Abstract #444], In: *ASTP 17th Annual Meeting*. Chicago; 1998.

Index

From: *Current Controversies in Bone Marrow Transplantation*
Edited by: B. Bolwell © Humana Press Inc., Totowa, NJ